2012
YEAR BOOK OF
OPHTHALMOLOGY®

The 2012 Year Book Series

Year Book of Anesthesiology and Pain Management™: Drs Chestnut, Abram, Black, Gravlee, Lien, Mathru, and Roizen

Year Book of Cardiology®: Drs Gersh, Cheitlin, Elliott, Gold, Graham, and Thourani

Year Book of Critical Care Medicine®: Drs Dries, Zanotti-Cavazzoni, Latenser, Martinez, Rincon, and Zwank

Year Book of Dermatology and Dermatologic Surgery™: Dr Del Rosso

Year Book of Diagnostic Radiology®: Drs Elster, Abbara, Oestreich, Offiah, Rosado de Christenson, Stephens, and Strickland

Year Book of Emergency Medicine®: Drs Hamilton, Bruno, Handly, Minczak, Mullin, Quintana, and Ramoska

Year Book of Endocrinology®: Drs Schott, Apovian, Clarke, Eugster, Meikle, Oetgen, Ovalle, Schteingart, and Toth

Year Book of Hand and Upper Limb Surgery®: Drs Yao, Adams, Isaacs, Lee, and Rizzo

Year Book of Medicine®: Drs Barker, Garrick, Gersh, Khardori, LeRoith, Panush, Talley, and Thigpen

Year Book of Neonatal and Perinatal Medicine®: Drs Fanaroff, Benitz, Donn, Neu, Papile, Polin, and Van Marter

Year Book of Neurology and Neurosurgery®: Drs Klimo, Minagar, Gandhi, House, Kevill, Liu, Mazia, Panagariya, Ragel, Riesenburger, Robottom, Schwendimann, Shafazand, Uhm, and Yang

Year Book of Obstetrics, Gynecology, and Women's Health®: Drs Dungan and Shulman

Year Book of Oncology®: Drs Arceci, Bauer, Chiorean, Gordon, Lawton, Murphy, Thigpen, and Tsao

Year Book of Ophthalmology®: Drs Rapuano, Cohen, Flanders, Hammersmith, Milman, Myers, Nagra, Nelson, Penne, Pyfer, Sergott, Shields, Talekar, and Vander

Year Book of Orthopedics®: Drs Morrey, Huddleston, Rose, Swiontkowski, and Trigg

Year Book of Otolaryngology-Head and Neck Surgery®: Drs Sindwani, Balough, Franco, Gapany, and Mitchell

Year Book of Pathology and Laboratory Medicine®: Drs Raab and Bissell

Year Book of Pediatrics®: Dr Stockman

Year Book of Plastic and Aesthetic Surgery™: Drs Miller, Gosman, Gurtner, Gutowski, Ruberg, Salisbury, and Smith

Year Book of Psychiatry and Applied Mental Health®: Drs Talbott, Ballenger, Buckley, Frances, Krupnick, and Mack

Year Book of Pulmonary Disease®: Drs Barker, Jones, Maurer, Spradley, Tanoue, and Willsie

Year Book of Sports Medicine®: Drs Shephard, Cantu, Feldman, Galea, Jankowski, Janssen, Lebrun, and Nieman

Year Book of Surgery®: Drs Copeland, Behrns, Daly, Eberlein, Fahey, Huber, Klodell, Mozingo, and Pruett

Year Book of Urology®: Drs Andriole and Coplen

Year Book of Vascular Surgery®: Drs Moneta, Gillespie, Starnes, and Watkins

2012
The Year Book of OPHTHALMOLOGY®

Editor-in-Chief
Christopher J. Rapuano, MD
Professor of Ophthalmology, Jefferson Medical College of Thomas Jefferson University; Director, Cornea Service; Co-Director, Refractive Surgery Department, Attending Surgeon, Wills Eye Institute, Philadelphia, Pennsylvania

Wills Eye®

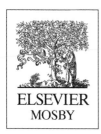

ELSEVIER
MOSBY

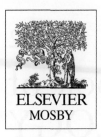

ELSEVIER
MOSBY

Vice President, Continuity: Kimberly Murphy
Editor: Yonah Korngold
Production Supervisor, Electronic Year Books: Donna M. Skelton
Electronic Article Manager: Mike Sheets
Illustrations and Permissions Coordinator: Dawn Vohsen

2012 EDITION

Composition by TNQ Books and Journals Pvt Ltd, India

Printed and bound by CPI Group (UK) Ltd, Croydon, CR0 4YY

Transferred to Digital Print 2012

Editorial Office:
Elsevier
1600 John F. Kennedy Blvd.
Suite 1800
Philadelphia, PA 19103-2899

International Standard Serial Number: 0084-392X
International Standard Book Number: 978-0-323-08886-2

Editorial Board

Table of Contents

Table of Contents

Journals Represented

Journals represented in this YEAR BOOK are listed below.
Acta Ophthalmologica
AJNR American Journal of Neuroradiology
American Journal of Medicine
American Journal of Ophthalmology
Annals of Neurology
Archives of Neurology
Archives of Ophthalmology
Archives of Pathology & Laboratory Medicine
BioMedical Central Ophthalmology
Brain
British Journal of Ophthalmology
Canadian Journal of Ophthalmology
Cornea
Drugs
Eye
Japanese Journal of Ophthalmology
Journal of Cataract & Refractive Surgery
Journal of Laryngology and Otology
Journal of Neurological Sciences
Journal of Oral and Maxillofacial Surgery
Journal of Pediatric Ophthalmology and Strabismus
Journal of Refractive Surgery
Journal of the American Association for Pediatric Ophthalmology and Strabismus
Leukemia Research
Nature
Neurology
New England Journal of Medicine
Ophthalmic Plastic and Reconstructive Surgery
Ophthalmology
Orbit
Retina
Stroke

STANDARD ABBREVIATIONS

The following terms are abbreviated in this edition: acquired immunodeficiency syndrome (AIDS), cardiopulmonary resuscitation (CPR), central nervous system (CNS), cerebrospinal fluid (CSF), computed tomography (CT), deoxyribonucleic acid (DNA), diopter (D), electrocardiography (ECG), health maintenance organization (HMO), human immunodeficiency virus (HIV), intensive care unit (ICU), intramuscular (IM), intravenous (IV), magnetic resonance (MR) imaging (MRI), ribonucleic acid (RNA), ultrasound (US), and ultraviolet (UV).

NOTE

The YEAR BOOK OF OPHTHALMOLOGY® is a literature survey service providing abstracts of articles published in the professional literature. Every effort is made to assure the accuracy of the information presented in these pages. Neither the editors nor the publisher of the YEAR BOOK OF OPHTHALMOLOGY® can be responsible for errors in the original materials. The editors' comments are their own opinions. Mention of specific products within this publication does not constitute endorsement.

To facilitate the use of the YEAR BOOK OF OPHTHALMOLOGY® as a reference tool, all illustrations and tables included in this publication are now identified as they appear in the original article. This change is meant to help the reader recognize that any illustration or table appearing in the YEAR BOOK OF OPHTHALMOLOGY® may be only one of many in the original article. For this reason, figure and table numbers will often appear to be out of sequence within the YEAR BOOK OF OPHTHALMOLOGY®.

1 Cataract Surgery

Characteristics of Traumatic Cataract Wound Dehiscence

Kloek CE, Andreoli MT, Andreoli CM (Harvard Med School, Boston, MA)
Am J Ophthalmol 152:229-233, 2011

Purpose.—To characterize the clinical course of cataract wound dehiscence.

Design.—Retrospective, comparative case series.

Methods.—Charts of open globe injuries (848 injuries in 846 patients) treated surgically at the Massachusetts Eye and Ear Infirmary between 2000 and 2009 were retrospectively reviewed. Time from original surgery to wound dehiscence, type of initial surgery, Ocular Trauma Score, age, gender, mechanism of injury, and visual acuity were analyzed.

Results.—Of 846 patients with 848 open globe injuries, 63 experienced cataract wound dehiscence. The majority of these cataract wounds (89%) were extracapsular cataract extraction (ECCE), with only 7 (11%) phacoemulsification wounds. The mean patient age in the wound rupture group was 78.2 years. Female patients comprised the majority (67%) of this subpopulation. The most common mechanisms of injury were fall (65%), blunt trauma (23%), and motor vehicle accident (7%). The median raw ocular trauma score was 47 in wound dehiscence patients. Visual acuity at presentation was light perception in the wound dehiscence group. The best postoperative visual acuity was significantly worse in the wound dehiscence group (hand motion) than in the remaining patients (20/40; *P* = .0002). When considering the phacoemulsification patients alone, these patients fared much better, with a median postoperative vision of 20/60.

Conclusions.—Despite recent advances in cataract surgery, wound dehiscence remains a significant source of visual disability, mainly in the geriatric population. Rupture ECCE wound patients have a poor visual prognosis. Fortunately, patients with phacoemulsification site dehiscence appear to regain the majority of their vision after open globe repair.

▶ This study examined the outcome of traumatic cataract wound dehiscence at a major ocular trauma center over a 9-year period. As expected, falls represented the majority of cases in this mostly geriatric patient population. The authors confirmed the findings of prior studies[1] that traditional large-incision extracapsular cataract extraction (ECCE) wounds are at risk for dehiscence from blunt trauma, even many years after surgery, and that small-incision phacoemulsification wounds are relatively resistant to trauma. In addition, final visual acuity after repair was poorer in the ECCE group, mainly due to a higher incidence of severe

2 / Ophthalmology

intraocular injury, including choroidal hemorrhage, uveal and vitreous prolapse, and retinal detachment. A previous case series published over 10 years ago showed better visual outcome after repair of ruptured ECCE wounds than the current study.[2] In that older series, a number of the dehisced wounds were within 8 weeks of surgery, and these patients had better final visual outcomes. Presumably, less force is required to rupture recent incisions.

Important points for the cataract surgeon are: Resistance to trauma is another advantage of small-incision phacoemulsification cataract extraction. Even patients with old, healed, large limbal incisions should be advised to wear impact-resistant glasses at all times, and surgeons should have a low threshold to explore these wounds in the setting of blunt trauma if dehiscence cannot be excluded on examination.

M. F. Pyfer, MD

References

1. Ball JL, McLeod BK. Traumatic wound dehiscence following cataract surgery: a thing of the past? *Eye (Lond)*. 2001;15:42-44.
2. Chowers I, Anteby I, Ever-Hadani P, Frucht-Pery J. Traumatic wound dehiscence after cataract extraction. *J Cataract Refract Surg*. 2001;27:1238-1242.

Cataract Surgery in Ranibizumab-Treated Patients With Neovascular Age-Related Macular Degeneration From the Phase 3 ANCHOR and MARINA Trials

Rosenfeld PJ, On behalf of the MARINA and ANCHOR Study Groups (Univ of Miami Miller School of Medicine, FL; et al)
Am J Ophthalmol 152:793-798, 2011

Purpose.—To investigate whether cataract surgery was beneficial in patients with neovascular age-related macular degeneration (AMD) receiving monthly ranibizumab injections in the ANCHOR (Anti-VEGF Antibody for the Treatment of Predominantly Classic Choroidal Neovascularization in AMD) and MARINA (Minimally Classic/Occult Trial of the Anti-VEGF Antibody Ranibizumab in the Treatment of Neovascular AMD) phase 3 trials.

Design.—Retrospective analysis.

Methods.—Patients were identified who underwent cataract surgery during the 2 pivotal trials. For this analysis, the best-corrected visual acuity (VA) just prior to cataract surgery was referred to as the redefined baseline VA. For the period after cataract surgery, endpoints included change in VA, time to first postsurgery injection, and total number of injections. Monthly follow-up visits after surgery were defined at 30-day intervals ± 15 days.

Results.—Three subgroups were identified: study eyes of ranibizumab-treated patients (758 eyes [23 undergoing surgery]), fellow eyes of ranibizumab-treated patients (758 eyes [28 undergoing surgery]), and eyes of non-ranibizumab patients (762 [16 undergoing surgery]). Three months postsurgery, the VA of ranibizumab-treated eyes improved by a mean of

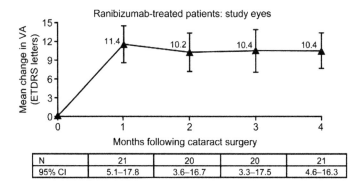

Ranibizumab-treated patients: study eyes

N	21	20	20	21
95% CI	5.1–17.8	3.6–16.7	3.3–17.5	4.6–16.3

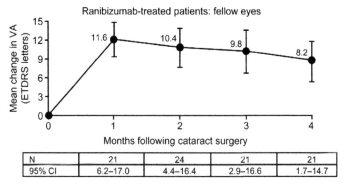

Ranibizumab-treated patients: fellow eyes

N	21	24	21	21
95% CI	6.2–17.0	4.4–16.4	2.9–16.6	1.7–14.7

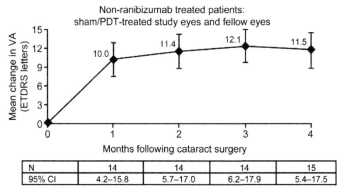

Non-ranibizumab treated patients: sham/PDT-treated study eyes and fellow eyes

N	14	14	14	15
95% CI	4.2–15.8	5.7–17.0	6.2–17.9	5.4–17.5

FIGURE.—Mean change in visual acuity (VA) from redefined baseline VA following cataract surgery in ranibizumab-treated and non–ranibizumab-treated patients in the ANCHOR and MARINA trials. (Top) Ranibizumab-treated eyes (pooled 0.3-mg and 0.5-mg dose cohorts). (Middle) Fellow eyes of ranibizumab-treated patients (pooled 0.3-mg and 0.5-mg dose cohorts). (Bottom) Non–ranibizumab-treated patients including a sham-/PDT-treated study eye or fellow eyes. In the MARINA trial, control patients received sham injections; in the ANCHOR trial, control patients received PDT plus sham injections. Redefined baseline VA is the VA documented just prior to cataract surgery. Error bars represent ± 1 standard error of the mean. ANCHOR = Anti-VEGF Antibody for the Treatment of Predominantly Classic Choroidal Neovascularization in AMD; CI = confidence interval; ETDRS = Early Treatment Diabetic Retinopathy Study; MARINA = Minimally Classic/Occult Trial of the Anti-VEGF Antibody Ranibizumab in the Treatment of Neovascular AMD; PDT = photodynamic therapy; VA = visual acuity. (Reprinted from Rosenfeld PJ, On behalf of the MARINA and ANCHOR Study Groups. Cataract surgery in ranibizumab-treated patients with neovascular age-related macular degeneration from the phase 3 ANCHOR and MARINA trials. Am J Ophthalmol. 2011;152:793-798, Copyright 2011, with permission from Elsevier.)

10.4 (± 3.4) letters compared to the redefined baseline (n = 20; 95% confidence interval +3.3 letters to +17.5 letters). The mean VA change from redefined baseline VA was not significantly different between the 3 groups at any of the evaluated time points postsurgery ($P > .44$ for all comparisons between each pair of the 3 groups at 1, 2, 3, and 4 months following surgery).

Conclusions.—In the phase 3 trials, cataract surgery appeared to be safe and beneficial for all eyes with AMD, including ranibizumab-treated eyes with neovascular AMD. An average VA improvement of more than 2 lines was typically observed (Fig).

▶ Management of patients with wet age-related macular degeneration (AMD) has changed dramatically in the last 10 years due to the introduction of effective therapy: first verteporfin photodynamic therapy and, more recently, anti–vascular endothelial growth factor (VEGF) treatment such as ranibizumab. Historically, cataract surgery was not recommended in patients with active wet AMD due to the typically poor visual prognosis of this progressive disease. However, if exudation is controlled with current treatment options, patients with visually significant cataract and wet AMD can now undergo cataract surgery with reasonable expectation for visual improvement.

This article examines the short-term visual outcome after cataract surgery for patients in the pivotal phase 3 trials of ranibizumab for wet AMD (the ANCHOR and MARINA trials). The average visual improvement after cataract surgery was about 10 letters on the ETDRS chart (Fig). To put this in perspective, that level of improvement was similar to the average gain in vision experienced by all ranibizumab-treated eyes in the 2 trials. This improvement was maintained for at least 4 months after surgery in treated wet AMD eyes. Untreated fellow eyes undergoing cataract surgery during the trials showed initial improvement followed by a slow decline in vision over the 4 months (Fig), but the reason for this was not studied. Limitations of the study are the relatively small number of patients (only 67 of 758 patients had cataract surgery during the trials) and short term follow-up (4 months).

M. F. Pyfer, MD

Evaluation of Posterior Lens Capsule by 20-MHz Ultrasound Probe in Traumatic Cataract
Tabatabaei A, Kiarudi MY, Ghassemi F, et al (Tehran Univ of Med Sciences, Iran)
Am J Ophthalmol 153:51-54, 2012

Purpose.—To investigate the accuracy of echography with a 20-MHz probe for evaluation of posterior lens capsule in traumatic cataract before surgery.

Design.—Prospective interventional case series.

Methods.—This study consisted of 43 eyes with traumatic cataract that were scheduled to undergo surgery. In all cases, cataract was dense enough to prevent visualization of the posterior lens capsule. Echography was performed using a 20-MHz probe to detect rupture of the posterior lens capsule. All patients subsequently underwent cataract extraction and intra-operative findings of the posterior lens capsule were compared with the preoperative echographic findings.

Results.—This study included 43 eyes of 43 patients (38 men and 5 women) with a mean age of 35.6 ± 15.3 years (range, 4-68 years). The trauma was either blunt (4 eyes) or sharp (39 eyes); there was closed globe injury in 2 eyes and open globe injury in 41 eyes. By 20-MHz echography, posterior border of the crsytalline lens was clearly visualized in all 43 eyes. By 20-MHz echographic imaging, rupture of the posterior lens capsule was identified in 17 eyes (39.5%). During cataract surgery, it was noted that 14 eyes (32.6%) had rupture of the posterior lens capsule. Sensitivity, specificity, positive predictive value, and negative predictive value were 93%, 86%, 76%, and 96%, respectively, for 20-MHz echography to detect rupture of the posterior lens capsule. Also, the positive likelihood ratio, negative likelihood ratio, and odds ratio were 6.7, 0.08, and 81, respectively.

Conclusion.—Echography with 20-MHz probe is an accurate imaging modality for detection of posterior lens capsule rupture in traumatic cataract preoperatively. This technique helps ophthalmologists have an appropriate surgical plan before operating (Fig).

▶ Cataract surgeons are frequently confronted with dense or hypermature cataracts that preclude visualization of the posterior lens capsule and other posterior eye structures. Brightness-mode (B-mode) ultrasound imaging using a 10-MHz probe is commonly employed in these situations to image the vitreous cavity and posterior retina-choroid to detect pathology such as retinal detachment preoperatively. In traumatic cataracts, the integrity of the posterior capsule is a key factor in predicting outcome and surgical planning. B-mode scan does not adequately visualize anterior structures such as the lens, including the posterior capsule.

This article demonstrates the effectiveness of 20-MHz ultrasound echography in imaging the posterior capsule to detect rupture preoperatively in dense traumatic cataracts (see Fig). The main limitation of this technique is the need for

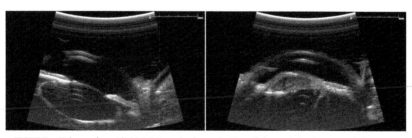

FIGURE.—Echography with 20-MHz probe for evaluation of the posterior lens capsule in traumatic cataract. (Left) An eye with an intact posterior lens capsule in echography, which was confirmed during surgery. (Right) An eye with ruptured posterior lens capsule demonstrating lack of normal integrity of the capsule. (Reprinted from Tabatabaei A, Kiarudi MY, Ghassemi F, et al. Evaluation of posterior lens capsule by 20-MHz ultrasound probe in traumatic cataract. *Am J Ophthalmol.* 2012;153:51-54, Copyright 2012, with permission from Elsevier.)

globe contact with a water bath, so that open globes cannot be safely imaged prior to repair. In contrast, gentle through-the-lid imaging using coupling gel for B-mode ultrasound can be used on a ruptured globe.

M. F. Pyfer, MD

Outcomes of cataract surgery in eyes with a low corneal endothelial cell density
Yamazoe K, Yamaguchi T, Hotta K, et al (Ichikawa General Hosp, Tokyo, Japan; Kameda Med Ctr, Tokyo, Japan)
J Cataract Refract Surg 37:2130-2136, 2011

Purpose.—To evaluate the surgical outcomes of cataract surgery in eyes with a low preoperative corneal endothelial cell density (ECD) and analyze factors affecting the prognosis.

Setting.—Tokyo Dental College, Ichikawa General Hospital, Chiba, Japan.

Design.—Noncomparative case series.

Methods.—Eyes with a preoperative ECD of less than 1000 cells/mm^2 that had cataract surgery between 2006 and 2010 were identified. Standard phacoemulsification with intraocular lenses was performed using the soft-shell technique. The rate of endothelial cell loss, incidence of bullous keratopathy, and risk factors were retrospectively assessed.

Results.—Sixty-one eyes (53 patients) with a low preoperative ECD were identified. Preoperative diagnoses or factors regarded as causing endothelial cell loss included Fuchs dystrophy (20 eyes), laser iridotomy (16 eyes), keratoplasty (10 eyes), traumatic injury (3 eyes), trabeculectomy (3 eyes), corneal endotheliitis (2 eyes), and other (7 eyes). The corrected distance visual acuity improved from 0.59 ± 0.49 logMAR preoperatively to 0.32 ± 0.48 logMAR postoperatively ($P < .001$). The mean ECD was 693 ± 172 cells/mm^2 and 611 ± 203 cells/mm^2, respectively ($P = .001$). The mean rate of endothelial cell loss was 11.5% ± 23.4%. Greater ECD loss was associated with a shorter axial length (AL) (<23.0 mm) and diabetes mellitus. Bullous keratopathy developed in 9 eyes (14.8%) and was associated with posterior capsule rupture.

Conclusions.—The results suggest that modern techniques for cataract surgery provide excellent visual rehabilitation in many patients with a low preoperative ECD. Shorter AL, diabetes mellitus, and posterior capsule rupture were risk factors for greater ECD loss and bullous keratopathy (Table 5).

▶ Cataract surgeons are frequently faced with coexisting conditions of corneal endothelial disease and visually significant cataract. Deciding which patients have a good prognosis with cataract surgery alone and which are likely to progress to pseudophakic bullous keratopathy (PBK), requiring a corneal grafting procedure, can be challenging. Modern phacoemulsification techniques, coupled

TABLE 5.—Risk Factors for Corneal Endothelial Cell Loss and Bullous Keratopathy

Subgroup	Eyes (n)	Mean Cell Loss (%)	P Value	Patients with BK	P Value
Age (y)			.748		1.000
≤69	19	11.0		3	
70−79	30	9.6		4	
80−90	12	16.8		2	
Sex			.414		.361
Male	12	19.6		3	
Female	49	9.6		6	
Preop CDVA (decimal)			.379		.475
≥20/50	30	14.2		3	
<20/50	32	8.6		6	
Axial length			.019*		.488
≤23.0 mm	33	19.4		6	
>23.0 mm	28	3.6		3	
Cataract grade			.228		.076
NS1−NS2	26	2.5		2	
NS3	22	15.7		3	
NS4−NS5	13	10.7		4	
Diabetes mellitus			.049*		.120
Absent	52	9.8		6	
Present	9	19.6		3	
Hypertension			.406		.462
Absent	38	10.2		7	
Present	23	14.0		2	
Capsule rupture/vitreous loss					.020*
Present	2	−		2	
Absent	59	11.5		7	

BK = bullous keratopathy; CDVA = corrected distance visual acuity; NS = nuclear sclerosis.
*Statistically significant.

with machines with sophisticated ultrasound modulation modes and fluidic control to minimize corneal endothelial stress, have led to a relaxation of the traditional guidelines for safety of corneal thickness—less than 640 μm or endothelial cell density (ECD) greater than 800 cells/mm.[2] In fact, many corneal specialists now recommend cataract surgery alone as an initial intervention in all patients with a sufficiently clear view through the cornea to permit safe surgery. If required later, lamellar endothelial grafting procedures such as Descemet's stripping automated endothelial keratoplasty are less complex in pseudophakic patients and less likely to alter corneal curvature than traditional penetrating keratoplasty.[1]

This retrospective analysis of patients undergoing cataract surgery with low preoperative ECD supports this viewpoint. Significant risk factors for subsequent onset of PBK above the overall rate of 15% in this study included diabetes (3 of 9 patients or 33%) and intraoperative posterior capsule rupture (2 of 2 patients or 100%) (Table 5). Not surprisingly, shorter axial length also led to greater loss of ECD. The association of diabetes with increased ECD loss has been noted in other studies, but the cause is unclear and merits further investigation given the high prevalence of this disease.

M. F. Pyfer, MD

Reference

1. Seitzman GD. Cataract surgery in Fuchs' dystrophy. *Curr Opin Ophthalmol.* 2005;16:241-245.

Capsular block syndrome associated with femtosecond laser–assisted cataract surgery
Roberts TV, Sutton G, Lawless MA, et al (Univ of Sydney, Australia)
J Cataract Refract Surg 37:2068-2070, 2011

We report intraoperative capsular block syndrome occuring during the first 50 femtosecond laser–assisted cataract surgeries performed in our facility. Two patients had uneventful combined laser fragmentation, capsulotomy, and corneal incision procedures. In both cases, following transfer to the operating room and manual removal of the laser-cut capsulotomy, posterior capsule rupture was noted during hydrodissection, resulting in posterior dislocation of the lens. Pars plana vitrectomy, removal of the crystalline lens, and sulcus implantation of an intraocular lens were performed in both patients with good visual outcomes. Femtosecond laser–assisted cataract surgery changes the intraoperative environment with the generation of intracapsular gas and laser–induced changes in the cortex. With awareness of the changed intraocular environment following laser lens fragmentation and capsulotomy and a modification of the surgical technique, no additional cases of intraoperative CBS have been seen in more than 600 laser–assisted cataract surgery procedures performed to date at our facility. Financial Disclosure: No author has a financial or proprietary interest in any material or method mentioned. Additional disclosure is found in the footnotes (Figs 1 and 2).

▶ The authors report 2 cases of posterior capsule rupture with lens subluxation during hydrodissection, presumably caused by capsular block syndrome (CBS), occurring among their first 50 femtosecond laser-assisted cataract surgeries (Figs 1 and 2).This is a much higher incidence rate than expected for this potentially serious intraoperative complication.

Femtosecond laser use during cataract surgery may increase the risk of posterior capsule rupture caused by CBS through several mechanisms, including a tighter seal of the anterior capsule margin to the underlying cortex, increased lenticular volume caused by gas bubble formation, or inadvertent damage to the posterior capsule by the laser during lens fragmentation.

Using a modified surgical technique, the authors had no further cases of CBS in the next 600 procedures. These modifications, designed to prevent excess fluid or gas pressure on the posterior capsule, are as follows:

1. Avoid overinflation of the anterior chamber with viscoelastic before hydrodissection.
2. Decompress the anterior chamber before and during hydrodissection by exerting pressure on the posterior lip of the corneal incision with the cannula.

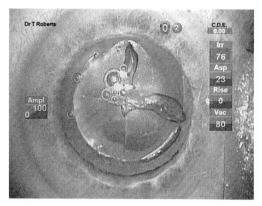

FIGURE 1.—Normal intracapsular gas bubble pattern following laser lens fragmentation and capsulotomy. (Reprinted from Journal of Cataract & Refractive Surgery. Roberts TV, Sutton G, Lawless MA, et al. Capsular block syndrome associated with femtosecond laser-assisted cataract surgery. *J Cataract Refract Surg*. 2011;37:2068-2070, Copyright 2011, with permission from ASCRS and ESCRS.)

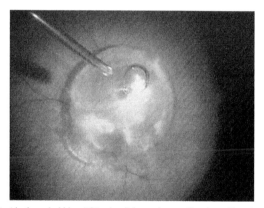

FIGURE 2.—Residual gas bubble within the dislocated crystalline lens. (Reprinted from Journal of Cataract & Refractive Surgery. Roberts TV, Sutton G, Lawless MA, et al. Capsular block syndrome associated with femtosecond laser-assisted cataract surgery. *J Cataract Refract Surg*. 2011;37:2068-2070, Copyright 2011, with permission from ASCRS and ESCRS.)

3. Decompress the lens capsule during hydrodissection by elevating the anterior capsule with the tip of the cannula during injection.

4. Inject the hydrodissection fluid slowly and titrate the volume based on the visible expanding fluid wave.

5. Use a blunt instrument to split the hemispheres before hydrodissection to allow trapped gas to come forward.

Only the last maneuver above is new for femto-assisted cataract surgery. The first 4 are common techniques used in standard cataract surgery to prevent complications during hydrodissection.

Use of the femtosecond laser during cataract surgery remains somewhat controversial, mainly because of the high cost/benefit ratio of the device.

However, I suspect it will become much more commonplace as costs decrease and new applications are developed that require the control and precision of the laser compared with current manual techniques. We can expect many more case reports and studies regarding this device to be published over the next few years.

M. F. Pyfer, MD

Assessment of a single-piece hydrophilic acrylic IOL for piggyback sulcus fixation in pseudophakic cadaver eyes
McIntyre JS, Werner L, Fuller SR, et al (Univ of Utah, Salt Lake City)
J Cataract Refract Surg 38:155-162, 2012

Purpose.—To evaluate a single-piece hydrophilic acrylic intraocular lens (IOL) designed for sulcus fixation in a piggyback configuration in post-mortem pseudophakic human eyes.

Setting.—John A. Moran Eye Center, University of Utah, Salt Lake City, Utah, USA.

Design.—Experimental study.

Methods.—Pseudophakic human cadaver eyes were imaged by high-frequency ultrasound (Artemis) to assess the overall position of the primary

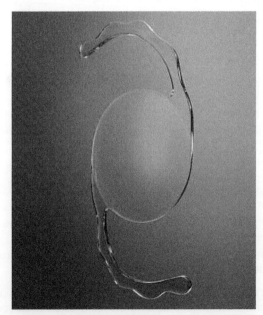

FIGURE 1.—Overall design of the study IOL (provided by Rayner Intraocular Lenses Ltd). (Reprinted from McIntyre JS, Werner L, Fuller SR, et al. Assessment of a single-piece hydrophilic acrylic IOL for piggyback sulcus fixation in pseudophakic cadaver eyes. *J Cataract Refract Surg.* 2012;38:155-162, Copyright 2012, with permission from ASCRS and ESCRS.)

IOL and the sulcus diameter. The piggyback IOL (Sulcoflex) was then injected into the ciliary sulcus of these eyes. After fixation in formalin, they were reevaluated by high-frequency ultrasound for assessment of IOL fixation, fit, centration, tilt, and clearance from the primary IOL and intraocular structures and analyzed after sectioning.

Results.—Data could be obtained from 11 eyes, all in which the primary IOL was located in the capsular bag. Different foldable IOLs and different degrees of Soemmerring ring formation were represented. The piggyback IOL could be injected and positioned in the ciliary sulcus and had overall appropriate centration and minimum or no tilt. Clearance between the 2 IOLs ranged from 232 to 779 μm, mostly depending on the thickness of the primary IOL. Direct assessment of the sulcus-fixated haptics showed no disturbances to the ciliary processes.

Conclusions.—The new IOL has large optic and overall diameters, smooth and undulating haptics, and a convex—concave optic profile. Results show that these characteristics minimize the possibility of interaction with

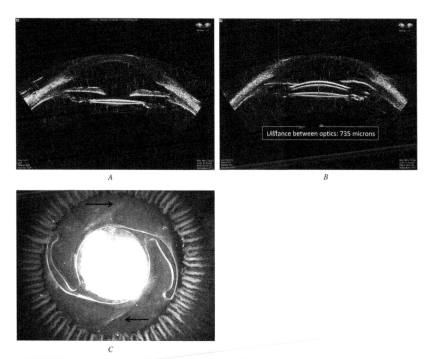

FIGURE 2.—Analysis of pseudophakic cadaver eyes before and after experimental implantation of the piggyback IOL; example 1. A: Preoperative ultrasound. B: Postoperative ultrasound. C: Postoperative Miyake-Apple posterior view; the in-the-bag IOL is a 1-piece hydrophobic acrylic IOL; Soemmerring ring formation = 0; the arrows show the haptics of the piggyback IOL. (Reprinted from McIntyre JS, Werner L, Fuller SR, et al. Assessment of a single-piece hydrophilic acrylic IOL for piggyback sulcus fixation in pseudophakic cadaver eyes. *J Cataract Refract Surg.* 2012;38:155-162, Copyright 2012, with permission from ASCRS and ESCRS.)

the primary IOL and uveal tissues, decreasing the likelihood of optical aberrations and pigmentary dispersion (Figs 1 and 2).

▶ This article presents a cadaver eye study of a novel 1-piece intraocular lens (IOL) design implanted in piggyback fashion in the iridociliary sulcus above a standard capsule fixated IOL (Fig 1). The postoperative position of the IOL was studied with anterior segment ultrasound biomicroscopy (UBM) and gross sectioning with standard microscopy (Fig 2). The results showed satisfactory secondary piggyback IOL positioning in all cases. The authors anticipate fewer complications with this design than with standard IOL models that are intended for in-the-bag placement due to several advantageous features: biocompatibility of the hydrophilic acrylic material, proper vaulting above the primary IOL due to convex-concave optic shape, and minimal iris chafe due to thin round-edge haptic and optic with posterior angulation.

I would anticipate broad potential applications of this IOL design if available in low plus and minus powers, with aspheric, toric, and multifocal features. Difficulties could still be encountered long term, such as decentration of the piggyback IOL due to migration of the haptics through a zonular defect. The next step should be human clinical trial, and we look forward to publication of these results in the future.

M. F. Pyfer, MD

In-the-Bag Capsular Tension Ring and Intraocular Lens Subluxation or Dislocation: A Series of 23 Cases
Werner L, Zaugg B, Neuhann T, et al (Univ of Utah, Salt Lake City; Augenklinik am Marienplatz, Munich, Germany)
Ophthalmology 119:266-271, 2012

Objective.—To describe clinical and pathologic findings from cases of in-the-bag capsular tension ring (CTR) and intraocular lens (IOL) subluxation or dislocation.

Design.—Retrospective case series with clinicopathologic correlation.

Participants.—Twenty-three explanted subluxated/dislocated capsular bags containing a CTR and an IOL explanted in Europe and submitted in fixative to the Berlin Eye Research Institute.

Methods.—Standard gross and light microscopy of specimens, complete histopathologic analyses of selected specimens done at the University of Utah, as well as questionnaire sent to explanting surgeons, and patient chart review, when available.

Main Outcome Measures.—Lens design, material, and abnormalities, capsular bag anomalies, patient demographic data, surgical dates, and presence or absence of known risk factors.

Results.—Patients were aged 76.31 ± 8.24 years at explantation, which was performed 81.5 ± 32.2 months after implantation. The IOLs in these cases were 3-piece hydrophobic acrylic (N = 11), 1-piece hydrophobic acrylic (n = 6), 3-piece silicone (n = 4), or 1-piece hydrophilic acrylic (n = 2) designs; all CTRs were made of poly(methyl methacrylate). Available information on associated ocular conditions included pseudoexfoliation (n = 17), glaucoma (n = 4), vitrectomy/retina surgery (n = 3), and trauma (n = 1). Complete histopathologic assessment in 3 specimens showed signs consistent with pseudoexfoliation, without available history related to this condition in one of the cases. Moderate/severe degrees of Soemmering's ring formation and capsulorhexis phimosis were observed or reported in 13 and 11 specimens, respectively. Fourteen eyes were implanted and explanted by the same surgeon, with an interval of 92.7 ± 23.4 months between the procedures. His rate of explantation because of subluxation/dislocation was 0.76% of the CTRs implanted during the time considered.

Conclusions.—Explantation because of postoperative subluxation or dislocation of CTR—IOL—capsular bag complexes occurred approximately 6.8 years after implantation in this series, providing further evidence that a fine line exists between zonular insufficiency that can be stabilized with the CTR alone and that requiring further support. Analyses of large series may help to define common factors associated with this complication, as well as surgical planning and employment of various endocapsular support devices to enhance postoperative zonular stabilization.

▶ This is the largest series of explanted in-the-bag intraocular lenses (IOLs) with a capsular tension ring (CTR) in place published to date. An earlier series of 86 subluxed in-the-bag IOLs had none with a CTR, leading the authors to speculate that the CTR is effective in preventing this late complication.[1] Obviously it is not completely effective. This series likely underestimates the true incidence of subluxation, since many of these lenses could be suture-fixated without explantation, especially in the presence of a CTR. As expected, the majority of cases here had pseudoexfoliation, a known risk factor for progressive zonular weakness. Also, a significant number showed extensive anterior capsule phimosis, despite the presence of a CTR. Early lysis of the phimotic ring with the yttrium aluminum garnet laser may help prevent further shrinkage and IOL subluxation, but this study did not examine this treatment.

M. F. Pyfer, MD

Reference

1. Davis D, Brubaker J, Espandar L, et al. Late in-the-bag spontaneous intraocular lens dislocation: evaluation of 86 consecutive cases. *Ophthalmology.* 2009;116: 664-670.

Improved Refractive Outcome for Ciliary Sulcus-Implanted Intraocular Lenses

Dubey R, Birchall W, Grigg J (The Univ of Sydney, Australia; Whangarei Hosp, New Zealand)
Ophthalmology 119:261-265, 2012

Objective.—To investigate the ideal correction of intraocular lens (IOL) power for sulcus implantation.

Design.—Retrospective, comparative case series.

Participants.—The records of 679 patients undergoing cataract surgery from June 2007 to June 2008 were reviewed.

Intervention.—Eyes in this series underwent phacoemulsification and IOL implantation with local anesthesia. Patients in our study population had their IOL power reduced by 0.5 or 1 diopter (D) from that calculated by the SRK-T formula for in-the-bag implantation. The IOL implanted was the foldable 3-piece acrylic Acrysof MA60AC (Alcon Laboratories Inc., Fort Worth, TX).

Main Outcome Measures.—In each case, the difference between actual spherical equivalent (SE) refraction and that predicted by biometry using the SRK-T formula was calculated.

Results.—Posterior capsule tears requiring implantation of IOL in the ciliary sulcus occurred in 36 eyes. When comparing eyes in which the power was reduced by 0.5 D with those in which the reduction was 1.0 D, those with a power reduction of 1.0 D had significantly less unexpected error (0.49 vs. 1.01 D SE). After stratifying eyes by axial length (AL), we found higher unexpected refractive error in short eyes (<22 mm AL). Likewise, eyes with a predicted IOL power >25 D had a greater postoperative refractive error.

Conclusions.—This is the first comparative clinical review examining adjustment of power of the sulcus-implanted IOL. We found that the IOL power should be adjusted according to the measured AL and predicted IOL power. For patients with a predicted IOL power from 18 to 25 D, power should be reduced by at least 1 D; for lenses >25 D, power should be reduced by 1.5 to 2 D.

▶ This elegant study challenges the conventional guideline for power adjustment on the fly when an intraocular lens (IOL) is placed in the ciliary sulcus rather than the capsular bag due to an unexpected capsular tear. The authors' retrospective analysis of 36 cases of sulcus-fixated IOLs indicates that improved refractive outcome is possible when the power reduction for sulcus fixation is scaled based on the intended IOL power (Table 4 in the original article). For the most frequent situation of IOL power between 18 and 25 diopters (D), a reduction of 1 D for sulcus fixation is more accurate. One limitation of this study is that most surgeons will attempt to capture the optic within the capsular bag if possible, even if the haptics are in the sulcus. Optic capture is desirable not only to put the optic closer to its intended location but to prevent tilt and iris contact. The power adjustment from this study does not apply in that case.

M. F. Pyfer, MD

Long-term visual outcome after cataract surgery: Comparison of healthy eyes and eyes with age-related macular degeneration
Mönestam E, Lundqvist B (Umeå Univ, Sweden)
J Cataract Refract Surg 38:409-414, 2012

Purpose.—To compare the long-term longitudinal visual acuity outcomes after cataract surgery in eyes with age-related macular degeneration (AMD) at surgery and eyes without comorbidity.
Setting.—University-based eye clinic.
Design.—Longitudinal cohort study.
Methods.—Patients having cataract surgery were evaluated over 1 year. A clinical eye examination and corrected distance visual acuity (CDVA) measurement were performed preoperatively and postoperatively as well as 5 and 10 years postoperatively for eligible patients. The patients were divided into functional groups depending on postoperative signs of macular degeneration and postoperative CDVA.
Results.—The study evaluated 810 patients. The rate of CDVA decline with age was faster in AMD patients than in patients without comorbidity. The slope of the visual acuity decline was similar in the 2 subgroups with AMD (almost normal CDVA and reduced CDVA postoperatively). After adjustment for age, there was a mean loss of 2.3 logMAR letters in patients with no comorbidity and 6.4 letters in patients with AMD at surgery for each decade of increasing age. More than 75% of AMD patients had better CDVA 10 years after surgery than before surgery.
Conclusions.—Patients with signs of AMD at cataract surgery had a longitudinally worse visual outcome than patients without clinical signs of AMD. However, there is no reason to discourage patients with concurrent visually significant cataract and AMD from having surgery because most AMD patients had better CDVA 10 years after surgery than before surgery (Fig 1).

▶ Does cataract surgery cause worsening of age-related macular degeneration (AMD)? Studies to date are inconclusive, with good evidence both for and against this hypothesis. This article does not claim to answer this question, but it does give us some real data that are reassuring when recommending cataract surgery for AMD patients.

The authors enrolled a fairly large cohort of 810 patients in Sweden undergoing cataract surgery and followed up with them for 10 years. The group included about 50% with no other pathology, 40% with AMD, and about 10% with other comorbid conditions such as diabetic retinopathy and glaucoma. Like most long-term studies in older patients, it suffers from significant attrition,

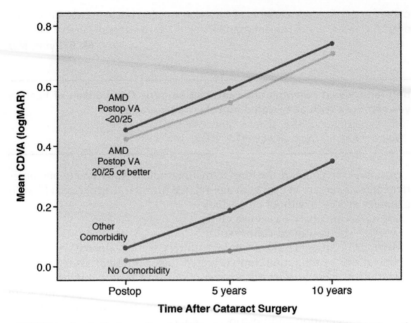

FIGURE 1.—Longitudinal age-adjusted CDVA outcomes in the 4 patient groups from 1 to 2 months postoperatively to 10 years after surgery for the 289 patients with 10-year data (CDVA = corrected distance visual acuity). (Reprinted from Mönestam E, Lundqvist B. Long-term visual outcome after cataract surgery: comparison of healthy eyes and eyes with age-related macular degeneration. *J Cataract Refract Surg.* 2012;38:409-414, Copyright 2012, with permission from ASCRS and ESCRS.)

so after 10 years, only 289 patients remained. However, 3 statistically valid observations are useful in counseling patients with AMD and cataract.

1. As might be expected, the rate of visual acuity decline over time is greater in patients with AMD than those without macular disease. But, somewhat surprisingly, this rate of vision loss (on a logMAR scale) is the same in patients with mild or more advanced AMD (Fig 1).

2. About 90% of patients with AMD had improved vision after cataract surgery.

3. After 10 years, more than 75% of patients with AMD still had better visual acuity after cataract surgery than before.

Patients with AMD often want to know if cataract surgery could make their vision worse. This study did not answer that question.

M. F. Pyfer, MD

Changes in the tear film and ocular surface after cataract surgery

Oh T, Jung Y, Chang D, et al (The Catholic Univ of Korea, Seoul)
Jpn J Ophthalmol 56:113-118, 2012

Purpose.—To evaluate changes in corneal sensitivity, tear film function, and ocular surface stability in patients after cataract surgery.

Methods.—This hospital-based prospective randomized trial included 48 eyes from 30 patients who underwent phacoemulsification. Slit-lamp examination, Schirmer test 1 (ST1), and measurement of corneal sensitivity and tear film breakup time (BUT) were performed for all patients 1 day before and 1 day, 1 month, and 3 months after surgery. In addition, conjunctival impression cytology from the temporal region of the conjunctiva was simultaneously performed.

Results.—Corneal sensitivity at the center and temporal incision sites had decreased significantly at 1 day postoperatively ($P = .021$, $P < .001$). However, the sensitivity had returned to almost the preoperative level 1 month postoperatively. The mean postoperative ST1 results were no different from preoperative values. On the other hand, BUT results had decreased significantly at 1 day postoperatively ($P = .01$) but had returned to almost the preoperative level 1 month postoperatively. Mean goblet cell density (GCD) had decreased significantly at 1 day, 1 month, and 3 months postoperatively ($P < .001$). In addition, decrease in GCD and cataract operative time were highly correlated ($r^2 = 0.65$).

Conclusions.—The decrease in GCD, which was correlated with operative time, had not recovered at 3 months after cataract surgery. Therefore, microscopic ocular surface damage during cataract surgery seems to be one of the pathogenic factors that cause ocular discomfort and dry eye syndrome after cataract surgery.

▶ Cataract surgeons are quite familiar with the temporary manifestation of dry eye syndrome in postsurgical patients. Symptoms can often be out of proportion to objective findings, such as fluorescein staining of the conjunctiva or Schirmer test score. This "nuisance" symptom often occurs despite an otherwise excellent outcome, and in my experience foreign body sensation after routine cataract surgery is one of the leading causes of patient dissatisfaction, often to the point of patients seeking a second opinion.

The authors' finding of reduced conjunctival goblet cell density (GCD) in proportion to surgical time is compelling, but clinically this may be less relevant, since the majority of cataract surgeons complete a routine case in 30 minutes or less. However, it is intriguing that GCD was found to be decreased significantly at 1 day postop and did not completely recover even at 3 months. Other studies have implicated toxicity of topical agents used perioperatively, such as anesthetics or povidone iodine. The authors did not mention these as a cause for decreased GCD. Further study with impression cytology taken just after surgical prepping and draping, or even a control group that underwent all preoperative steps including the prep but without surgery, would help further elucidate the cause for decreased GCD. Until these studies are done, it is prudent for cataract surgeons to protect the ocular surface during surgery, minimize operative time, and aggressively treat even mild dry eyes before and after surgery.

M. F. Pyfer, MD

Severe Adverse Events after Cataract Surgery Among Medicare Beneficiaries
Stein JD, Grossman DS, Mundy KM, et al (Univ of Michigan, Ann Arbor; Duke Univ, Durham, NC)
Ophthalmology 118:1716-1723, 2011

Purpose.—To determine rates and risk factors associated with severe postoperative complications after cataract surgery and whether they have been changing over the past decade.

Design.—Retrospective longitudinal cohort study.

Participants.—A total of 221 594 Medicare beneficiaries who underwent cataract surgery during 1994—2006.

Methods.—Beneficiaries were stratified into 3 cohorts: those who underwent initial cataract surgery during 1994—1995, 1999—2000, or 2005—2006. One-year rates of postoperative severe adverse events (endophthalmitis, suprachoroidal hemorrhage, retinal detachment) were determined for each cohort. Cox regression analyses determined the hazard of developing severe adverse events for each cohort with adjustment for demographic factors, ocular and medical conditions, and surgeon case-mix.

Main Outcome Measures.—Time period rates of development of severe postoperative adverse events.

Results.—Among the 221 594 individuals who underwent cataract surgery, 0.5% (1086) had at least 1 severe postoperative complication. After adjustment for confounders, individuals who underwent cataract surgery during 1994—1995 had a 21% increased hazard of being diagnosed with a severe postoperative complication (hazard ratio [HR] 1.21; 95% confidence interval [CI], 1.05—1.41) relative to individuals who underwent cataract surgery during 2005—2006. Those who underwent cataract surgery during 1999—2000 had a 20% increased hazard of experiencing a severe complication (HR 1.20; 95% CI, 1.04—1.39) relative to the 2005—2006 cohort. Risk factors associated with severe adverse events include a prior diagnosis of proliferative diabetic retinopathy (HR 1.62; 95% CI, 1.07—2.45) and cataract surgery combined with another intraocular surgical procedure on the same day (HR 2.51; 95% CI, 2.07—3.04). Individuals receiving surgery by surgeons with the case-mix least prone to developing a severe adverse event (HR 0.52; 95% CI, 0.44—0.62) had a 48% reduced hazard of a severe adverse event relative to recipients of cataract surgery performed by surgeons with the case-mix most prone to developing such outcomes.

Conclusions.—Rates of sight-threatening adverse events after cataract surgery declined during 1994—2006. Future efforts should be directed to identifying ways to reduce severe adverse events in high-risk groups.

▶ This study examined a large database of cataract surgery Medicare billing data. The authors sampled three 1-year periods between 1994 and 2006 to determine trends in the incidence of severe adverse events (AEs) after surgery, specifically, endophthalmitis, suprachoroidal hemorrhage, and rhegmatogenous or traction retinal detachment. Since only billing claims' data were available, clinical features such as postoperative vision could not be analyzed.

The findings of a reduced incidence of these sight-threatening AEs for each time period are compelling, indicating increased safety in cataract surgery over the 10-year period. As one might expect, patients with proliferative diabetic retinopathy and those undergoing combined procedures had higher rates of AEs. It is tempting to speculate that improvements in phaco machines, surgical devices, and medications, along with a trend toward smaller incisions during the study period, were largely responsible for the improvement. However, this is impossible to determine in the context of this study. Nonetheless, it is reassuring that we are heading in the right direction.

M. F. Pyfer, MD

Impact of Resident Participation in Cataract Surgery on Operative Time and Cost
Hosler MR, Scott IU, Kunselman AR, et al (Penn State College of Medicine, Hershey, PA; et al)
Ophthalmology 119:95-98, 2012

Objective.—To investigate the impact of resident participation in cataract surgery on operative time and cost.

Design.—Retrospective chart review.

Participants.—All patients who underwent phacoemulsification cataract surgery by an attending or resident surgeon of the Penn State Hershey Eye Center between July 1, 2004, and June 30, 2007.

Methods.—Operating room records of all phacoemulsification surgeries performed at a single academic center between July 1, 2004, and June 30, 2007, were reviewed.

Main Outcome Measures.—Operative case length in minutes and cost of operating room time.

Results.—The primary surgeon was an attending physician in 474 cases and a senior resident physician in 473 cases. Phacoemulsification surgeries took an average of 12 minutes 41 seconds longer per eye when performed by a senior resident compared with an attending surgeon (95% confidence interval [CI], 1 minute 48 seconds to 23 minutes 35 seconds; $P = 0.027$). Resident cases averaged 63 minutes in July, and decreased to an average of 27 minutes in June. Every month from July through December of the academic year, the monthly mean operative case length for resident cases was significantly longer than the mean operative case length for attending cases (*P*<0.05), except November, when the difference was borderline significant (95% CI, −23 seconds to 23 minutes 9 seconds; *P* = 0.057). From January through June, there was no difference. Using the nonsupply cost of running the operating room at our institution ($8.30 per operating minute), resident participation added $105.40 to the average phacoemulsification case. This cost totaled $8293.23 per resident per year.

Conclusions.—Resident participation is associated with significantly increased phacoemulsification operative times and costs during the first half, but not the second half, of the academic year. The time and cost per resident may be important to consider when allocating resources for preclinical training.

▶ Training residents to perform phacoemulsification cataract surgery is an essential part of ophthalmology residency. Traditionally, the mentor-apprentice model is followed, in which residents observe, then assist, and finally perform surgery under close supervision by an experienced attending surgeon. A recent trend in cataract surgery training involves increased use of formalized wet-lab training and surgical simulators early in residency. Anecdotally these measures have led to higher skill level for beginning postgraduate year 4 residents as they begin to operate as the primary surgeon under supervision.

This study examines the cost of resident-performed cataract surgery in the form of operative time. At a single training site, with a small number of attendings, senior residents in this program achieved operative times on average similar to experienced surgeons after 6 months of experience (after performing about 40 cases). The authors then estimate the extra expense of having residents perform cataract surgery at about $8000 per resident per year, based on per-minute operating room charges. The cost of extra materials or possible second procedures due to complications is not included, but would likely increase that cost substantially.

M. F. Pyfer, MD

Determination of Valid Benchmarks for Outcome Indicators in Cataract Surgery: A Multicenter, Prospective Cohort Trial
Hahn U, Krummenauer F, Kölbl B, et al (The OcuNet Cataract Benchmark Trial Group, Duesseldorf, Germany; Med Faculty of the Private Univ of Witten/ Herdecke, Germany)
Ophthalmology 118:2105-2112, 2011

Objective.—To evaluate a systematic approach to derive valid benchmarks for 2 outcome indicators intended to ascertain quality in cataract surgery and to propose benchmark levels drawn from the study results.
Design.—Prospective, multicenter cohort trial.
Participants.—A total of 1685 patients (206−239 eyes per trial site) were recruited consecutively at 7 study sites. The patients featured age-related

cataracts and were undergoing unilateral cataract surgery in the period between January 2007 and August 2008.

Methods.—Only patients with uncomplicated age-related cataracts were included. Cataract surgery was performed by phacoemulsification. The SN60AT (Alcon, Inc., Fort Worth, TX) intraocular lens (IOL) was used as a study lens. The IOL power was calculated using the SRK-T formula with a standardized A constant. Biometry was performed with the IOL Master (Carl Zeiss Meditex, Jena, Germany). Only highly experienced senior surgeons were involved.

Main Outcome Measures.—The outcome indicators 1 month and 3 months after surgery were the respective achievement of: (1) maximum absolute deviation of 0.5 diopter (D) between target refraction and post-operative spherical equivalent (primary end point, refractive accuracy); (2) best-corrected visual acuity of at least 0.8 (secondary end point, visual acuity outcome).

Results.—In the pooled data, maximum absolute deviation of ± 0.5 D from target refraction was achieved in 80% (95% confidence interval, 78%−82%) of cases. Visual acuity of 0.8 or more was reached in 87% (95% confidence interval, 80%−93%) of cases. The results from the trial centers differed significantly in the outcomes of the primary and secondary end points (*P*<0.001).

Conclusions.—The study quantified benchmark levels for 2 outcome indicators in a standardized cataract surgery procedure. External confounding factors such as the comorbidity of patients, which cannot be influenced by the surgeon, were excluded. The derived benchmarks selectively illustrate the quality of the surgery and are superior to success rates published in the literature from unspecific data collections. This method is more suited for improving outcome quality by benchmarking. General methodologic problems are discussed, leading to recommendations for future study designs (Table 5).

▶ Establishing benchmarks for outcome quality in any surgical procedure is a complex process, but it is a growing trend as payers seek to measure the effectiveness of payments for care. Cataract surgery is no exception.

This study examined over 1500 routine cataract surgical procedures at a group of high-volume clinics in Germany. Unlike previous large population studies of cataract surgery outcomes (Table 5), the authors excluded patients with preexisting pathology that could affect vision, including corneal and retinal disease. They also standardized the procedures to a single intraocular lens model, biometry technique, and intraocular lens formula. Doing so, the authors propose 2 quality benchmarks: postoperative refraction within a half diopter of target, and best corrected visual acuity of 20/25 or better. They were able to achieve this in an impressive 80% and 87% of patients, respectively.

I agree with the authors that any outcome metric for cataract surgery must control for comorbid factors and either quantify them in a complex formula or exclude patients with these conditions from measurement altogether. One important metric of effectiveness in cataract surgery that the authors did not

TABLE 5.—Literature Results for Postoperative Visual and Refractive Outcome Indicators

	Data Source	Interval Between Surgery and Data Collection	Relative Frequencies for Postoperative Best-Corrected Visual Acuity ≥0.5			Relative Frequencies for Absolute Deviation Target Refraction Postoperative Spherical Equivalent (D)	
			All Patients	Patients with Comorbidities	Patients without Comorbidities	≤0.5	≤1
2002[17]	UK, 1 postgraduate teaching hospital	3 wks	86.9%		95.4%	44.6%	72.3%
2002[13]	Swedish National Cataract Register (SNCR)	Mean interval, 38 d	84%	72%	95%		79.2%
2007[15]	UK, 1 teaching hospital		93%			65.7%	82.1%
2007[21]	Swedish National Cataract Register (SNCR)	Mean interval, 48 d				58.4%	83.8%
2009[22]	UK Cataract National Database (UK CND)	Median, 35 d	91.4%	82%	94.6%		
2009[6]	UK, 2 hospitals	4 wks				60.2%	87%
2010	Germany, 7 high-volume study centers (OcuNet)	3 mos			98.5%	80.3%	97.3%

D = diopter; UK = United Kingdom.
Editor's Note: Please refer to original journal article for full references.

address is the patients' subjective improvement in visual function or quality of life. Subjective rating or patient questionnaire data will very likely play a role in cataract outcome metrics when adopted, and these should be included in future research.

M. F. Pyfer, MD

Femtosecond Laser Capsulotomy and Manual Continuous Curvilinear Capsulorrhexis Parameters and Their Effects on Intraocular Lens Centration
Kránitz K, Takacs A, Miháltz K, et al (Semmelweis Univ Budapest, Hungary; et al)
J Refract Surg 27:558-563, 2011

Purpose.—To measure and compare sizing and positioning parameters of femtosecond laser capsulotomy with manual continuous curvilinear capsulorrhexis (CCC).

Methods.—Femtosecond capsulotomies (Alcon-LenSx Lasers Inc) and CCC were carried out in 20 eyes of 20 patients, respectively. Intraocular lens (IOL) decentration, circularity, vertical and horizontal diameters of capsulotomies, and capsule overlap were measured with Adobe Photoshop (Adobe Systems Inc) 1 week, 1 month, and 1 year after surgery. Between-group differences of parameters and predictors of IOL decentration were determined with repeated measures analysis of variance, chi-square test, and logistic regression analyses.

Results.—Vertical diameter of CCC was statistically significantly higher in the first week and month. Significantly higher values of capsule overlap over 1 year and circularity in the first week showed more regular femtosecond capsulotomies. Horizontal IOL decentration was statistically significantly higher in the CCC group over 1 year. A significant difference was noted between the two groups in dichotomized horizontal decentration values at 0.4 mm with chi-square test after 1 week and 1 year ($P=.035$ and $P=.016$, respectively). In univariable general estimating equation models, type of capsulorrhexis ($P<.01$) and capsule overlap ($P=.002$) were significant predictors of horizontal decentration. Vertical diameter showed significant correlation to the overlap in the CCC group (1 week: $r=-0.91$; 1 month: $r=-0.76$, $P<.01$; 1 year: $r=-0.62$, $P<.01$), whereas no significant correlation was noted in the femtosecond group ($P>.05$).

Conclusions.—More precise capsulotomy sizing and centering can be achieved with femtosecond laser. Properly sized, shaped, and centered femtosecond laser capsulotomies resulted in better overlap parameters that help maintain proper positioning of the IOL (Fig 2).

▶ The introduction of femtosecond laser devices to perform part of the cataract surgical procedure is controversial but will almost certainly lead to a profound change in the way most procedures are performed in the future. Phacoemulsification was not widely accepted until improved machines made the procedure

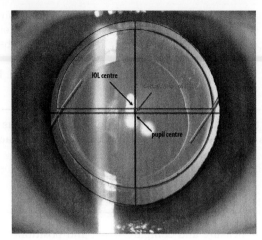

FIGURE 2.—Decentration of the IOL from the pupil center. (Reprinted from Kránitz K, Takacs A, Miháltz K, et al. Femtosecond laser capsulotomy and manual continuous curvilinear capsulorrhexis parameters and their effects on intraocular lens centration. *J Refract Surg.* 2011;27:558-563, with permission from SLACK Incorporated.)

safer and easier, and foldable intraocular lenses (IOLs) were developed to take advantage of smaller incisions. I believe femtosecond laser-assisted cataract surgery will undergo a similar evolution, along with a concomitant reduction in cost of the device.

This article is one of several by the authors examining the outcome of femtosecond laser-assisted cataract surgery versus standard manual with regard to parameters such as IOL centration, tilt, and continuous curvilinear capsulorrhexis (CCC) overlap. The significant result here is that horizontal IOL centration (Fig 2) was better in the femtosecond laser group than the manual CCC group for up to 1 year postop. At 1 year, one-third of the CCC group had horizontal IOL decentration greater than 0.4 mm, compared to none in the femtosecond group. This amount of decentration is sufficient to cause a reduction in optical image quality in aspheric or multifocal IOLs.

We can certainly expect more studies on femtosecond laser-assisted cataract surgery to be published over the next few years.

M. F. Pyfer, MD

A four-year prospective study on intraocular pressure in relation to phacoemulsification cataract surgery
Falck A, Hautala N, Turunen N, et al (Oulu Univ Hosp, Finland)
Acta Ophthalmol 89:614-616, 2011

Aim of Study.—To follow up prospectively the intraocular pressure (IOP) of healthy eyes with senile cataract undergoing phacoemulsification surgery over a duration of 4 years.

Patients and Methods.—Thirty-five patients entering first eye cataract surgery had IOP measured by applanation tonometry pre-operatively and on day 1, at 1 month, 6 months, 1 year, 2 years and 4 years after surgery at 9 a.m. and again at 2 p.m. in the Department of Ophthalmology, Oulu University Hospital. Thirty-four patients attended the 1-year checkup, and the 2- and 4-year results are available for 31.

Results.—The pre-operative IOP was 16.0 (SD 4.3, range 6−25) mmHg in the morning and 16.4 (SD 4.0, range 8−25.5) mmHg in the afternoon. On the first postoperative day, the IOP was 2.1 ± 5.6 mmHg higher than before surgery (p = 0.029). At 1 month, the IOP morning measurement had decreased 2.8 ± 3.6 mmHg, and in the afternoon, the decrease was 3.0 ± 2.7 mmHg from the pre-operative level. At 6 months, the decrease was 3.3 ± 2.7 mmHg in the morning and 3.6 ± 2.7 mmHg in the afternoon, at 1 year, 3.2 ± 3.0 mmHg and 3.5 ± 3.2 mmHg, at 2 years, 3.2 ± 2.4 mmHg and 3.1 ± 2.8 mmHg, and at the 4-year postoperative checkup, 3.6 ± 3.4 mmHg and 3.6 ± 2.7 mmHg, respectively (p = 0.000 for all time-points).

Conclusions.—IOP decreases by about 3 mmHg (16−23% from the pre-operative IOP level) after phacoemulsification and remains at this reduced level with no trend towards an increase during 4 years.

▶ This small study shows that in normal eyes undergoing routine phacoemulsification cataract surgery, the well-known side effect of reduced intraocular pressure (IOP) is achieved by 1 month postoperatively and is maintained for at least 4 years. The authors excluded patients with pseudo-exfoliation syndrome or with any coexisting pathology, including ocular hypertension or glaucoma. Previous studies have found even greater reduction of IOP in eyes with these conditions.[1] The authors and others[2] speculate that the IOP reduction is due to anatomic changes after surgery, such as greater anterior chamber depth and volume with a wider open angle. This study supports that conclusion. Mechanical washout of the trabecular meshwork from anterior chamber irrigation during surgery is less likely, because this effect would be expected to diminish over time.

M. F. Pyfer, MD

References

1. Mathalone N, Hyams M, Neiman S, Buckman G, Hod Y, Gever O. Long-term intraocular pressure control after clear corneal phacoemulsification in glaucoma patients. *J Cataract Refract Surg.* 2005;31:479-483.
2. Shingleton BJ, Pasternack JJ, Hung JW, O'Donoghue MW. Three and five year changes in intraocular pressures after clear corneal phacoemulsification in open angle glaucoma patients, glaucoma suspects, and normal patients. *J Glaucoma.* 2006;15:494-498.

Prevention of capsular bag opacification with a new hydrophilic acrylic disk-shaped intraocular lens
Kavoussi SC, Werner L, Fuller SR, et al (Univ of Utah, Salt Lake City)
J Cataract Refract Surg 37:2194-2200, 2011

Purpose.—To evaluate capsular bag opacification with a new disk-shaped single-piece hydrophilic acrylic intraocular lens (IOL) suspended between 2 haptic rings connected by a pillar of the haptic material and with a commercially available single-piece hydrophobic acrylic IOL in rabbits.

Setting.—John A. Moran Eye Center, University of Utah, Salt Lake City, Utah, USA.

Design.—Experimental study.

Methods.—The study IOL was implanted in the right eyes of 5 New Zealand rabbits and the control IOL in the left eyes. Slitlamp examination was performed at weeks 1 through 5. After the rabbits were humanely killed, the globes were enucleated and examined by ultrasound. Capsular bag opacification scoring from the posterior aspect (Miyake-Apple view) was then performed, followed by histopathology.

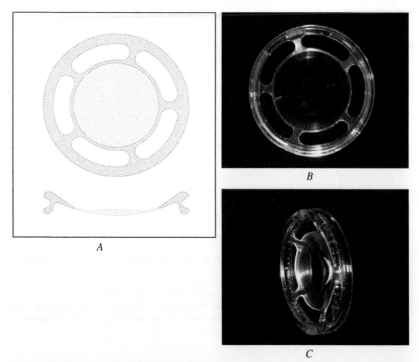

FIGURE 1.—A: Overall design of the study IOL (*top*: front view; *bottom*: side view). The 6.0 mm optic is depicted in blue and the haptic element in pink. B and C: Gross photographs of the study IOL (B: front view; C: side view). For interpretation of the references to color in this figure legend, the reader is referred to web version of this article. (Reprinted from Kavoussi SC, Werner L, Fuller SR, et al. Prevention of capsular bag opacification with a new hydrophilic acrylic disk-shaped intraocular lens. *J Cataract Refract Surg.* 2011;37:2194-2200, Copyright 2011, with permission from ASCRS and ESCRS.)

Results.—Trace honeycomb posterior capsule opacification (PCO) was noted in some study eyes. All control eyes developed moderate to marked PCO, which was more pronounced at the level of the optic—haptic junction. The mean PCO score was 0.4 ± 0.22 (SD) in the study group and 3.4 ± 0.54 in the control group ($P = .000179$, paired t test). Minimal proliferative cortical material was confined to the space between the anterior and posterior rings of the study IOL haptics. Anterior capsule opacification was absent in study eyes and mild in control eyes. There was no contact between the anterior capsule and the anterior surface of study IOLs.

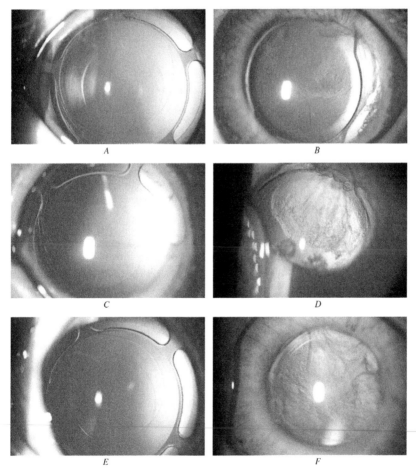

FIGURE 2.—Both eyes of rabbits 1, 2, and 3 at 5 weeks (A, C, and E: right eyes with study IOLs; B, D, and F: left eyes with control IOLs). Eyes with study IOLs showed clear anterior and posterior capsules while eyes with control IOLs developed diffuse PCO, starting at the optic—haptic junctions (slitlamp photographs). (Reprinted from Kavoussi SC, Werner L, Fuller SR, et al. Prevention of capsular bag opacification with a new hydrophilic acrylic disk-shaped intraocular lens. *J Cataract Refract Surg.* 2011;37:2194-2200, Copyright 2011, with permission from ASCRS and ESCRS.)

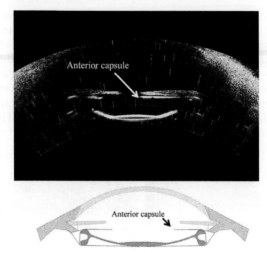

FIGURE 3.—Right eye of rabbit 2. Ultrasound examination confirmed that the anterior capsule remained at a distance from the anterior optic surface, as hypothesized before the in vivo study and according to the bottom schematic drawing. (Reprinted from Kavoussi SC, Werner L, Fuller SR, et al. Prevention of capsular bag opacification with a new hydrophilic acrylic disk-shaped intraocular lens. *J Cataract Refract Surg.* 2011;37:2194-2200, Copyright 2011, with permission from ASCRS and ESCRS.)

Conclusion.—The peripheral rings of the study IOL, by expanding the capsular bag and preventing IOL surface contact with the anterior capsule, appear to prevent opacification of the capsular bag (Figs 1-3).

▶ This article describes an innovative foldable intraocular lens (IOL) design that proved remarkably effective at preventing both anterior capsule opacification and posterior capsule opacification compared to a standard control hydrophobic acrylic IOL in the rabbit model (Fig 2). This is especially impressive given the highly reactive nature of the rabbit eye. The new lens design (Fig 1) incorporates features of a capsular tension ring to expand the capsular bag for 360 degrees and is designed to keep the anterior capsule rim elevated away from the posterior capsule as well as the IOL optic (Fig 3). The novel peripheral ring sequesters residual lens epithelial cells in the capsular fornix. It may eventually prove to be as important a development for posterior capsule opacification prevention as the now popular square-edged optic. This design also looks promising as the basis for a new accommodating IOL if modified with a dual optic configuration. I look forward to hearing more about this IOL as it progresses toward human trials.

M. F. Pyfer, MD

Impact on visual function from light scattering and glistenings in intraocular lenses, a long-term study

Mönestam E, Behndig A (Norrlands Univ Hosp, Umeå, Sweden)
Acta Ophthalmol 89:724-728, 2011

Purpose.—To investigate the impact on visual function from light scattering and glistenings in intraocular lenses (IOLs) in patients who had cataract surgery 10 years previously.

Setting.—Eye clinic, Norrlands university hospital, Umeå, Sweden.

Methods.—One hundred and three patients, who had phacoemulsification with implantation of Acrysof® MA60BM IOLs 10 years previously, were evaluated with best corrected visual acuity (VA), and low contrast visual acuity (LCVA) 10% and 2.5%. The light scattering from the IOLs was measured by Scheimpflug photography. The degree of glistenings was also quantified at the slit-lamp. Eyes with coexisting pathology that could affect VA and LCVA were excluded.

Results.—The patients were divided into various groups according to the degree of light scattering and grade of glistenings. In two subsets of patients, paired data from the patients' eyes were analysed. It was not possible to detect any significant impact on visual function, best corrected visual acuity (BCVA) and LCVA 10% and 2.5% in eyes with a more pronounced light scattering or a higher grade of glistenings seen at the slit-lamp. The correlation between IOL dioptric power and both the total light scattering of the IOL, and the subjective grading of the intensity of the glistenings at the slit-lamp was statistically significant ($r_P = 0.25$; $p = 0.012$; $r_S = 0.23$; $p = 0.019$, respectively).

Conclusion.—Most patients in this case series operated 10 years previously had severe glistenings and a high level of light scattering from their intraocular lenses. No detectable impact on BCVA, LCVA 10% and 2.5% was found.

▶ The presence of so-called glistenings in intraocular lenses (IOLs) is disconcerting to most ophthalmologists, since the slit lamp appearance can be dramatic. Although they may occur in any IOL, they are most common in hydrophobic acrylic lenses and appear to increase in density over time. There have been case reports of IOL exchange due to presumed visual symptoms from severe glistenings. The exact cause of glistenings is not well understood, although they have been characterized as microscopic water vacuoles within the lens material.

This study from Sweden examined over 100 patients 10 years after implantation of a 3-piece hydrophobic acrylic IOL, the Alcon Acrysof® MA60BM. All patients had mild to severe glistenings graded on slit lamp examination. Grade of glistenings was found to correlate with the power (thus thickness) of the IOL. Scheimpflug photography using the Pentacam HR confirmed the glistenings quantitatively with light scattering, but surprisingly no reduction in visual acuity or low-contrast vision was found. This is reassuring since this lens material has been used in many thousands of patients throughout the world.

M. F. Pyfer, MD

Theoretical Performance of Intraocular Lenses Correcting Both Spherical and Chromatic Aberration

Weeber HA, Piers PA (AMO Groningen B.V, Netherlands)
J Refract Surg 28:48-52, 2012

Purpose.—To assess the performance and optical limitations of intraocular lenses (IOLs) correcting both longitudinal spherical aberration (LSA) and longitudinal chromatic aberration (LCA) compared to standard spherical and aspheric IOLs.

Methods.—Using a set of 46 white light, pseudophakic eye models representing a population of cataract patients, retinal image quality was assessed for three IOL designs—standard spherical IOLs; aspheric IOLs, correcting a fixed amount of LSA; and aspheric refractive/diffractive IOLs, correcting a fixed amount of LSA and LCA. Depth of field and tolerance to IOL misalignments were also assessed.

Results.—The improvement factor, based on the area under the radial polychromatic modulation transfer function (pMTF) curve of the IOL, correcting both average LSA and LCA over the aspheric IOL was 1.19 ± 0.12, and over the spherical IOL was 1.43 ± 0.29. Within the range of ± 1.00 diopter of defocus, pMTF of the IOL correcting both LSA and LCA was equal or higher than both the spherical and aspheric IOLs. The IOL could be decentered up to 0.6 to 0.8 mm before the performance degraded below that of a spherical IOL.

Conclusions.—This is the first study that evaluates IOLs correcting both LSA and LCA in the presence of corneal higher order aberrations. Intraocular lenses that correct both LSA and LCA improve simulated retinal image quality over spherical IOLs and IOLs that correct LSA alone, without sacrificing depth of field or tolerance to decentration. Correction of LCA in combination with LSA shows the potential to improve visual performance.

▶ From those who developed the first intraocular lens (IOL) to correct spherical aberration[1] now comes word that they are working on a new IOL design to correct chromatic aberration as well. Flash back to 2002: unless you were involved in wavefront-corrected excimer laser refractive surgery, most cataract surgeons paid little attention to spherical aberration (SA). Today, chances are the IOLs you use every day are designed to reduce SA, with a measurable benefit to our patients' vision, especially for those with larger pupils or in low-light situations.

This article describes optical testing of a novel IOL design that corrects both spherical and chromatic aberration. Chromatic aberration results from different wavelengths of light encountering slightly different refractive power, which in white light leads to a defocused image. It turns out that chromatic aberration of the aphakic eye (mostly corneal) varies little among patients, so a single average correction value can be used. The chromatic aberration of the IOL itself must also be corrected, which changes as a function of IOL power. An ingenious design is discussed, combining monofocal refractive and diffractive components to achieve a total IOL power with the intended spherical and chromatic aberration to offset that of the average eye. One potential problem with the proposed design is the loss inherent in diffractive lenses, but the authors do not address this issue. Theoretically, based on the modulation transfer function (MTF) of the IOL in the model eye, chromatic aberration correction provides about as much improvement in image quality over the current aspheric IOL as the aspheric IOL adds to the old standard spherical IOL.

The authors hint that the best image quality would result from adding chromatic aberration correction to a customized IOL that minimizes other ocular higher-order aberrations besides SA, such as coma and trefoil. We look forward to a time in the not-too-distant future when IOL surgery can be fully customized or adjustable, similar to wavefront-driven corneal refractive surgery. I am certain that these advanced IOLs will incorporate features to correct not only lower and higher order refractive errors, but also chromatic aberration, as illustrated in this article.

M. F. Pyfer, MD

Reference

1. Holladay JT, Piers PA, Koranyi G, van der Mooren M, Norrby NE. A new intraocular lens design to reduce spherical aberration of pseudophakic eyes. *J Refract Surg.* 2002;18:683-691.

Cataract Surgery After Trabeculectomy: The Effect on Trabeculectomy Function

Husain R, Liang S, Foster PJ, et al (Singapore at Natl Eye Ctr and Singapore Eye Res Inst; Univ College London Inst of Ophthalmology, England, UK; et al)
Arch Ophthalmol 130:165-170, 2012

Objective.—To determine whether the timing of cataract surgery after trabeculectomy has an effect on trabeculectomy function in terms of intraocular pressure control.

Methods.—This was a cohort study nested within a randomized clinical trial. There were 235 participants with glaucoma who had a single previous trabeculectomy augmented with either intraoperative 5-fluorouracil or placebo. Cataract surgery with intraocular lens implantation was performed on participants judged to have significant lens opacity. Cox regression was performed to evaluate the effect of time between trabeculectomy and cataract surgery on the time to trabeculectomy failure, after adjusting for other relevant risk factors. The main outcome measure was time to failure of trabeculectomy, defined as an intraocular pressure of greater than 21 mm Hg.

Results.—Of the 235 participants, 124 (52.7%) underwent subsequent cataract surgery. The median time from trabeculectomy to cataract surgery for these patients was 21.7 months (range, 4.6-81.9 months). The median follow-up period was 60 months (range, 28-84 months) for the cataract surgery group and 48 months (range, 12-84 months) for the non—cataract surgery group. Cox regression showed that the time from trabeculectomy to cataract surgery was significantly associated with time to trabeculectomy failure (hazard ratio, 1.73 [95% CI, 1.05-2.85]; $P = .03$). The adjusted declining hazard ratios for risk of subsequent trabeculectomy failure when cataract surgery was performed 6 months, 1 year, and 2 years after trabeculectomy were 3.00 (95% CI, 1.11-8.14), 1.73 (95% CI, 1.05-2.85), and 1.32 (95% CI, 1.02-1.69), respectively.

Conclusions.—Cataract surgery after trabeculectomy increases the risk of trabeculectomy failure, and this risk is increased if the time between trabeculectomy and cataract surgery is shorter.

▶ Cataracts and glaucoma frequently occur together and require surgical intervention. Significant glaucoma that fails medical or laser treatment is often managed with surgical trabeculectomy using adjunctive intraoperative antimetabolites, either mitomycin-C (MMC) or 5-fluorouracil (5FU). Modern cataract surgery using topical anesthesia with a clear corneal incision does not involve conjunctival manipulation and is felt to have a low risk for causing bleb failure after successful trabeculectomy.

This study found a substantially higher risk for bleb failure if cataract surgery is performed less than 1 year after the trabeculectomy. Failure was defined as intraocular pressure (IOP) above 21 mmHg without use of medications. Bleb needling was permitted in the trial before failure, but additional antimetabolite injections were not.

This study is relevant to current practice, since all but 2 of the 124 cataract surgeries were done with temporal clear corneal small-incision phacoemulsification. However, most U.S. surgeons use intraoperative MMC during trabeculectomy rather than 5FU, as in this study. Also, more than 50% of cases had no antimetabolite, which is known to increase the risk for late bleb failure. Nevertheless, in light of these results, it seems prudent to wait at least 1 year after successful trabeculectomy before performing cataract surgery. If cataract extraction is anticipated sooner for visual rehabilitation, then combined surgery should be considered, or cataract surgery should be performed prior to trabeculectomy if short-term medical IOP control is adequate. Since cataract surgery alone often leads to decreased IOP, this approach may even avoid the need for subsequent trabeculectomy in some cases.

M. F. Pyfer, MD

Comparison of prediction error: Labeled versus unlabeled intraocular lens manufacturing tolerance
Zudans JV, Desai NR, Trattler WB (Florida Eye Inst, Vero Beach; Eye Inst of West Florida, Largo, FL; Ctr for Excellence in Eye Care, Miami, FL)
J Cataract Refract Surg 38:394-402, 2012

Purpose.—To compare the prediction error between intraocular lenses (IOLs) available in 0.25 diopter (D) increments with a labeled manufacturing tolerance and IOLs available in 0.50 D increments without a labeled manufacturing tolerance.

Setting.—Community-based multidisciplinary outpatient ophthalmic practices.

Design.—Comparative case series.

Methods.—Eyes with cataract had implantation of an IOL available in 0.25 D increments and labeled with a manufacturing tolerance of ±0.11 D (labeled group) or an IOL available in 0.50 D increments without a labeled manufacturing tolerance (unlabeled group). Postoperatively, the prediction error was calculated and compared between groups.

Results.—By the SRK/T formula, the mean error of prediction after optimization was −0.03 D ± 0.35 (SD) in the labeled group and −0.05 ± 0.46 D in the unlabeled group (*P* =.64). The mean absolute error of prediction was statistically significantly smaller in the labeled group (0.26 ± 0.23 D) than in the unlabeled group (0.37 ± 0.28 D) (*P* =.04). The mean and absolute errors were not statistically significantly different with the Holladay 1 or Hoffer Q formula. Sixty-three percent of patients in the labeled group and 43% in the unlabeled group (*P* =.03) were within ±0.25 D of the prediction error; 84% and 69%, respectively, were within ±0.50 D (*P* =.06).

Conclusion.—The IOLs available in 0.25 D increments with a labeled manufacturing tolerance of ±0.11 D increased the percentage of patients within ±0.25 D of the targeted refraction to a statistically significant and clinically meaningful level compared with unlabeled IOLs available in 0.50 D increments (Fig 4).

▶ This study lends credence to the assertion that use of intraocular lenses (IOLs) labeled in 0.25 D increments and manufactured to tight tolerance can improve

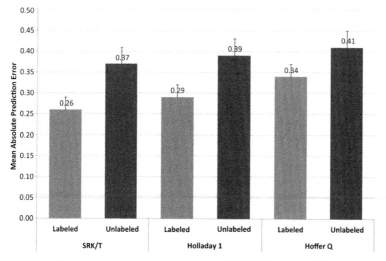

FIGURE 4.—Mean absolute prediction error based on SRK/T, Holladay 1, and Hoffer Q formulas. (Reprinted from Zudans JV, Desai NR, Trattler WB. Comparison of prediction error: labeled versus unlabeled intraocular lens manufacturing tolerance. *J Cataract Refract Surg.* 2012;38:394-402, Copyright 2012, with permission from ASCRS and ESCRS.)

the accuracy of refractive outcomes after cataract surgery. Current accurate biometry using partial coherence interferometry for axial length (Zeiss IOL Master or Haag-Streit Lenstar) coupled with optimized lens constants and consistent reproducible surgical technique have improved the refractive predictability of cataract surgery. Effective lens position uncertainty still leaves room for improvement, but intraoperative measurements with new devices may help reduce this source of error as well.

This is the first article that I am aware of that demonstrates reduced refractive prediction error using IOLs available in 0.25 D increments (Fig 4). As a retrospective study that excluded any patient with worse than 20/25 best correct visual acuity or with more than 1 D of astigmatism, it may suffer from selection bias. Also, I would like to see a comparison of uncorrected postoperative vision, not just refractive error, since that is how patients judge their result.

M. F. Pyfer, MD

Evaluating teaching methods of cataract surgery: Validation of an evaluation tool for assessing surgical technique of capsulorhexis
Smith RJ, McCannel CA, Gordon LK, et al (Univ of California at Los Angeles)
J Cataract Refract Surg 38:799-806, 2012

Purpose.—To develop and assess the validity of an evaluation tool to quantitatively assess the capsulorhexis portion of cataract surgery performed by residents.

Setting.—University of California at Los Angeles (UCLA), Department of Ophthalmology, Jules Stein Eye Institute, Los Angeles, California, USA.

Design.—Masked prospective case series.

Methods.—Ophthalmology faculty members at UCLA were surveyed and literature was reviewed to develop a grading tool comprising 12 questions to evaluate surgical technique, including 4 from the Global Rating Assessment of Skills in Intraocular Surgery and 2 from the International Council of Ophthalmology's Ophthalmology Surgical Competency Assessment Rubric. Video clips of continuous curvilinear capsulorhexis (CCC) performed by 2 postgraduate year (PGY) 3 residents, 2 PGY 4 residents, and 2 advanced surgeons were independently graded in a masked fashion by a 7-member faculty panel.

Results.—Four questions had low interobserver variability and a significant correlation with surgical skill level (intraclass correlation coefficient >0.75; $P<.05$, analysis of variance; 42 observations). The 4 questions were visual Likert-scale questions grading flow of operation, set up for regrasp, commencement of flap and formation, and circular completion of the CCC.

Conclusions.—Surgical performance can be validly measured using an evaluation tool. However, not all evaluation questions produced reliable results. The reliability and accuracy of the measurements appear to depend on the form and content of the question. Studies to optimize assessment tools identifying the best questions for evaluating each step of cataract surgery may help ophthalmic educators more precisely measure outcomes for improving teaching interventions.

▶ Most active US cataract surgeons have been trained in a supervised setting with experienced mentors using the traditional surgical apprenticeship-type teaching model (oversimplified by medical trainees in the adage "See one, do one, teach one"). We are all in some sense indebted to our teachers and obliged to return the favor by mentoring students of our craft. In fact, this arrangement is formalized in the Hippocratic oath taken by all physicians upon graduation from medical training. However, those of us who teach residents are painfully aware of the limitations of this system when it comes to providing a structured introduction to cataract surgery and giving objective feedback on progress and technique.

This study attempts to validate a rating system for the continuous curvilinear capsulorhexis maneuver that is essential for successful phacoemulsification cataract surgery. Using masked expert observers watching video clips, the authors showed objective validity, high repeatability, and low variability of the measurement for 4 questions (of 12 tested) graded on a continuous numeric (Likert) scale.

Instead of measuring experience by simply counting cases, scientifically valid rating systems for surgical performance will allow accurate assessment of surgical proficiency and outcomes. This approach can be extended to other steps of the cataract surgical procedure and to other procedures as well. A validated rating system for surgical technique would help both residents in training and their mentors. I encourage our professional organizations such as the American Academy of Ophthalmology and the Accreditation Council for Graduate Medical Education to help develop and disseminate these tools for use in ophthalmology residency training programs nationwide.

M. F. Pyfer, MD

2 Refractive Surgery

Angle-supported phakic intraocular lens for correction of moderate to high myopia: Three-year interim results in international multicenter studies
Knorz MC, Lane SS, Holland SP (Univ of Heidelberg, Mannheim, Germany; Associated Eye Care, Stillwater, MN; Univ of British Columbia, Vancouver, Canada)
J Cataract Refract Surg 37:469-480, 2011

Purpose.—To evaluate the safety and effectiveness of an angle-supported phakic intraocular lens (pIOL) for correction of moderate to high myopia.

Setting.—Ophthalmology centers in the United States, Canada, and the European Union.

Design.—Cohort study.

Methods.—This study comprised patients with moderate to high myopia (range −6.00 to −16.50 diopters [D]) who had implantation of the AcrySof Cachet pIOL. Outcome measures included uncorrected distance visual acuity (UDVA), corrected distance visual acuity (CDVA), predictability, stability of the manifest refraction spherical equivalent (MRSE), adverse events, and endothelial cell density (ECD).

Results.—Pooled interim data from 360 patients assessed for up to 3 years postoperatively are presented. Of the 104 patients who reached the 3-year visit, the UDVA was 20/40 or better in 101 (97.1%) and 20/20 or better in 48 (46.2%). The CDVA was 20/32 or better in 103 (99.0%) of the 104 patients and 20/20 or better in 84 patients (80.8%). The mean MRSE was −0.24 D ± 0.55 (SD) (range −2.00 to 1.63 D). The residual refractive error was within ± 0.50 D of target in 82 patients (78.8%) and within ± 1.00 D in 95 patients (91.3%). The annualized percentage loss in central ECD and peripheral ECD from 6 months to 3 years was 0.41% and 1.11%, respectively. No pupil ovalization, pupillary block, or retinal detachment was observed.

Conclusions.—Three-year findings from pooled global studies showed that the angle-supported pIOL provided favorable refractive correction and predictability and acceptable safety in patients with moderate to high myopia (Table 3).

▶ Phakic intraocular lenses (IOLs) have been Food and Drug Administration—approved in the United States for more than 5 years but are still not popular. The main concern with the implantable Collamer lens posterior chamber phakic intraocular lens is cataract formation, both soon after surgery and long term. The

TABLE 3.—Adverse Event Incidence* (N = 360)

Event	n	%
Raised IOP requiring treatment	10	2.8
Cataract formation	7	1.9
Secondary surgical intervention	6	1.7
Synechiae	6	1.7
Hospitalization for raised IOP[†]	5	1.4
Photorefractive keratectomy[†]	2	0.6
Preventative iridotomy[†]	1	0.3
Prophylactic treatment by argon laser[‡]	1	0.3
Photodisruption of cyst with YAG laser[‡]	1	0.3
Laser coagulation of a retinal tag[†]	1	0.3
New suturing[‡,§]	1	0.3
Corneal haze	1	0.3
CDVA loss of >0.2 logMAR	1	0.3

CDVA = icorrected distance visual acuity; IOP = intraocular pressure.
*Incidence rates are based on the number of eyes with an event divided by the number of eyes having intraocular lens implantation.
[†]Resulting from residual ophthalmic viscosurgical device used at surgery. Events were not related to the intraocular lens but were related to the surgical procedure.
[‡]Surgical treatments not monitored as an International Organization for Standardization control rate.
[§]One patient had secondary surgical intervention and new suturing.

main issue with the Verisyse iris clip anterior chamber phakic IOL is the unfamiliar surgical technique and the "trickiness" of the procedure. The angle-supported foldable phakic anterior chamber IOL described in this report is straightforward to insert through a small incision and stays away from the crystalline lens; however, there are haptics in the angle with their associated issues.

Inclusion criteria for this study included an anterior chamber depth (measured from the corneal epithelium) of at least 3.2 mm. Endothelial cell counts needed to be greater than 2000 cells per square millimeter for patients older than 45 years to greater than 2800 cells per square millimeter for patients over 18 years old. The size of the lens was determined by the white-to-white measurement plus 1.0 mm. Iridectomies were not required. The lens was placed through a 3.0- to 3.5-mm corneal incision. Diamox was given at the end of surgery.

Overall, the 3-year results were very good. Only 104 (29%) of the original 360 patients were examined at this time gate. Two IOL exchanges were performed to improve the IOL power, 5 IOLs were explanted, 2 eyes underwent photorefractive keratectomy, and 1 eye underwent cataract surgery (Table 3). There was minimal endothelial cell loss. Fortunately, there were no episodes of pupillary block or pupil ovalization, which have been issues with other designs of phakic anterior chamber IOLs. This phakic anterior chamber IOL seems straightforward to insert and safe and effective at 3 years. Time will tell whether it will become more popular than the other phakic IOLs.

C. J. Rapuano, MD

Pediatric Refractive Surgery and Its Role in the Treatment of Amblyopia: Meta-analysis of the Peer-reviewed Literature

Alió JL, Wolter NV, Piñero DP, et al (Vissum/Instituto Oftalmológico de Alicante, Avda Denia, Spain; et al)
J Refract Surg 27:364-374, 2011

Purpose.—To provide an overview of the visual outcomes after pediatric refractive surgery in anisometropic amblyopia and to analyze the relationship of these outcomes with age and type of refractive surgery.

Methods.—Systematic searches in PubMed, Embase, and Web of Science databases without data restrictions and a search by surveillance of the literature regarding pediatric refractive surgery were performed. Only studies reporting individual data of pediatric cases (age 1 to 17 years) undergoing photorefractive keratectomy (PRK), laser epithelial keratomileusis (LASEK), and LASIK were included. A total of 15 articles including data from a total of 213 amblyopic eyes were considered: LASIK in 95 eyes and surface ablation in 118 eyes. Changes in uncorrected (UDVA) and corrected distance visual acuity (CDVA) were investigated as well as their relation with age and ablation type.

Results.—A significant increase in logMAR UDVA and CDVA was found in the overall sample of amblyopic eyes after surgery ($P<.001$). A significant correlation was found between age and preoperative CDVA ($r=0.34$, $P<.001$) as well as between age and the change in CDVA after surgery ($r=-0.38$, $P<.001$). The change in UDVA was significantly superior for eyes undergoing surface ablation compared to those undergoing LASIK ($P=.04$). Corneal haze was the predominant complication, which was reported in 5.3% of LASIK cases and 8.5% of surface ablation cases.

Conclusions.—Laser refractive surgery is an effective option for improving the visual acuity in children with an amblyopic eye in association with anisometropia.

▶ The main strength of a meta-analysis is its numbers. Its weakness is that sometimes you're adding apples and oranges to achieve greater numbers.

This meta-analysis found 15 studies on results of surface ablation and laser-assisted in situ keratomileusis (LASIK) for the treatment of refractive amblyopia in children aged 1 to 17 years. Just under half of the eyes had LASIK, and the rest had surface ablation. On average, uncorrected and best-corrected vision improved in both groups, but there was greater improvement in the surface ablation group compared with the LASIK group (Table 3 in the original article).

The use of refractive surgery in children is quite controversial; however, in patients in whom conventional therapy is failing, refractive surgery appears to be a reasonable option. I believe a large multicentered trial is warranted to address this issue.

C. J. Rapuano, MD

Phakic intraocular lens implantation for treatment of anisometropia and amblyopia in children: 5-year follow up
Alió JL, Toffaha BT, Laria C, et al (Instituto Oftalmologico de Alicante, Spain)
J Refract Surg 27:494-501, 2011

Purpose.—To evaluate the safety and efficacy during 5-year follow-up of phakic intraocular lens (PIOL) implantation to correct high anisometropia in amblyopic children who were non-compliant with traditional medical treatment including spectacles or contact lenses.

Methods.—Retrospective study of 10 eyes of 10 children with high anisometropia who underwent PIOL implantation (9 with an iris-supported IOL and 1 with a posterior chamber IOL). Patient age at the time of implantation ranged from 2 to 15 years. Mean preoperative spherical equivalent refraction was −10.14 ± 6.96 diopters (D) (range: +8.00 to −18.00 D). Mean logMAR corrected distance visual acuity (CDVA) was 0.84 ± 0.52. Postoperative data at 6, 24, and 60 months were evaluated.

Results.—Corrected distance visual acuity improved in all children. At 24 months, logMAR CDVA was 0.39 ± 0.35 and at 5 years was 0.36 ± 0.38 (range for both: 0.1 to 1.0) ($P = .01$). Improvement of more than three logMAR lines of CDVA was achieved in all children except for one (one line improvement) who was implanted with a posterior chamber PIOL. No loss of CDVA was detected in any patient. Five years after surgery, endothelial cell count was >2000 cells/mm^2 in eight (80%) patients; for the remaining two patients, one reported frequent eye rubbing and the other suffered ocular trauma.

Conclusions.—Phakic IOL implantation in children with anisometropic amblyopia showed a positive long-term impact on visual acuity.

▶ Anisometropia can cause severe visual loss from amblyopia. Although amblyopia is often treatable with nonsurgical methods, such as refractive correction, patching, and atropinization, treatment is not successful in some patients. In these patients, refractive surgery is an option. Refractive surgery can be in the form of corneal surgery or lens-based surgery. Corneal refractive surgery is still somewhat controversial for pediatric anisometropic amblyopia. However, corneal refractive surgery is not appropriate in some eyes because of the severity of the refractive error or the corneal thickness. In these eyes, a phakic intraocular lens (IOL) can be considered. As is true for phakic IOLs in adults, the main concerns are not refractive accuracy or quality of vision or even short-term complications (such as endophthalmitis), but rather long-term complications, including endothelial cell loss, glaucoma, iritis, and cataract. These long-term issues are understandably of even more concern in children.

This series reports on 5-year results of phakic IOLs in 10 eyes of 10 pediatric patients. Nine had iris-clip anterior chamber phakic IOLs and 1 had a posterior chamber phakic IOL. The authors' preference was an iris-clip phakic IOL; however, 1 eye required a posterior chamber phakic IOL due to anatomic considerations. Overall, the results were fairly good. Best corrected vision statistically significantly improved. According to the authors, most of this improvement because of improved magnification and retinal spot size issues, although vision continued to improve over the 5-year period, possibly indicating some improvement in the amblyopia. One eye had trauma, requiring repositioning of the phakic IOL. No eyes developed glaucoma or cataract in the follow-up time period. My primary concern is still endothelial cell loss. Although the authors state that 8 of the 9 eyes (excluding the 1 that had trauma) had a cell count of greater than 2000 cells per square millimeter at 5 years, there was a mean endothelial cell loss of 10.24% over the 5-year period (Table 3 in the original article). Physiologic endothelial cell loss is estimated to be 0.6% cells per square millimeter per year or 3% over 5 years. If triple the rate of endothelial cell loss continues, many of these patients will develop corneal edema, requiring treatment relatively early in their lives.

C. J. Rapuano, MD

Intracorneal inlay to correct presbyopia: Long-term results
Yılmaz ÖF, Alagöz N, Pekel G, et al (Beyoğlu Eye Training and Res Hosp, Istanbul, Turkey; et al)
J Cataract Refract Surg 37:1275-1281, 2011

Purpose.—To evaluate the long-term visual results of Acufocus ACI-7000 (now Kamra) intracorneal inlay implantation in presbyopic phakic patients.

Setting.—Beyoğlu Eye Training and Research Hospital, Istanbul, Turkey.

Design.—Clinical trial.

Methods.—This study comprised patients with emmetropic or post-laser in situ keratomileusis (LASIK) presbyopia. Patients had an uncorrected near visual acuity (UNVA) of 20/40 or worse, correctable to 20/25 or better at distance. The inlay was implanted on the stromal bed after the LASIK flap was relifted or a flap created. The inlay was centered on the presurgical position of the first Purkinje reflex. The main outcome measures were distance and near vision and the complication rate.

Results.—The study enrolled 39 patients aged 45 to 60 years. At the 4-year follow-up, all patients (N = 22) had 2 or more lines of improvement in UNVA with no significant loss in distance vision. The mean final UNVA was 20/20 (Jaeger [J1]); 96% of patients could read J3 or better. The uncorrected distance acuity was 20/40 or better in all eyes. Five patients had cataract progression, and 2 had a change in refractive status. No eye with an intracorneal inlay had intraoperative complications during cataract extraction. Four inlays were explanted during the study. There were no severe corneal complications that affected final vision.

Conclusion.—Intracorneal inlay implantation was an effective, safe, and reversible procedure for the long-term surgical treatment of presbyopia (Fig 1).

▶ One-year results of this Kamra (previously Acufocus) corneal inlay for presbyopia have been good (Fig 1). This study looked at 4-year results in 22 patients

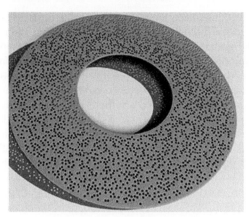

FIGURE 1.—The intracorneal implant. (Reprinted from Yılmaz OF, Alagöz N, Pekel G, et al. Intracorneal inlay to correct presbyopia: long-term results. *J Cataract Refract Surg.* 2011;37:1275-1281, with permission from Elsevier.)

(of the 39 patients enrolled). Here too the visual results were quite good, with 55% of eyes achieving 20/20 uncorrected distance vision and 55% of eyes achieving uncorrected J-1 for near vision; 77% of eyes were 20/25 uncorrected for distance and 96% of eyes were J-3 uncorrected for near. Whether J-3 is good enough for the procedure to gain wide acceptance is still unknown.

At 4 years, the refractive results appear stable. Five of the 22 eyes developed visually significant cataracts (which seems a bit high for a study population with a mean age of 52 years, range 46-60 years). Two eyes underwent cataract surgery, which fortunately was uncomplicated and the vision results were excellent.

There were no cases of corneal melting or corneal stromal fibrosis. Dry eyes and epithelial ingrowth developed in several eyes, but at the same rate as in fellow eyes that had undergone laser in situ keratomileusis without a Kamra implant, and none required treatment.

Four eyes had the Kamra implant explanted: 1 for a button-hole flap, 1 for a thin flap, and 2 for refractive shifts. After explantation, the corneas were clear and the refractions returned to their preoperative state. Overall, the 4-year results of this limited number of eyes seem pretty good. Hopefully, these results will hold true once this inlay is more widely available.

C. J. Rapuano, MD

Reading performance after implantation of a small-aperture corneal inlay for the surgical correction of presbyopia: Two-year follow-up
Dexl AK, Seyeddain O, Riha W, et al (Paracelsus Med Univ, Salzburg, Austria)
J Cataract Refract Surg 37:525-531, 2011

Purpose.—To evaluate the change in reading-performance parameters after implantation of the Kamra small-aperture intracorneal inlay over a 2-year follow-up.

Setting.—University Eye Clinic, Paracelsus Medical University, Salzburg, Austria.

Design.—Cohort study.

Methods.—This study comprised naturally emmetropic presbyopic patients. Bilateral reading acuity, reading distance, reading speed, and the smallest log-scaled sentence were evaluated in a standardized testing procedure using the Salzburg Reading Desk. The minimum postoperative follow-up was 24 months.

Results.—The study enrolled 32 patients. The reading desk results showed a significant improvement in each parameter tested. After a mean follow-up of 24.2 months ± 0.8 (SD), the mean reading distance changed from the preoperative value of 48.1 ± 5.5 cm to 38.9 ± 6.3 cm ($P < .0001$), the mean reading acuity at best distance improved from 0.3 ± 0.14 logRAD to 0.24 ± 0.11 logRAD ($P < .000001$), and the mean reading speed increased from 142 ± 13 words per minute (wpm) to 149 ± 17 wpm ($P = .029$). One patient lost 1 line, and 1 patient had no change. The improvement was up to 6 log-scaled lines (mean improvement 2.7 ± 1.6 lines) in the other 30 patients.

Conclusions.—After implantation of the small-aperture intracorneal inlay, there was an improvement in all tested reading performance parameters in emmetropic presbyopic patients; the improvement was the result of an increased depth of field. These 2-year results indicate that the inlay is an effective treatment for presbyopia.

▶ Why should this corneal inlay work while many others over the last 50 years have not? (1) Biocompatible material, (2) very thin (5 μm) inlay, (3) thousands of microscopic fenestrations allow nutrients to pass through it, and (4) it is intended to aid reading vision through the pin-hole effect in the same way that increasing the F stop in a camera increases depth of focus.

This inlay is placed after creation of a 170-μm to 200-μm femtosecond laser-created flap or pocket. Centration is KEY to maintain excellent distance visual acuity. Given that the diameter of the inlay is 3.8 mm and the diameter of the central hole is 1.6 mm, centration can be very tricky.

The authors make an excellent point that measuring reading acuity, and not simply near visual acuity, is very important when treating presbyopic patients. Picking out 1 letter at a time up close is very different from reading word after word. They used the Salzburg Reading Desk to measure size of type read, the reading speed, and reading distance. The 2-year results in this small group (32 patients) were quite good. I believe it has great potential for the treatment of presbyopia. It is currently undergoing US Food and Drug Administration trials.

C. J. Rapuano, MD

Aspheric wavefront-guided LASIK to treat hyperopic presbyopia: 12-month results with the VISX platform

Jackson WB, Tuan KM, Mintsioulis G (Univ of Ottawa Eye Inst, Ontario, Canada)

J Refract Surg 27:519-529, 2011

Purpose.—To evaluate an aspheric ablation profile to improve near vision in presbyopic patients with hyperopia and to outline the key factors of success.

Methods.—A prospective, nonrandomized, clinical trial of 66 eyes of 33 hyperopic patients who underwent customized bilateral refractive surgery, which included an aspheric presbyopia treatment shape and wavefront-driven hyperopic treatment, was studied. Surgeries were performed using the VISX STAR S4 or STAR S4 IR excimer laser system (Abbott Medical Optics). Mean preoperative refractive error was +1.77 ± 0.56 diopters (D) sphere (range: 0.75 to 3.50 D) with 0.41 ± 0.34 D cylinder (range: 0.00 to 1.50 D). All patients received full distance refractive correction. No patients received monovision or were intentionally left with residual myopia. Patient satisfaction results were evaluated using a questionnaire with a 5-point scale.

Results.—Sixty eyes completed 6-month and 50 eyes completed 12-month postoperative follow-up. At 6 months, mean corrected distance visual acuity (CDVA) was 20/20 ± 1 line (range: 20/25 to 20/10). Mean gain in distance-corrected near visual acuity (DCNVA) was 2.7 ± 1.7 lines with a maximum of 6 lines of near. Spectacle dependence for tasks, such as reading and computer use, was reduced. At 12 months, 100% of patients had achieved binocular simultaneous uncorrected vision of 20/25 or better and J3. Refraction was stable over 12 months. Contrast sensitivity reduction was clinically insignificant (1 step or 0.15 logCS). Negative spherical aberration highly correlated with postoperative improvement of DCNVA. Patients who had a larger amount of preoperative hyperopia or a greater decrease of preoperative DCNVA were more likely to have overall satisfaction.

Conclusions.—The aspheric ablation designed to expand near functional vision was effective and stable over 12 months. The wavefront-customized hyperopic treatment significantly reduced spectacle dependence.

▶ The patients enrolled in this study all had surgery between 2004 and 2006. Although the clinical results were fairly good, the authors stopped performing this presbyopia laser in situ keratomileusis (LASIK) procedure in 2008. The question is why? I believe there are several reasons. The first reason is that while the uncorrected distance vision was excellent (20/20 to 20/25), the near goal (which was achieved most of the time) was J-3. J-3 is not good enough for most people to be eye-glasses independent.

The second reason is that there was a statistically significant decrease in contrast sensitivity. The authors state they do not believe this was "clinically significant." The decrease in contrast sensitivity is to be expected. The presbyopia LASIK ablation improves distance and near uncorrected vision by increasing depth of focus, which decreases clarity and contrast. Although this decrease may not have been thought to be clinically significant during this trial, because these older patients develop cataracts, it may certainly become clinically significant. The third reason is that many patients require 3 to 6 months for the brain to adapt to the aspheric shape before benefits of correction can be fully appreciated. That may be too long for most people to wait.

C. J. Rapuano, MD

Femtosecond laser versus mechanical microkeratome laser in situ keratomileusis for myopia: Metaanalysis of randomized controlled trials
Zhang Z-H, Jin H-Y, Suo Y, et al (Shanghai First People's Hosp Affiliated to Shanghai Jiaotong Univ, China; et al)
J Cataract Refract Surg 37:2151-2159, 2011

Purpose.—To examine differences in efficacy, accuracy, safety, and changes in aberrations between femtosecond and mechanical microkeratome laser in situ keratomileusis (LASIK) for myopia.
Setting.—Department of Ophthalmology, Shanghai First People's Hospital Affiliated to Shanghai Jiaotong University, Shanghai, China.
Design.—Evidence-based manuscript.
Methods.—Data sources, including PubMed, Medline, EMBASE, and Cochrane Controlled Trials Register, were searched to identify potentially relevant prospective randomized controlled trials. Primary outcome measures were efficacy (uncorrected distance visual acuity $\geq 20/20$), accuracy (± 0.50 diopter mean spherical equivalent), and safety (loss of ≥ 2 lines of corrected distance visual acuity). Aberrations and postoperative complications were secondary outcomes.
Results.—Seven prospective randomized controlled trials describing a total of 577 eyes with myopia were included in this metaanalysis. At 6 months or more follow-up, no significant differences were found in the efficacy (odds ratio [OR], 1.17; 95% confidence interval [CI], 0.40 to 3.42; $P=.78$), accuracy (OR, 1.69; 95% CI, 0.68 to 4.20; $P=.26$), or safety (OR, 7.37; 95% CI, 0.37 to 147.61; $P=.19$). In eyes that had femtosecond LASIK, the postoperative total aberrations (mean difference -0.03 µm; 95% CI, -0.05 to -0.01; $P=.002$) and spherical aberrations (mean difference -0.02 µm; 95% CI, -0.03 to -0.01; $P<.00001$) were significantly lower.
Conclusions.—According to the metaanalysis, femtosecond LASIK did not have an advantage in efficacy, accuracy, and safety measures over mechanical microkeratome LASIK in the early and midterm follow-up, although it might induce fewer aberrations.

▶ This meta-analysis included 7 (of the 139 potentially relevant studies identified) prospective randomized controlled trials. These studies were published between 2005 and 2010, meaning the surgeries were performed at least 1 to 2 years prior to that and often longer. While these results are interesting, significant advances have been made in both femtosecond laser and mechanical microkeratome technology since these studies were conducted. In fact, the only femtosecond laser used in these studies included in this meta-analysis was the Intralase. Of the 7 studies, 5 used the Hansatome as the mechanical microkeratome.

Overall, the results between the 2 groups were equivalent. The mechanical microkeratome group had more total higher-order aberrations and spherical aberrations than the femtosecond laser group, although due to reporting inconsistencies the authors state, "We should interpret the aberration results with caution." Three trials looked at flap thickness. The femtosecond laser group had a lower mean deviation from intended flap thickness and smaller standard deviation. Whether these results would hold true for new microkeratomes is not known. There was statistically significantly more diffuse lamellar keratitis in the femtosecond laser group ($P = .01$), but again, whether this would hold true for newer versions of the Intralase or other femtosecond lasers is also unknown. It is comforting to know that if there is in fact a difference in the results of LASIK with these 2 flap-making modalities, it is probably quite small.

C. J. Rapuano, MD

Outcomes of custom laser in situ keratomileusis: Dilated wavescans versus undilated wavescans
Virasch VV, Stwalley D, Kymes SM, et al (Rush Univ Med Ctr, Chicago, IL; Washington Univ School of Medicine, St Louis, MO)
J Cataract Refract Surg 37:1847-1851, 2011

Purpose.—To evaluate refractive outcomes of custom laser in situ keratomileusis (LASIK) based on undilated and pharmacologically dilated wavefront aberrometry with the Visx laser system.

Setting.—Clinical refractive practice, St. Louis, Missouri, USA.

Design.—Comparative case series.

Methods.—Eyes that had LASIK using dilated wavescans (study group) were evaluated for the reason for use of dilated scans; age; preoperative refractive error; preoperative root mean square (RMS), coma, trefoil, and spherical aberration values; postoperative uncorrected distance visual acuity (UDVA); postoperative refractive error; percentage of iris-registration capture; and enhancement rate. The study group was compared with a control group that had LASIK using undilated wavescans.

Results.—The study group comprised 52 eyes (31 patients) and the control group, 104 eyes (55 patients). At 1 month, the mean postoperative UDVA was 20/21 in the study group and 20/22 in the control group and at 3 months, 20/22 and 20/20, respectively. At 1 month, the mean postoperative spherical equivalent (SE) was +0.07 diopter (D) ± 0.49 (SD) in the study group and +0.14 ± 0.30 D in the control group and at 3 months, −0.01 ± 0.44 D and +0.02 ± 0.23 D, respectively; there was no statistically significant difference between groups at either timepoint. There was no statistically significant difference in preoperative RMS or postoperative coma, trefoil, or spherical

TABLE 2.—Between-Group Comparison of Postoperative and Aberration Outcomes

Parameter	Study Group	Control Group	P Value
Mean 1 mo postop UDVA	20/21	20/22	—
Mean 1 mo postop SE (D)	+0.07 ± 0.49	+0.14 ± 0.30	.04
Mean 3 mo postop UDVA	20/22	20/20	—
Mean 3 mo postop SE (D)	−0.01 ± 0.44	+0.02 ± 0.23	.13
Mean preop RMS (μm)	0.45 ± 0.15	0.36 ± 0.15	.17
Mean physician adjustment (D)	−0.23	−0.41	—
IR capture rate (%)	86.5	95.2	—
Enhancement rate (%)	6.0	1.9	.89
Mean coma (μm)	0.24 ± 0.15	0.22 ± 0.13	.58
Mean trefoil (μm)	0.20 ± 0.09	0.15 ± 0.10	.28
Mean spherical aberration (μm)	0.20 ± 0.17	0.13 ± 0.11	.14

IR = iris registration; RMS = root mean square; SE = spherical equivalent; UDVA = uncorrected distance visual acuity.

aberration between the groups. Although the study group had a slightly higher enhancement rate, the difference was not statistically significant.

Conclusion.—Compared with custom LASIK based on undilated wavescans, use of dilated wavescans for custom LASIK resulted in comparable postoperative outcomes (Table 2).

▶ I am sure many refractive surgeons who use the Visx platform have been frustrated on occasion by the inability to get accurate, usable wavefront maps in certain patients. I know I have. It is more often from excessive accommodation where the wavescan refraction is much more myopic than the manifest refraction or the cycloplegic refraction performed in the office. It is less often from a pupil smaller than 5 to 6 mm in diameter. In such cases I often wondered about using dilating/cycloplegic drops to obtain the wavescan measurements. I haven't used them because (1) Visx recommends (and the Food and Drug Administration studies were based on) obtaining the wavescan map in an undilated eye, and (2) I did not know whether the results would be accurate. Although my first reason has not changed, this study, while not huge, indicates no ill effect on refractive results when using dilating/cycloplegic drops. It should be noted that all the laser in situ keratomileusis procedures were performed on undilated eyes at least 3 days after the wavescan maps were obtained.

What are the concerns about obtaining a wavescan map in a dilated state? The first concern is that the centration of the pupil can shift, causing a decentered ablation. No decentered ablations were noted in this study. The second concern is that a large pupil may result in a difference in higher order aberrations, perhaps from lenticular changes. No difference in coma, trefoil, or spherical aberration was found in this study (Table 2). In patients where the wavescan map does not appear to be accurate or usable, I have used conventional treatments in the past. From now on, I will offer them an off-label treatment using a dilated wavescan.

C. J. Rapuano, MD

Effect of Preoperative Pupil Size on Quality of Vision after Wavefront-Guided LASIK

Chan A, Manche EE (Stanford Univ School of Medicine, CA)

Ophthalmology 118:736-741, 2011

Purpose.—To evaluate the effect of preoperative pupil size on quality of vision after wavefront-guided LASIK.

Design.—Prospective study.

Participants.—One hundred two eyes.

Intervention.—LASIK for mild to moderate myopia or astigmatism (preoperative manifest spherical equivalent, -3.99 ± 1.42 diopters).

Main Outcome Measures.—Questionnaires evaluating specific visual symptoms before and after surgery. Each eye was evaluated before surgery, and 1 week and 1, 3, 6, and 12 months postoperatively. Pupils were stratified according to size: small (≤ 5.5 mm), medium ($5.6-6.4$ mm), or large (≥ 6.5 mm). Mesopic pupil size and preoperative and postoperative variables were evaluated using an analysis of variance. A regression model was also performed to determine the correlation between mean spherical equivalent and cylinder and visual symptoms.

Results.—In the early postoperative period, there was no difference between the 3 groups with regard to any of the symptoms. At the final 12-month postoperative visit, patients with medium pupils experienced less glare at night than small pupils ($P = 0.02$), medium pupils had less halos than small or large pupils ($P = 0.001$ and $P = 0.02$, respectively), and medium pupils experienced greater satisfaction in visual improvement than small pupils ($P = 0.014$).

Conclusions.—Twelve months after wavefront-guided LASIK surgery, large pupil size does not positively correlate with any postoperative visual symptoms.

▶ The debate continues. Is pupil size related to visual disturbance, such as glare and haloes, especially at night, after refractive surgery? Older literature typically concluded that patients with larger pupils tended to have more complaints of vision issues, especially at night, whereas the more recent literature has generally not found a correlation. Residual refractive error, regardless of pupil size, has often been shown to be associated with unwanted visual symptoms.

This study looked at 102 eyes of 51 patients with mild to moderate myopia (up to 6 diopters), with a reasonable range of pupil diameters (from 4 to 8 mm), with about one-third at 4 to 5.5 mm, one-third at 5.6 to 6.4 mm and one-third at 6.5 to 8.0 mm. All eyes underwent wavefront-guided laser-assisted in situ keratomileusis (LASIK) with a WaveScan abberrometer (VISX) laser. Wavefront treatments with the VISX laser are US Food and Drug Administration approved only when data through a 6-mm pupil are obtained, and can't be done at all when the pupil size during the wavefront measurement is less than 5.0 mm. I wonder how many eyes were treated with data from a pupil size less than 6 mm when the full benefit of the wavefront treatment is not likely to be realized.

Some eyes had flaps made with a Hansatome and other eyes with an Intra-lase femtosecond laser, although the authors do not give the numbers or separate the results for these 2 techniques. It would be interesting to know if there were differences in quality of vision between these 2 types of LASIK flaps. The authors conclude that there was no correlation between large pupil size and postoperative visual symptoms at 1 year. They do note that residual refractive error had the most effect (statistically significant) on glare symptoms at night in eyes with large pupils. While I agree that I have fewer complaints from patients regarding quality of vision issues after surface ablation and LASIK using wavefront-guided treatments than conventional treatments, the small size of this study and the fact that there were no pupil sizes greater than 8 mm make the results interesting but do not close the door on this important issue.

C. J. Rapuano, MD

Post–Laser Assisted in Situ Keratomileusis Epithelial Ingrowth and Its Relation to Pretreatment Refractive Error
Mohamed TA, Hoffman RS, Fine IH, et al (Assiut Univ Hosps, Egypt; Oregon Health Science Univ)
Cornea 30:550-552, 2011

Purpose.—To assess the incidence of epithelial ingrowth after laser in situ keratomileusis and its correlation with myopic or hyperopic treatment.

Methods.—This retrospective study analyzed 1000 consecutive LASIK procedures performed by 3 surgeons using identical surgical technique with a Hansatome microkeratome. Eyes that developed epithelial ingrowth were evaluated using the Machat grading system. Patients were subdivided into 2 groups (myopic or hyperopic) based on the preoperative refractive error.

Results.—The total incidence of epithelial ingrowth was 4.7%. The incidence after primary treatment was 3.9%. The incidence after enhancement was 12.8%. The total incidence of epithelial ingrowth was 3% in the myopic group compared with 23% in the hyperopic group. After primary myopic treatment, there was a 3% incidence of epithelial ingrowth compared with 17% after primary hyperopic treatment. The incidence after enhancement was 7% in the myopic group and 43% in the hyperopic group.

Conclusions.—Patients undergoing hyperopic laser in situ keratomileusis have a greater incidence of epithelial ingrowth than those undergoing myopic treatment. In addition, enhancement procedures have a higher incidence than primary procedures.

▶ While this large study did not produce any earth-shattering findings, it does emphasize several important points for both surgeons and patients.

One, epithelial ingrowth after laser-assisted in situ keratomileusis (LASIK) isn't rare. Using their grading system, approximately 3% of eyes had non-visually significant ingrowth, 1% had ingrowth requiring removal in 2 to 3 weeks, and approximately 1% had significant ingrowth requiring urgent treatment. The fact that 2% of patients require surgical treatment of epithelial ingrowth after LASIK is something patients need to understand.

Two, epithelial ingrowth is much more common (approximately 5 times) after hyperopic treatments than after myopic treatments. Hyperopic patients should be aware of this.

Three, epithelial ingrowth is more than twice as common after flap lift enhancement than after primary LASIK surgery. Surgeons (and patients) need to know this when deciding whether to perform a flap lift enhancement or a surface ablation enhancement on a LASIK flap.

C. J. Rapuano, MD

Mitomycin C—Assisted Photorefractive Keratectomy in High Myopia: A Long-Term Safety Study
Gambato C, Miotto S, Cortese M, et al (Univ of Padua, Italy)
Cornea 30:641-645, 2011

Purpose.—To evaluate the long-term corneal safety of topical mitomycin C (MMC) used during photorefractive keratectomy to prevent haze formation in highly myopic eyes.

Methods.—Twenty-eight patients with bilateral high myopia underwent photorefractive keratectomy. One eye was randomly assigned to intraoperative 0.02% MMC and the fellow eye to conventional treatment. Each eye was checked at baseline and at 5 years after surgery using in vivo corneal confocal microscopy.

Results.—At baseline, the endothelial cell density was 2970 ± 295 cells per square millimeter in the MMC-treated eyes and 2839 ± 323 cells per square millimeter in the control eyes. At 5 years, it was 2803 ± 307 and 2780 ± 264 cells per square millimeter, respectively ($P = 0.27$). The number of corneal nerve fibers was 3.9 ± 1.6 in the MMC-treated eyes and 4.4 ± 1.3 in the control eyes. At 5 years, it was 3.0 ± 1.6 and 2.7 ± 1.3, respectively ($P = 0.15$). The density of corneal nerves was 9600 ± 2915 $\mu m/mm^2$ in the MMC-treated eyes and 11,352 ± 3898 $\mu m/mm^2$ in the control eyes. At 5 years, the density was higher in the MMC-treated eyes (6790 ± 2447 $\mu m/mm^2$) than in the control eyes (6024 ± 2977 $\mu m/mm^2$) ($P = 0.003$). The number of nerve beadings at baseline was 12.9 ± 1.7/ 100 μm in the MMC-treated eyes and 12.3 ± 2.0/100 μm in the control eyes. At 5 years, it was 9.9 ± 2.6/100 and 9.4 ± 2.9/100 μm, respectively ($P = 1.00$). At 5 years, corneal nerve branching and tortuosity were similar in the 2 groups ($P = 0.88$ and 0.54, respectively). Epithelium thickness remained statistically unchanged ($P = 0.69$).

Conclusions.—Intraoperative use of topical 0.02% MMC compared with standard treatment does not induce significant long-term corneal changes, as assessed by in vivo corneal confocal microscopy (Table 1).

▶ There is no debate that mitomycin C (MMC) on the sclera (eg, after pterygium excision) has rare but serious complications such as scleral melt. There

TABLE 1.—Descriptive Statistics of Confocal Microscopy Parameters for MMC-Treated Eyes and Steroid-Treated Eyes (5 Years)

Parameter	Preoperative		Postoperative (5 Yrs)	
	MMC	Steroid	MMC	Steroid
Fibers (n/image), mean ± SD (range)	3.9 ± 1.6 (2–9)	4.4 ± 1.3 (1–7)	3.0 ± 1.6 (1–7)	2.7 ± 1.3 (1–6)
Density (μm/mm^2), mean ± SD (range)	9600 ± 2916 (3293–15375)	11352 ± 3898 (3714–17087)	6790 ± 2447 (2238–12455)*	6024 ± 2977 (2329–11921)
Beadings (n/100 mm), mean ± SD (range)	12.9 ± 1.7 (10–16)	12.3 ± 2.0 (9–17)	9.9 ± 2.6 (5–14)	9.4 ± 2.9 (5–15)
Branching, n (%)				
Order 0	1 (3.6)	3 (10.7)	1 (3.6)	3 (10.7)
Order 1	17 (60.7)	14 (50.0)	18 (64.2)	17 (60.7)
Order 2	10 (35.7)	11 (39.3)	9 (32.1)	8 (28.6)
Tortuosity, n (%)				
Grade 1	14 (50.0)	15 (53.6)	12 (42.8)	12 (42.8)
Grade 2	11 (39.3)	11 (39.3)	14 (50.0)	13 (46.4)
Grade 3	3 (10.7)	2 (7.1)	2 (7.2)	3 (10.7)

*Values statistically different between the 2 groups ($P < 0.05$).

is also no debate that MMC drops to treat conjunctival tumors are toxic to the corneal surface and can result in permanent limbal stem cell changes. There is still, however, debate on the safety of intraoperative MMC during surface ablation. Most research on the subject has focused on the health of the endothelium. The majority of studies have found no deleterious effects of MMC on endothelial cell counts, but a few have. Not many studies have looked at the effects of MMC on other corneal cells.

This is a superb study for several reasons: (1) a reasonable number of patients, 28; (2) one eye was randomly assigned to receive intraoperative MMC (2 minutes on a surgical sponge), while the other eye received intraoperative topical steroids; (3) all patients had moderately high myopia (−7 to −14.25 D, mean 9.25 D in both groups), with essentially equal refractions in both eyes; (4) confocal microscopy was used; and (5) all eyes were evaluated preoperatively and 5 years postoperatively. The MMC-treated eyes received no topical steroids in the postoperative period. As most surgeons use steroids after surface ablation for weeks to months, whether they also use MMC or not, this aspect of this study is different from most surgeons' current practices.

The clinical results at 5 years revealed equal uncorrected vision in both groups. No MMC-treated eyes had corneal haze, whereas 4 eyes (14.3%) had 1+ haze in the control group. Endothelial cell loss was equal in the 2 groups consistent with physiological loss over 5 years. All other parameters evaluated, including number of corneal nerve fibers, density of corneal nerves, number of corneal nerve beadings, corneal nerve branching and tortuosity, and epithelial thickness, were the same or better in the MMC group (Table 1).

I have been using MMC 0.02% for 12 seconds after most surface ablation procedures with excellent clinical results for years. Studies such as this one reinforce my impression that it is safe and effective. Whether 12 seconds is better or worse than 2 minutes is still unknown.

C. J. Rapuano, MD

Meta-analysis of clinical outcomes comparing surface ablation for correction of myopia with and without 0.02% mitomycin C
Chen SH, Feng YF, Stojanovic A, et al (Wenzhou Med College, Zhejiang, China)
J Refract Surg 27:530-541, 2011

Purpose.—To evaluate the current clinical evidence of safety and efficacy of intraoperative topical application of 0.02% mitomycin C (MMC) used for up to 2 minutes after surface ablation for correction of myopia.

Methods.—A comprehensive literature search was conducted of Cochrane Library, MEDLINE, and EMBASE to identify relevant trials comparing surface ablation for correction of myopia with and without MMC. A meta-analysis was performed on the results of the reports and statistical analysis was performed.

Results.—Eleven clinical trials were identified with MMC used in 534 eyes and no MMC in 726 eyes. Surface ablations with MMC led to significantly less corneal haze in photorefractive keratectomy, whereas the results were comparable in laser epithelial keratomileusis (LASEK) and epithelial laser in situ keratomileusis (epi-LASIK). Although proportionately more eyes in the MMC group achieved uncorrected distance visual acuity 20/25 or better and less frequently lost ≥2 lines of corrected distance visual acuity, the difference was not statistically significant.

Conclusions.—Our meta-analysis suggests that the topical intraoperative application of 0.02% MMC may reduce haze and improve visual acuity after surface ablation for correction of myopia. However, the advantage of using MMC in LASEK and epi-LASIK is unclear.

▶ The strength of meta-analyses is that they increase the power of smaller studies. To do so, however, you need to find comparable studies. This meta-analysis found that mitomycin C reduced corneal haze after photorefractive keratectomy (PRK). Although it did not find similar convincing evidence for laser epithelial keratomileusis and epithelial laser in situ keratomileusis, most surgeons treat all 3 forms of surface ablation similarly. The authors were not able to stratify the benefits of mitomycin C by degree of myopia. Some surgeons only use mitomycin C above a certain level of myopia (eg, greater than −3.00 diopters or −4.00 diopters) or stromal ablation depth (eg, greater than 50 to 65 μm). Others titrate the application time depending on the level of myopia (eg, between 12 seconds and 60 seconds). I personally continue to use mitomycin C 0.02% for 12 seconds for all my surface ablation patients with over −3.00 or −4.00 diopters of myopia.

C. J. Rapuano, MD

Live or Let Die: Epithelial Flap Vitality and Keratocyte Proliferation Following LASEK and Epi-LASIK in Human Donor and Porcine Eyes
Angunawela RI, Winkler von Mohrenfels C, Kumar A, et al
J Refract Surg 27:111-118, 2011

Purpose.—To determine the relationship between epithelial flap vitality and stromal keratocyte proliferation following two epithelial refractive techniques: epi-LASIK and laser epithelial keratomileusis (LASEK).

Methods.—Human corneas were maintained in organ culture and underwent standard -6.00-diopter ablation. Rates of stromal keratocyte proliferation were detected 1 week postoperative using a Ki67 antibody specific to proliferating cells. Images were captured with a laser scanning confocal microscope and analyzed by a masked observer. Epithelial flap vitality was determined with propidium iodide using fresh porcine corneas. Epithelial flaps were created with Gebauer Epikeratome epi-LASIK or alcohol-assisted LASEK method. Flaps treated with 100% alcohol and uninjured corneas were used as controls.

Results.—The number of proliferating keratocytes was greatest at 1 week in the epi-LASIK corneas (P<.001). Cell vitality was greatest in the epi-LASIK flaps and declined in the LASEK and 100% alcohol flaps (P<.001).

Conclusions.—In this in vitro setting, epi-LASIK results in an epithelial flap with significantly more live cells. There is also a greater number of proliferating stromal cells following epi-LASIK at 1 week. Based on these in vitro observations, epi-LASIK may result in greater levels of haze compared to LASEK.

▶ Reported here are really 2 separate in vitro studies. One was in human corneas kept in organ culture for 1 week; the authors found more proliferating keratocytes in the epi-LASIK eyes than in the LASEK eyes. The second study was in pig eyes in which the authors found epithelial cell vitality was much better after epi-LASIK than LASEK. They concluded that the "healthier" epithelium, combined with the greater number of proliferating keratocytes after epi-LASIK, may increase the risk of postoperative haze after epi-LASIK compared with LASEK.

It is a big jump from small in vitro studies to human clinical results, especially in light of the fact that most human studies to date have found no difference in haze between LASEK and epi-LASIK. I personally have found the greatest correlation of haze with the time it takes for healthy re-epithelialization to occur after surface ablation. A few extra days, and the risk of haze goes up. I changed from LASEK to epi-LASIK many years ago because the epithelium seemed more injured from the alcohol than the epi-tome and didn't heal as well. I switched from epithelium on to epithelium off epi-LASIK because of unpredictable recovery of the epithelium when I left it on. I do like epithelium off epi-LASIK because the smooth epithelial defect heals about 1 day faster than mechanical photorefractive keratectomy in my hands.

C. J. Rapuano, MD

Effect of preemptive topical diclofenac on postoperative pain relief after photorefractive keratectomy
Mohammadpour M, Jabbarvand M, Nikdel M, et al (Tehran Univ of Med Sciences, Iran)
J Cataract Refract Surg 37:633-637, 2011

Purpose.—To assess the prophylactic effect of preoperative application of topical diclofenac on postoperative pain control in patients having photorefractive keratectomy (PRK).

Setting.—Farabi Eye Hospital, Tehran University of Medical Sciences, Tehran, Iran.

Design.—Randomized masked clinical trial.

Methods.—In this paired-eye study, patients having bilateral PRK received 1 drop of diclofenac 0.1% in 1 eye and 1 drop of placebo in the fellow eye 2 hours before PRK. Postoperatively, both arms of the trial (both eyes of each patient) received topical diclofenac every 6 hours for 2 days. One day and 2 days postoperatively, patients were asked to rate the perceived pain in each eye using an 11-point verbal numerical rating scale. A trained examiner noted the eye-specific responses.

Results.—All 70 patients (140 eyes) completed the study and were included in the statistical analysis. Twenty-four hours after PRK, patients reported pain scores that were clinically and statistically significantly lower in the eyes pretreated with diclofenac than in the fellow eyes (0.97 versus 2.09) (*P*=.018). Pain scores at 2 days did not differ significantly (*P*=.877).

Conclusion.—Administration of a single drop of topical diclofenac 0.1% 2 hours before PRK seemed to increase the efficacy of postoperative pain management in a clinically and statistically significant manner.

▶ One of the 3 main downsides to surface ablation is pain (the others being slow visual recovery and haze). Over the years, numerous techniques to reduce pain after surface ablation have emerged. Creating the smallest epithelial defect needed to perform the ablation (by using epi—laser assisted in situ keratomileusis, alcohol or transepithelial photorefractive keratectomy [PRK]), cooling the corneal surface immediately after the laser ablation, using a bandage soft contact lens postoperatively, using narcotic and neuropathic pain medications postoperatively, and postoperative topical nonsteroidal anti-inflammatory drugs (NSAIDS) have all greatly reduced postoperative surface ablation pain compared with the early days of PRK in the 1990s. But even less pain would be better (assuming of course it did not cause additional side effects).

These authors wanted to know if one NSAID drop preoperatively (in addition to the standard postoperative NSAIDs) would help the pain after surface ablation. They performed a very straightforward, masked study giving 1 eye a drop of NSAID (diclofenac) and the fellow eye a placebo drop 2 hours before surface ablation. All eyes received a bandage soft contact lens and postoperative antibiotics and steroids. All eyes also received diclofenac 4 times a day for 2 days postoperatively. A masked observer asked patients about pain 1 day and 2 days postoperatively. On a 0 to 10 scale, the eyes that received the preoperative NSAID drop had a pain score of approximately 1, while the eyes that received the placebo drop had a pain score of approximately 2 on postoperative day 1 (*P* = .018). On postoperative day 2, both groups had a similar pain score of between 0.8 and 0.9. The authors did not find any untoward effects of the extra dose of NSAID.

Is a 1-point difference on a 0- to 10-diopter scale of pain for 1 day a real life difference? If I am the one in pain, it sure might be. Given its low downside risk, I am now using NSAIDs preoperatively in my surface ablation patients.

C. J. Rapuano, MD

Oral gabapentin for photorefractive keratectomy pain
Kuhnle MD, Ryan DS, Coe CD, et al (Walter Reed Army Med Ctr, Washington, DC; et al)
J Cataract Refract Surg 37:364-369, 2011

Purpose.—To compare the efficacy of oral gabapentin versus placebo for the control of severe pain after photorefractive keratectomy (PRK).

Setting.—Center for Refractive Surgery, Walter Reed Army Medical Center, Washington, DC, USA.

Design.—Randomized masked clinical trial.

Methods.—This single-center clinical trial comprised active-duty United States Army soldiers aged 21 years or older having bilateral PRK for myopia with or without astigmatism. Patients received gabapentin 300 mg or placebo 3 times daily for 7 days beginning 2 days before and continuing for 4 days after surgery. Current and maximum pain levels were assessed using the Visual Analog Pain scale 2 hours after surgery and then daily on days 1 through 4. Repeated-measures analysis of variance (ANOVA) was used to compare the current and maximum pain scores over time between the gabapentin group and the placebo group. The Fisher exact test was used to determine whether there was a difference in severe pain (>7/10) between the 2 groups.

Results.—Forty-two patients received gabapentin and 41 patients, placebo. The repeated-measures ANOVA showed no significant difference between the 2 groups in current pain ($P = .84$) or in maximum pain over time ($P = .35$). Oxycodone—acetaminophen use in the gabapentin group was significantly higher than in the placebo group 1 day postoperatively ($P = .034$).

Conclusion.—When added to a standardized postoperative pain regimen, gabapentin use led to no additional improvement in PRK pain control compared with a placebo at the dose and the time intervals tested.

► The 2 main reasons laser in situ keratomileusis is much more popular than surface ablation around the world are (1) more postoperative pain and 2) slower visual recovery after surface ablation. This study evaluated the use of gabapentin (eg, Neurontin) after photorefractive keratectomy (PRK) to reduce postoperative pain. Neurontin is US Food and Drug Administration approved to treat post-herpes zoster neuralgia, where it can be extremely effective in controlling devastating pain and often "giving patients their lives back." It is reasonable to assume it could work for post-PRK pain.

This small but well-designed, double-masked study did not find any difference in pain during the first 4 postoperative days. Interestingly, the gabapentin group used more escape oxycodone-acetaminophen on postoperative day 1.

They also found more pain in patients younger than 30 years compared with those older than 30. There was 1 other unexpected finding. They used 0.02% mitomycin C in patients with laser ablations greater than 70 μm. They found significantly less pain in eyes that received mitomycin C. I don't know why this should be and neither did the authors.

C. J. Rapuano, MD

Infectious keratitis in 18 651 laser surface ablation procedures

de Rojas V, Llovet F, Martínez M, et al (Instituto Oftalmológico Europeo, Spain)
J Cataract Refract Surg 37:1822-1831, 2011

Purpose.—To evaluate the incidence, culture results, risk factors, treatment strategies, and visual outcomes of infectious keratitis after surface ablation.
Setting.—Multicenter study in Spain.
Design.—Case series.
Methods.—The medical records of patients who had surface ablation between January 2003 and December 2009 were reviewed to identify cases of infectious keratitis. The incidence, risk factors, clinical course, days to diagnosis, medical and surgical treatment, and visual outcome were recorded. Main outcome measures were incidence of infectious keratitis after surface ablation, culture results, response to treatment, and visual outcomes.
Results.—The study reviewed the records of 9794 patients (18 651 eyes). Infectious keratitis after surface ablation was diagnosed in 39 eyes of 38 patients. The onset of infection was early (within 7 days after surgery) in 28 cases (71.79%). Cultures were positive in 13 of 27 cases in which samples were taken. The most frequently isolated microorganism was *Staphylococcus* species (9 cases). The final corrected distance visual acuity (CDVA) was 20/20 or better in 23 cases (58.97%), 20/40 or better in 36 cases (92.30%), and worse than 20/40 in 3 cases (7.69%).
Conclusions.—The incidence of infectious keratitis after surface ablation was 0.20%. Infectious keratitis is a potentially vision-threatening complication. Prompt and aggressive management with an intensive regimen of fortified antibiotic agents is strongly recommended. Proper management can preserve useful vision in most cases.

▶ This study is from the same large, multicenter private practice group in Spain that in 2010 reported a 0.035% infection rate (72 in 204 586) after laser in situ keratomileusis (LASIK). This study of infection after surface ablation demonstrated an infection rate of 0.2%—almost 6 times higher than after LASIK. This is very likely due to the moderately large epithelial defect and extended use of a bandage soft contact lens after surface ablation. These reasons are consistent with the higher incidence of infections within the first week after surface ablation (72%) compared with the first week after LASIK (62%). Cultures were performed in 27 of the 39 eyes identified as infected. Thirteen of these 27 cultures were positive. It is possible that some of these eyes had sterile and not infected infiltrates. Fortunately, all of these infiltrates resolved rapidly with aggressive antibiotic therapy.

Although there appears to be a higher incidence of infectious keratitis after surface ablation than with LASIK, the infections are easier to manage as there is no LASIK flap to contend with. Even so, the visual results were similarly very good when comparing this study after surface ablation with the same group's previous study after LASIK. This study reinforces the excellent safety record of surface ablation.

C. J. Rapuano, MD

Long-term outcome of central toxic keratopathy after photorefractive keratectomy
Neira W, Holopainen JM, Tervo TM (Helsinki Univ Central Hosp, Finland)
Cornea 30:1207-1212, 2011

Purpose.—To describe long-term postoperative results of 5 eyes that had central toxic keratopathy after photorefractive keratectomy (PRK).

Method.—In a period of 2 months, 74 eyes were subjected to refractive surgery (21 by PRK and 53 by laser in situ keratomileusis) in 2006. Laser ablations were performed with a VISX S4 (VISX, Santa Ana, CA) excimer laser. Five eyes of 5 different patients in the PRK group experienced a corneal stromal thinning associated with a central opacification (haze), hyperopic shift, and central striae in the first postoperative week. Follow-up examinations were at 1 month and at 2, 6, and 12 months and included uncorrected visual acuity, best spectacle-corrected visual acuity (BCVA), manifest refraction, biomicroscopy, and ultrasound pachymetry. At the last follow-up, confocal microscopy was performed in 3 eyes.

Results.—Corneal thickness measured by ultrasound pachymetry at the first month postoperatively showed an unexpected stromal thinning of 48 ± 39 μm (range, 19-116 μm) compared with the expected postoperative value. At the last postoperative follow-up, corneal thickness had gained 44 ± 22 μm (range, 20-80 μm) compared with the thickness obtained at 1 month. Uncorrected visual acuity, BCVA, haze, and corneal thickness improved in the first postoperative months and stabilized after 6 months.

Conclusions.—Central toxic keratopathy is not related to laser in situ keratomileusis (LASIK) only. The presence of 5 cases after PRK in a short period (2 months) associated with a period of simultaneous change of both postoperative medications and postoperative bandage lens practice suggests a link with an unknown pharmacological response leading to stromal dehydration.

▶ The evolution of the condition now termed central toxic keratopathy (CTK) has an interesting history. The diagnosis is generally made within 2 to 4 days after surgery in eyes with central haze, stromal thinning, striae, and a hyperopic shift from excessive corneal flattening. It was first thought to be a severe form of diffuse lamellar keratitis (DLK) after laser in situ keratomileusis (LASIK); however, classic DLK is inflammatory and responds to topical steroids, whereas CTK does not. Additionally, classic DLK occurs only after LASIK, whereas CTK can also occur after surface ablation (and has also been described after other laser procedures such as selective laser trabeculoplasty). CTK is now thought to be a sterile, noninflammatory corneal reaction, whose pathophysiology remains unclear.

This case series describes 1 year of follow-up of CTK in 4 eyes and 6 months of follow-up in 1 eye. The 4 myopic eyes had a hyperopic shift 1 month postoperatively, which improved in 2 eyes at last follow-up. The 1 hyperopic eye had a myopic shift, which improved at 1 year follow-up (Table 1 in the original article). The authors stress that any enhancement surgery should be delayed at least 12 to 18 months after the initial procedure as spontaneous recovery is common. They also suggest rinsing bandage soft contact lenses prior to use and delaying topical nonsteroidal and steroid drops until after the epithelial defect has resolved and the bandage contact lens is removed. Interesting thoughts, but they are without any evidence of effect. I have not been rinsing the contact lens prior to placement after surface ablation and used topical nonsteroidal anti-inflammatory drugs for several days and topical steroids beginning the day of surgery in hundreds of eyes for over 10 years without any episodes of CTK. We need to determine the reason for CTK before we can effectively combat or prevent it.

C. J. Rapuano, MD

Laser-assisted subepithelial keratectomy and photorefractive keratectomy for post-penetrating keratoplasty myopia and astigmatism in adults

Huang PYC, Huang PT, Astle WF, et al (Univ of Calgary, Alberta, Canada; Alberta Children's Hosp, Calgary, Canada)
J Cataract Refract Surg 37:335-340, 2011

Purpose.—To evaluate whether laser-assisted subepithelial keratectomy (LASEK) and photorefractive keratectomy (PRK) achieve effective targeted correction and the extent of post-treatment corneal haze after corneal transplantation.

Setting.—Nonhospital surgical facility, Calgary, Alberta, Canada.

Design.—Evidence-based manuscript.

Methods.—This study evaluated visual acuity, refractive error correction, and potential complications after LASEK or PRK to eliminate refractive error differences after penetrating keratoplasty in adults. A Nidek EC-5000 or Technolas 217 excimer laser was used in all treatments.

Results.—At last follow-up (mean 20.50 months post laser), the mean spherical equivalent (SE) decreased from -2.71 diopters (D) $\pm$ 4.17 (SD) to -0.54 ± 3.28 D in the LASEK group and from -4.87 ± 3.90 D to -1.82 ± 3.34 D in the PRK group. The mean preoperative uncorrected distance visual acuity (UDVA) was 1.63 ± 0.53 and 1.45 ± 0.64, respectively, and the mean postoperative UDVA, 0.83 ± 0.54 and 0.90 ± 0.55, respectively. The improvement in SE and UDVA was statistically significant in both groups ($P<.01$). The mean haze (0 to 3 scale) at the last follow-up was 0.46 ± 0.708 in the LASEK group and 0.58 ± 0.776 in the PRK group.

Conclusions.—The UDVA improved and refractive errors were effectively reduced after LASEK or PRK in eyes with previous PKP. There was no significant difference in the change in SE, UDVA, or corrected distance visual acuity between LASEK and PRK. Some patients had evidence of corneal haze, although the difference between the groups was not significant.

▶ Thirty-two eyes of 32 patients underwent photorefractive keratectomy (PRK), and 60 eyes of 54 patients underwent laser-assisted subepithelial keratectomy (LASEK) after penetrating keratoplasty (PK). Interestingly, mean preoperative spherical equivalent was −4.9 diopters (D) in the PRK group and −2.7 D in the LASEK group. It is impossible to tell from the article, but most, if not all, of the sutures were removed at least 3 to 4 months before the laser refractive surgery. No mitomycin C was used in any of these eyes. Fluorometholone drops were used for 3.5 months postoperatively.

Postoperative sphere and cylinder improved in both groups, and haze was very similar in both groups.

Postgraft (PK and deep anterior lamellar keratoplasty) refractive error can be very frustrating for the surgeon and especially for patients. Suture removal, glasses, and contact lenses often help, but not always. Laser in situ keratomileusis is often problematic due to flap or graft wound issues. Surface ablation has been associated with significant postoperative haze after PK in some patients. This large study shows good safety, refractive, and haze results with surface ablation after PK. An unanswered question is whether mitomycin C could potentially improve the results.

C. J. Rapuano, MD

Photorefractive keratectomy with mitomycin-C after corneal transplantation for keratoconus

Hodge C, Sutton G, Lawless M, et al (Sydney Univ, Australia)
J Cataract Refract Surg 37:1884-1894, 2011

Purpose.—To evaluate the efficacy of photorefractive keratectomy (PRK) for residual refractive error after penetrating keratoplasty (PKP) for keratoconus.

Setting.—Private ophthalmic clinic.

Design.—Case series.

Method.—Consecutive patients who had PRK augmented with topical mitomycin-C (MMC) after PKP for keratoconus were retrospectively reviewed. Patients were divided into a a low cylinder group (refractive cylinder ≤6.00 D) and a high cylinder group (refractive cylinder >6.00 D). Visual acuity, refraction, and keratometry were analyzed preoperatively and 1, 3, 6, and 12 months postoperatively.

Results.—The study comprised 47 eyes (41 patients). The spherical equivalent (SE) decreased from −4.24 D ± 3.23 (SD) preoperatively to −0.71 ± 1.03 D 12 months postoperatively in the low cylinder group and from −4.19 ± 3.54 D to −2.45 ± 3.42 D, respectively, in the high cylinder group. The refractive cylinder decreased from −4.27 ± 1.4 D to −1.71 ± 1.55 D, respectively, in the low cylinder group and from −7.78 ± 1.21 D

TABLE 2.—Preoperative and Postoperative Topography Results

| | | Mean (D) ± SD | | | |
| | | | Postoperative[†] | | |
Group	Preoperative*	1 Month	3 Months	6 Months	12 Months
Low cylinder					
Sphere	46.15 ± 2.99	42.11 ± 4.21	44.97 ± 5.50	42.33 ± 3.06	43.14 ± 2.83
Cylinder	5.18 ± 2.61	2.63 ± 0.60	4.86 ± 4.19	3.46 ± 2.67	3.73 ± 3.30
High cylinder					
Sphere	46.83 ± 2.99	43.79 ± 2.06	42.89 ± 1.93	43.28 ± 1.92	43.51 ± 1.65
Cylinder	9.09 ± 3.04	5.48 ± 1.69	4.78 ± 2.56	5.30 ± 5.25	7.17 ± 5.07

*30 eyes, low cylinder group; 16 eyes, high cylinder group.
[†]At 1 month, 5 eyes, low cylinder group and 4 eyes, high cylinder group; at 3 months, 10 eyes and 6 eyes, respectively; at 6 months, 16 eyes and 6 eyes, respectively; at 12 months, 17 eyes and 9 eyes, respectively.

to −4.6 ± 2.54 D, respectively, in the high cylinder group. By the last follow-up, 8.3% of patients had lost 2 lines of corrected distance visual acuity. There were no cases of corneal haze greater than 2+ or of graft rejection.

Conclusions.—Penetrating keratoplasty with adjunctive MMC decreased several refractive variables in patients with previous PKP. These results compare well with those in the published literature and suggest PRK is as effective as, and probably safer than, laser in situ keratomileusis in treating refractive error in these cases (Table 2).

▶ The success rate for penetrating keratoplasty for keratoconus is among the highest of all indications for corneal transplantation—over 95% of patients achieve 20/40 or better best corrected vision at 1 to 2 years. Unfortunately, that best corrected vision often includes significant myopia and astigmatism. Most of these refractive errors are correctible with glasses or contact lenses. For patients who are glasses and contact lens intolerant, refractive surgery can be performed. Relaxing incisions and wedge resections for astigmatism are only moderately predictable. Laser in situ keratomileusis (LASIK) has been done after penetrating keratoplasty (PKP), but there is a reasonably high risk of flap complications, and it may destabilize the corneal transplant wound. Photorefractive keratectomy (PRK) was performed in the early days of excimer laser surgery but was quickly stopped due to the high rate of significant corneal haze in the PKP.

These authors report good results for PRK with mitomycin-C after PKP. They applied mitomycin-C for 15 to 60 seconds depending on the level of correction treated. In eyes with less than or equal to 6.00 diopters of astigmatism, there was a 60% reduction in cylinder and an 83% reduction in spherical equivalent. In eyes with greater than 6.00 diopters astigmatism, there was a 41% reduction in cylinder and 42% reduction in spherical equivalent (Table 2). Results appeared more stable in the lower astigmatism group than in the higher astigmatism group. Importantly, 2 eyes developed greater than grade 2 haze. Interestingly, there was no difference in haze between the low-astigmatism group and the high-astigmatism group. One eye did require a repeat corneal transplant due to significant persistent haze. There were no cases of graft rejection related to the PRK procedure.

The authors did not state how long after the PKP the PRKs were performed. PKPs in keratoconus patients can remain clear for decades. However, after 10 to 20 years, the PKP wounds tend to become progressively ectatic with increasing levels of cylinder. Treating an eye with high (presumably relatively stable) refractive error 1 to 2 years after PKP is probably very different from treating a relatively unstable refractive error from an ectatic wound 20 years after a PKP.

C. J. Rapuano, MD

Laser-assisted in situ keratomileusis or photorefractive keratectomy after descemet stripping automated endothelial keratoplasty
Ratanasit A, Gorovoy MS (Gorovoy MD Eye Specialists, Ft Myers, FL)
Cornea 30:787-789, 2011

Purpose.—To report the outcomes of laser-assisted in situ keratomileusis (LASIK) and photorefractive keratectomy (PRK) after Descemet stripping automated endothelial keratoplasty (DSAEK).

Methods.—A retrospective case series was conducted on 5 postoperative unilateral DSAEK cases that underwent LASIK or PRK. DSAEK was performed for Fuchs corneal dystrophy and pseudophakic bullous keratopathy. Postoperative uncorrected visual acuity (UCVA), best spectacle-corrected visual acuity (BSCVA), and current graft status were ascertained for the 5 eyes included in the study.

Results.—All eyes had clear grafts at the most recent postoperative visit. Three eyes underwent LASIK, and 2 eyes had PRK 11 to 17 months after DSAEK. UCVA ranged from 20/80 to 20/200 before refractive surgery (BSCVA: 20/20 to 20/30). Postoperative UCVA improved to 20/20-20/40, and BSCVA was unchanged at 20/20 to 20/30. No patient lost vision.

Conclusions.—Refractive error after DSAEK may be safely treated with LASIK or PRK. PRK is equally as effective as LASIK. All grafts remain clear, and all the eyes have significantly improved UCVA.

▶ Descemet stripping automated endothelial keratoplasty (DSAEK) tends to induce a certain degree of hyperopia. On average it is about 1.5 to 1.75 diopters at 1 to 2 months postoperatively and approximately 1.00 diopter at 9 to 12 months postoperatively. Most patients wear glasses if needed. This case series reports on laser in situ keratomileusis (LASIK) or photorefractive keratectomy (PRK) in 5 eyes after DSAEK. Four eyes were hyperopic and 1 eye was myopic (after an intraocular lens exchange). Three eyes underwent uncomplicated LASIK. Two eyes underwent PRK, as they had previously undergone LASIK. Interestingly, both of these eyes underwent DSAEK for Fuchs' dystrophy. Why they had undergone LASIK in light of their Fuchs' dystrophy is not discussed. These 2 eyes were treated for hyperopic astigmatism with adjunctive mitomycin-C applied for 15 seconds. LASIK and PRK worked quite well in this small series. There was no damage to the DSAEK with a follow-up of 1 to 2.5 years. It is good to know that both LASIK and PRK can be used successfully after DSAEK.

C. J. Rapuano, MD

Small incision corneal refractive surgery using the small incision lenticule extraction (SMILE) procedure for the correction of myopia and myopic astigmatism: results of a 6 month prospective study

Sekundo W, Kunert KS, Blum M (Phillips Univ of Marburg, Germany; Helios Hosp Erfurt, Germany)
Br J Ophthalmol 95:335-339, 2011

Aim.—This 6 month prospective multi-centre study evaluated the feasibility of performing myopic femtosecond lenticule extraction (FLEx) through a small incision using the small incision lenticule extraction (SMILE) procedure.

Design.—Prospective, non-randomised clinical trial.

Participants.—Ninety-one eyes of 48 patients with myopia with and without astigmatism completed the final 6 month follow-up. The patients' mean age was 35.3 years. Their preoperative mean spherical equivalent (SE) was -4.75 ± 1.56 D.

Methods.—A refractive lenticule of intrastromal corneal tissue was cut utilising a prototype of the Carl Zeiss Meditec AG VisuMax femtosecond laser system. Simultaneously two opposite small 'pocket' incisions were created by the laser system. Thereafter, the lenticule was manually dissected with a spatula and removed through one of incisions using modified McPherson forceps.

Main Outcome Measures.—Uncorrected visual acuity (UCVA) and best spectacle corrected visual acuity (BSCVA) after 6 months, objective and manifest refraction as well as slit-lamp examination, side effects and a questionnaire.

Results.—Six months postoperatively the mean SE was -0.01 D $\pm$ 0.49 D. Most treated eyes (95.6%) were within ± 1.0 D, and 80.2% were within ± 0.5 D of intended correction. Of the eyes treated, 83.5% had an UCVA of 1.0 (20/20) or better, 53% remained unchanged, 32.3% gained one line, 3.3% gained two lines of BSCVA, 8.8% lost one line and 1.1% lost ≥ 2 lines of BSCVA. When answering a standardised questionnaire, 93.3% of patients were satisfied with the results obtained and would undergo the procedure again.

Conclusion.—SMILE is a promising new flapless minimally invasive refractive procedure to correct myopia.

▶ The first all femtosecond laser corneal refractive surgery involved creating a complete laser-assisted in situ keratomileusis (LASIK)-type flap and a corneal lenticule with a femtosecond laser. The flap was completely lifted, the lenticule removed, and the flap replaced. This procedure is called FLEx-femtosecond lenticule extraction. This procedure includes the pros and cons of LASIK, such as neurotrophic dry eye syndrome, flap striae, epithelial ingrowth, and straightforward flap lift enhancements.

This article describes a small incision version of the FLEx surgery, where instead of lifting an entire LASIK flap, 2 peripheral incisions are used to remove the lenticule. It is termed *small incision lenticule extraction* (SMILE). The authors make the point that it is much more difficult to remove the lenticule in SMILE than in FLEx. The surgeon needs to separate the plane over the top of the lenticule before separating the base. Certainly, refinements in this technique will be made, but I believe it has great promise.

C. J. Rapuano, MD

3   Glaucoma

Laminar and Prelaminar Tissue Displacement During Intraocular Pressure Elevation in Glaucoma Patients and Healthy Controls
Agoumi Y, Sharpe GP, Hutchison DM, et al (Dalhousie Univ, Halifax, Canada)
Ophthalmology 118:52-59, 2011

Objective.—To determine the response of the anterior lamina cribrosa and prelaminar tissue to acute elevation of intraocular pressure (IOP) in glaucoma patients and healthy subjects.

Design.—Prospective case-control series.

Participants and Controls.—Patients with open-angle glaucoma (n = 12; mean age ± standard deviation [SD], 66.8 ± 6.0 years), age-matched healthy controls (n = 12; mean age ± SD, 67.1 ± 6.2 years), and young controls (n = 12; mean age ± SD, 36.1 ± 11.7 years).

Methods.—One eye was imaged with spectral-domain optical coherence tomography to obtain 12 high-resolution radial scans centered on the optic disc. Imaging was repeated at precisely the same locations with an ophthalmodynamometer held perpendicular to the globe via the inferior lid to raise the IOP. A line joining Bruch's membrane opening in 4 radial scans was used as reference in the baseline and elevated IOP images. The vertical distance from the reference line to the anterior prelaminar tissue surface and anterior laminar surface was measured at equidistant points along the reference line in the 2 sets of images. The difference between the 2 sets of corresponding measurements were used to determine laminar displacement (LD) and prelaminar tissue displacement (PTD).

Main Outcome Measures.—Laminar displacement and PTD.

Results.—Intraocular pressure elevation among patients, age-matched controls, and young controls was similar (mean ± SD, 12.4 ± 3.2 mmHg). The mean ± SD LD and PTD were 0.5 ± 3.3 μm and 15.7 ± 15.5 μm, respectively. The LD was not statistically different from 0 ($P = 0.366$), but PTD was ($P < 0.001$). The mean ± SD LD was similar among the groups ($-0.5 ± 3.7$ μm, $0.2 ± 2.0$ μm, and $2.0 ± 3.6$ μm, respectively; $P = 0.366$), whereas the mean ± SD PTD was different ($6.8 ± 13.7$ μm, $20.8 ± 17.5$ μm, and $19.6 ± 11.8$ μm, respectively; $P = 0.045$). In all subjects, the PTD was greater than LD. In multivariate regression analyses, LD was negatively associated with optic disc size ($P = 0.007$), whereas PTD was positively associated with the degree of IOP elevation ($P = 0.013$).

Conclusions.—In glaucoma patients and controls, the anterior laminar surface is noncompliant to acute IOP elevation. Acute optic disc surface

Glaucoma

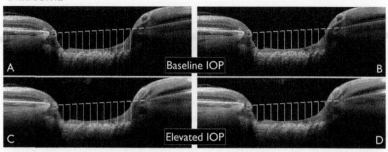

Control

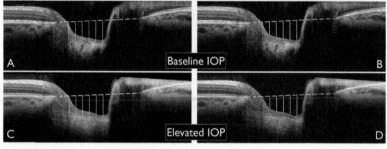

FIGURE 2.—Radial spectral-domain optical coherence tomography scans in (**Top**) a glaucoma patient and (**Bottom**) an age-matched healthy control subject. A reference line connecting Bruch's membrane opening was used in (**A** and **B**) corresponding baseline intraocular pressure (IOP) images and (**C** and **D**) elevated IOP images. Vertical lines at equidistant points along the reference line were extended to (**A** and **C**) the anterior laminar surface and (**B** and **D**) the prelaminar tissue surface. The mean difference in corresponding vertical lines was termed *laminar displacement* and *prelaminar tissue displacement*, respectively. IOP = intraocular pressure. (Reprinted from Agoumi Y, Sharpe GP, Hutchison DM, et al. Laminar and prelaminar tissue displacement during intraocular pressure elevation in glaucoma patients and healthy controls. *Ophthalmology.* 2011;118:52-59, Copyright 2011, with permission from the American Academy of Ophthalmology.)

changes represent compression of prelaminar tissue and not laminar displacement (Figs 2 and 3).

▶ The pathophysiology of glaucomatous damage remains incompletely understood. The so-called mechanical theory suggests that backward bowing of the lamina cribrosa by pressure causes crimping and damage to retinal ganglion cell axons.

In this article, glaucoma and control eyes were subject to pressure elevation, and the changes in the position of the anterior aspect of the lamina cribrosa and the prelaminar tissue were measured with optical coherence tomography. Interestingly, with about an average pressure elevation of 12 mm Hg, compression of prelaminar tissue was seen but almost no displacement of the laminar tissue. The compression was more evident in controls; glaucoma eyes showed less change in prelaminar thickness.

Other studies, with patients having greater pressure elevations and in monkeys using other imaging techniques, have reported changes in the position

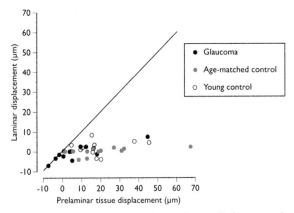

FIGURE 3.—Scatterplot showing the relationship between laminar displacement and prelaminar tissue displacement in glaucoma patients, agematched control subjects, and young control subjects. In each case, the magnitude of prelaminar tissue displacement was greater than laminar displacement. Diagonal line, slope = 1. (Reprinted from Agoumi Y, Sharpe GP, Hutchison DM, et al. Laminar and prelaminar tissue displacement during intraocular pressure elevation in glaucoma patients and healthy controls. *Ophthalmology.* 2011;118:52-59, Copyright 2011, with permission from the American Academy of Ophthalmology.)

of the lamina. At physiologic pressures in humans, this study did not find changes in laminar position. The reduced compression of the prelaminar tissue in glaucoma eyes subjected to pressure elevation may be the results of chronic glaucomatous structural changes to the tissue or may, although not reported by the authors, be related to the volume of the tissue in glaucomatous eyes. However, the prelaminar compression versus laminar movement in response to pressure elevation is notable, and may represent loss of axoplasmic volume or blood volume. These are important insights that may direct future studies and understanding of the pathophysiology.

J. S. Myers, MD

YAG Laser Peripheral Iridotomy for the Prevention of Pigment Dispersion Glaucoma: A Prospective, Randomized, Controlled Trial

Scott A, Kotecha A, Bunce C, et al (Moorfields Eye Hosp, London, UK)
Ophthalmology 118:468-473, 2011

Purpose.—To test the hypothesis that neodymium:yttrium—aluminum—garnet (Nd:YAG) laser peripheral iridotomy (LPI) significantly reduces the incidence of conversion from pigment dispersion syndrome (PDS) with ocular hypertension (OHT) to pigmentary glaucoma (PG).

Design.—Prospective, randomized, controlled 3-year trial.

Participants.—One hundred sixteen eyes of 116 patients with PDS and OHT.

Intervention.—Patients were assigned randomly either to Nd:YAG LPI or to a control group (no laser).

Main Outcome Measures.—The primary outcome measure was conversion to PG within 3 years, based on full-threshold visual field (VF) analysis using the Ocular Hypertension Treatment Study criteria. Secondary outcome measures were whether eyes required topical antiglaucoma medications during the study period and the time to conversion or medication.

Results.—Fifty-seven patients were randomized to undergo laser treatment and 59 were randomized to no laser (controls). Age, gender, spherical equivalent refraction, and intraocular pressure at baseline were similar between groups. Outcome data were available for 105 (90%) of recruited subjects, 52 in the laser treatment group and 53 in the no laser treatment group. Patients were followed up for a median of 35.9 months (range, 10–36 months) in the laser arm and 35.9 months (range, 1–36 months) in the control arm. Eight eyes (15%) in the laser group and 3 eyes (6%) in the control group converted to glaucoma in the study period. The proportion of eyes started on medical treatment was similar in the 2 groups: 8 eyes (15%) in the laser group and 9 eyes (17%) in the control group. Survival analyses showed no evidence of any difference in time to VF progression or commencement of topical therapy between the 2 groups. Cataract extraction was performed on 1 patient in the laser group and in 1 patient in the control group during the study period (laser eye at 18 months; control eye at 34 months).

Conclusions.—This study suggests that there was no benefit of Nd:YAG LPI in preventing progression from PDS with OHT to PG within 3 years of follow-up (Fig 2, Table 1).

▶ Laser peripheral iridotomy (LPI) has been shown to convert the concave iris typically associated with pigment dispersion syndrome to a more planar configuration. The pathophysiology of pigment dispersion syndrome likely involves

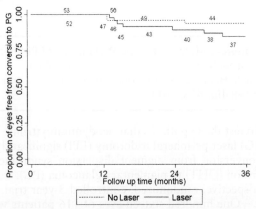

FIGURE 2.—Kaplan-Meier survival analysis showing proportion of patients converting to pigmentary glaucoma on the basis of visual fields in the laser and control arms. PG = pigmentary glaucoma. (Reprinted from Scott A, Kotecha A, Bunce C, et al. YAG laser peripheral iridotomy for the prevention of pigment dispersion glaucoma: a prospective, randomized, controlled trial. *Ophthalmology.* 2011;118:468-473, Copyright 2011, with permission from the American Academy of Ophthalmology.)

TABLE 1.—Inclusion and Exclusion Criteria

Inclusion Criteria	Exclusion Criteria
Pigmented angles with at least 1other feature of the following 3: Krukenberg's spindle Midperipheral iris transillumination defects Backward-bowing iris configuration Reliable, full visual field tested using the Humphrey Field Analyzer 24-2 full-threshold strategy: ≤15% false positives/negatives ≤30% fixation losses Normal Glaucoma hemifield test results AGIS score 0 IOP ≥21 mmHg (off treatment) VA of 20/40 or better	Other diseases capable of producing visual field loss Any systemic medication that could alter IOP (i.e., glucocorticoids, cardiac glycosides, β-adrenergic blockers) Recent ocular trauma, infection, inflammation, surgery

AGIS = Advanced Glaucoma Intervention Study; IOP = intraocular pressure; VA = visual acuity.

both an abnormal iris composition that predisposes to pigment release and an anatomic predisposition through irido-zonular contact. Therefore, performing LPI in patients with pigment dispersion syndrome may relieve irido-zonular contact and ultimately reduce pigment dispersion and conversion to pigmentary glaucoma.

A retrospective study of newly diagnosed cases of pigment dispersion syndrome among patients identified through the Rochester Epidemiology Project found that the most significant risk factor for conversion to pigmentary glaucoma was intraocular pressure > 21 mm Hg at initial examination.[1] This study focuses on the high-risk population with pigment dispersion and ocular hypertension via a randomized, controlled trial of neodymium:yttrium—aluminum—garnet (Nd:YAG) LPI to prevent pigmentary glaucoma.

Fifty-seven patients were randomly assigned to undergo laser treatment, and 59 patients were controls (see Table 1 for inclusion/exclusion criteria). Median follow-up was about 3 years. Visual field conversion was determined by the criteria used in the Ocular Hypertension Treatment Study. Fifteen percent of patients in the laser group and 6% in the control group converted to pigmentary glaucoma by visual field progression. Medical treatment was initiated in 15% and 17% of the laser and control groups, respectively. Odds for conversion were 3 times higher in the laser group than in the control group.

This study suggests that Nd:YAG LPI is of little benefit in preventing conversion of pigment dispersion syndrome to pigmentary glaucoma in a patient population seemingly at high risk of conversion. By targeting those most likely at risk of conversion, the authors provide important evidence in a well-designed study. Nonetheless, it's possible that the onset of ocular hypertension indicates the horse is already out of the barn in these patients. Maybe ocular hypertension in the presence of pigment dispersion syndrome is a harbinger of pathologic processes that already occurred in the outflow apparatus and are irreversible. Perhaps LPI in patients with pigment dispersion syndrome but no ocular hypertension would be more effective at limiting conversion to pigmentary glaucoma.

Unfortunately, our understanding of the natural history of pigment dispersion syndrome is subject to scarce and sometimes conflicting information. Ultimately, more evidence is needed to determine why patients convert to pigmentary glaucoma and whether LPI may have a role in preventing conversion among patients with minimal outflow damage and appropriate intraocular pressure.

S. J. Fudemberg, MD

Reference

1. Siddiqui Y, Ten Hulzen RD, Cameron JD, Hodge DO, Johnson DH. What is the risk of developing pigmentary glaucoma from pigment dispersion syndrome? *Am J ophthalmol.* 2003;135:794-799.

Continuous intraocular pressure monitoring with a wireless ocular telemetry sensor: initial clinical experience in patients with open angle glaucoma
Mansouri K, Shaarawy T (Univ of Geneva, Switzerland)
Br J Ophthalmol 95:627-629, 2011

The authors report their initial clinical results with a novel wireless ocular telemetry sensor (OTS) (Sensimed AG, Switzerland) for continuous intraocular pressure (IOP) monitoring in patients with open angle glaucoma. This was a prospective, observational cohort of 15 patients. The OTS is a disposable silicone contact lens with an embedded micro-electromechanical system, which measures changes in corneal curvature induced by variations in IOP. An antenna, mounted around the eye, receives the data, which are then transmitted to a recorder. A signal was recorded in all patients. Thirteen (87%) patients completed 24-h IOP monitoring: one patient discontinued IOP monitoring due to device intolerance, and incomplete recordings were obtained in a second patient due to technical device malfunction. In 9/13 (69%) patients, the highest signals were recorded during the nocturnal period. No serious adverse events were recorded. The OTS shows good safety and functionality to monitor IOP fluctuations in patients over 24 h. This technology has the potential to provide hitherto unobtainable data on the chronobiology of IOP, possibly leading to improved care of glaucoma patients (Figs 1, 2, and 4).

▶ Intraocular pressure (IOP) monitoring is central to the management of glaucoma. However, for most patients with glaucoma, we have IOP measurements of only a few minutes out of an entire year. Thus, pressure spikes may be occurring at night, on weekends, or at other times that are unobserved.

Continuous IOP monitoring has long been a dream of glaucoma specialists. This report describes a new device based on a pressure transducer mounted inside a silicone contact lens, with a wireless antenna system to pick up signals from the unit (Fig 1).

The results show that continuous outpatient pressure measurement is possible with this unit, although more data, including more corroboration with Goldmann

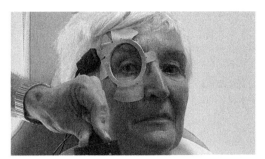

FIGURE 1.—The wireless sensor is in place. A soft patch containing the antenna is applied around the eye and transmits the information via wire to the recorder that the patient wears in a pocket fixed around the neck and waist. The patient can continue to wear her spectacles during monitoring (patient consent was obtained for publication of this photograph). (Reprinted from Mansouri K, Shaarawy T. Continuous intraocular pressure monitoring with a wireless ocular telemetry sensor: initial clinical experience in patients with open angle glaucoma. *Br J Ophthalmol.* 2011;95:627-629, Copyright 2011, with permission from BMJ Publishing Group Ltd.)

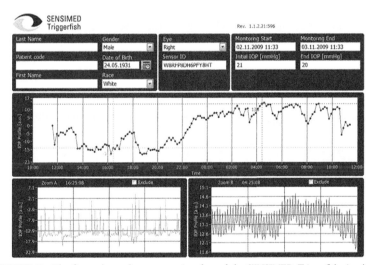

FIGURE 2.—The figure shows the computer interface of the SENSIMED Triggerfish signal when downloaded to the physician's computer at the end of the 24-h IOP monitoring. In the centre, the IOP curve over 24 h is shown. Each point on the graph represents 60 s of IOP measurement, repeated every 600 s. The user can place one of two cursors on any point in time and see the detailed measurements in the smaller windows at the bottom (each corresponding to a period of 60 s), where spikes due to blinking as well as ocular pulsations are clearly visible. A characteristic short-term signal drop is occasionally noticed and correlates well with exposure to sunlight during outdoor activities. The effect of blinking is visible in the detailed profile as a fraction-of-a-second peak (Zoom A). Ocular pulsations could be seen in all curves. In Zoom B, showing the registration signal during 60 s at night, it can be seen that the ocular pulsation frequency is in line with that of cardiac activity. The patient is asleep and no blinkings are seen. The patient instils his topical prostaglandin drops (PG) at around 22:00. (Reprinted from Mansouri K, Shaarawy T. Continuous intraocular pressure monitoring with a wireless ocular telemetry sensor: initial clinical experience in patients with open angle glaucoma. *Br J Ophthalmol.* 2011;95:627-629, Copyright 2011, with permission from BMJ Publishing Group Ltd.)

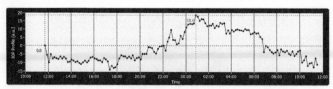

FIGURE 4.—The graph shows the 24-h IOP curve of a 79-year-old female POAG patient under treatment with a PG, with GAT IOPs of 14 mm Hg (baseline) and 16 mm Hg (end of 24-h SENSIMED Triggerfish monitoring). The curve reveals a stable profile during the afternoon hours with a trough at 17:30. The signal then increases continuously during evening hours with significant fluctuations throughout the nighttime. A peak is observed at 01:00. This patient was under a topical treatment with twice-daily α-2-adrenergic agonist (instilled around 17:00 and 09:30, following day) and once-daily PG drops (instillation time not recorded by patient). (Reprinted from Mansouri K, Shaarawy T. Continuous intraocular pressure monitoring with a wireless ocular telemetry sensor: initial clinical experience in patients with open angle glaucoma. *Br J Ophthalmol.* 2011;95:627-629, Copyright 2011, with permission from BMJ Publishing Group Ltd.)

IOP, are needed. This type of measurement may dramatically increase our understanding of the physiology of IOP in normal eyes and the pathophysiology of glaucoma. Hitherto, unmeasured IOP spikes may explain why selected patients get worse, or more complex patterns of IOP variability may prove to be more deleterious to ganglion cell survival. It is possible that widespread study of continuous IOP measurement may lead to great advances within the field of glaucoma.

J. S. Myers, MD

Assessment of Bleb Morphologic Features and Postoperative Outcomes After Ex-PRESS Drainage Device Implantation Versus Trabeculectomy
Good TJ, Kahook MY (Univ of Colorado School of Medicine, Aurora)
Am J Ophthalmol 151:507-513, 2011

Purpose.—To investigate bleb morphologic features and postoperative outcomes after Ex-PRESS drainage device (Alcon Laboratories) implantation versus trabeculectomy.

Design.—Retrospective, consecutive case-control series.

Methods.—Information was collected from the charts of 35 consecutive Ex-PRESS procedures and 35 consecutive trabeculectomy procedures with at least 2 years of follow-up. Intraocular pressure (IOP), bleb morphologic features, reduction of dependence on medication, visual recovery, number of postoperative visits, and postoperative complication rates were compared between groups.

Results.—Average follow-up was 28 months (standard deviation, 3.23 months). Mean IOP measurements were similar after 6 months, then became slightly higher in the Ex-PRESS group at 1 year and at the final follow-up ($P = .004$ and $P = .008$, respectively). Final percent IOP lowering was similar between groups ($P = .209$). Unqualified success was achieved in 77.14% of Ex-PRESS and 74.29% of trabeculectomy procedures at last follow-up ($P = 1.00$). An additional 5.71% and 8.57% reached qualified success for Ex-PRESS and trabeculectomy surgeries, respectively ($P = .99$). Evaluation by the Moorfields Bleb Grading System revealed less vascularity

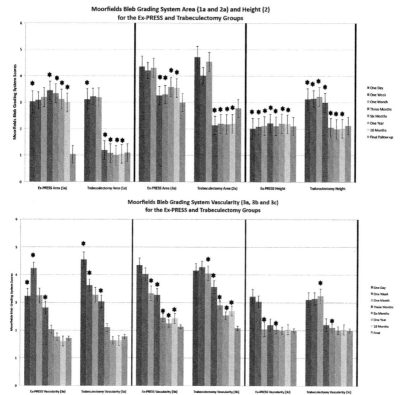

FIGURE 1.—Bar graph showing Moorfields Bleb Grading System data for the Ex-PRESS (Alcon Laboratories, Fort Worth, Texas, USA) and trabeculectomy patients for the duration of postoperative follow-up. The black asterisks above the bars represent P values that are statistically significant and different between the Ex-PRESS group and the trabeculectomy group. Scoring was carried out according to standard Moorfields Bleb Grading System protocol (http://www.blebs.net/html/Protocol.html) using reference photographs of the various aspects of the bleb (http://www.blebs.net/html/Images.html). All photographs were evaluated in masked fashion without indication of type of procedure or timeline when photographs were obtained for each patient. Six criteria are assessed that pertain to the 3 main aspects of the bleb: (1) area, (2) height, and (3) vascularity. (1) Bleb area is assessed based on maximal bleb area and central demarcation area. A score of 1 to 5 is given based on extension, from 0% to 100% extension. Graph 1a compares the central demarcation area with the total conjunctival area, and graph 2a compares the peripheral margins with the total conjunctival area. The chart above shows that the Ex-PRESS group had higher scores for both graph 1a and graph 2a from 3 months to 18 months of follow-up, with similar scoring at the final follow-up. (2) Bleb height, labeled as criteria 2, represents the highest point of the bleb and is graded from 1 to 4 against reference photographs, with 1 being the least height and 4 being the greatest height. Our data found the Ex-PRESS group to have lesser bleb height in the early postoperative period until 6 months of follow-up and then greater bleb height from 6 months to 18 months of follow-up. Both groups were similar in bleb height at final follow-up. (3) Bleb vascularity has 3 criteria, each of which is scored from 1 to 5, with 1 corresponding to avascular and 5 corresponding to severe vessel inflammation. Graph 3a represents the vascularity at the central demarcation area of the bleb, graph 3b represents the vascularity at the peripheral part of the bleb, and graph 3c represents the vascularity at the peripheral, nonbleb conjunctiva. Our data show that the Ex-PRESS group overall had less vascularity, with the most pronounced difference in bleb vascularity at the peripheral part of the bleb. (Reprinted from Good TJ, Kahook MY. Assessment of bleb morphologic features and postoperative outcomes after ex-PRESS drainage device implantation versus trabeculectomy. *Am J Ophthalmol.* 2011;151:507-513, Copyright 2011, with permission from Elsevier.)

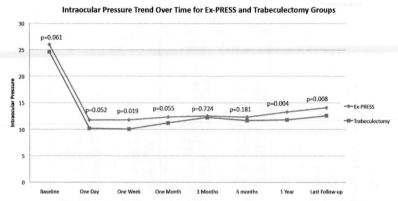

FIGURE 2.—Graph showing average intraocular pressure (IOP) and *P* values for the Ex-PRESS (Alcon Laboratories, Fort Worth, Texas, USA) and trabeculectomy patients at each follow-up. The diamonds represent the Ex-PRESS group and squares represent the trabeculectomy group. Both groups have upward trending IOPs after 6 months of follow-up, but the Ex-PRESS group IOP trend is more significant, as indicated by the *P* value comparison of the 2 groups. (Reprinted from Good TJ, Kahook MY. Assessment of bleb morphologic features and postoperative outcomes after ex-PRESS drainage device implantation versus trabeculectomy. *Am J Ophthalmol.* 2011;151:507-513, Copyright 2011, with permission from Elsevier.)

and height but more diffuse area associated with the Ex-PRESS blebs, although these differences were absent at study completion. There were fewer cases of early postoperative hypotony and hyphema and quicker visual recovery in the Ex-PRESS group. The Ex-PRESS group required fewer postoperative visits compared with the trabeculectomy group (*P* < .000).

Conclusions.—Success of Ex-PRESS surgery, as defined in our study, was similar to trabeculectomy. Final IOP measurements were slightly lower after trabeculectomy compared with Ex-PRESS. Differences in some postoperative outcomes faded with follow-up. There remains a need for long-term prospective studies comparing these 2 procedures (Figs 1 and 2).

▶ The Ex-PRESS drainage device is a small metal tube that is inserted underneath the trabeculectomy flap in place of performing the scleral punch, such as with a Kelly Descemet punch. The Ex-PRESS was originally intended as a subconjunctival shunt without a flap; this was abandoned because of flat chambers and hypotony. Proponents feel that the Ex-PRESS simplifies surgery, results in fewer complications, increases success rates, and produces better-looking blebs.

This retrospective article did not find evidence to show better outcomes in terms of intraocular pressure or final bleb morphology. The authors did see reduced follow-up and early postoperative complications, but these findings are the least solid in terms of confidence, given the retrospective, nonrandomized methodology, which may inadvertently introduce bias.

The Ex-PRESS shunt is an innovation that simplifies the procedure. Its use results in significantly increased procedure costs and leaves the patient with a foreign body that has been reported to, in some cases, erode or cause other late complications. Prospective, randomized studies are underway to see if there is evidence to suggest its widespread adoption.

J. S. Myers, MD

A Randomized Trial of Brimonidine Versus Timolol in Preserving Visual Function: Results From the Low-pressure Glaucoma Treatment Study

Krupin T, on behalf of the Low-Pressure Glaucoma Study Group (Northwestern Univ and the Chicago Ctr for Vision Res, IL; et al)
Am J Ophthalmol 151:671-681, 2011

Purpose.—To compare the alpha2-adrenergic agonist brimonidine tartrate 0.2% to the beta-adrenergic antagonist timolol maleate 0.5% in preserving visual function in low-pressure glaucoma.

Design.—Randomized, double-masked, multicenter clinical trial.

Methods.—Exclusion criteria included untreated intraocular pressure (IOP) >21 mm Hg, visual field mean deviation worse than −16 decibels, or contraindications to study medications. Both eyes received twice-daily monotherapy randomized in blocks of 7 (4 brimonidine to 3 timolol). Standard automated perimetry and tonometry were performed at 4-month intervals. Main outcome measure was field progression in either eye, defined as the same 3 or more points with a negative slope ≥−1 dB/year at $P < 5\%$, on 3 consecutive tests, assessed by pointwise linear regression. Secondary outcome measures were progression based on glaucoma change probability maps (GCPM) of pattern deviation and the 3-omitting method for pointwise linear regression.

Results.—Ninety-nine patients were randomized to brimonidine and 79 to timolol. Mean (± SE) months of follow-up for all patients was 30.0 ± 2. Statistically fewer brimonidine-treated patients (9, 9.1%) had visual field progression by pointwise linear regression than timolol-treated patients (31, 39.2%, log-rank 12.4, $P = .001$). Mean treated IOP was similar for brimonidine- and timolol-treated patients at all time points. More brimonidine-treated (28, 28.3%) than timolol-treated (9, 11.4%) patients discontinued study participation because of drug-related adverse events ($P = .008$). Similar differences in progression were observed when analyzed by GCPM and the 3-omitting method.

Conclusion.—Low-pressure glaucoma patients treated with brimonidine 0.2% who do not develop ocular allergy are less likely to have field progression than patients treated with timolol 0.5% (Figs 2 and 3).

▶ The only known treatment for glaucoma is intraocular pressure reduction. Animal models have suggested that many compounds, including brimonidine, may be protective of the optic nerve separate from any intraocular pressure reduction. This study investigated if brimonidine might be neuroprotective beyond intraocular pressure reduction in low-pressure glaucoma.

This prospective, randomized, multicenter study, in which my department participated, was rigorously designed and conducted. Patients were randomly assigned to brimonidine 0.2% or timolol, with extra patients being assigned to the brimonidine group, as it was anticipated that allergy and side effects would lead to increased drop outs from this group.

Similar, although modest, intraocular pressure reductions were seen in both groups. More dropouts were seen in the brimonidine group, but no differences

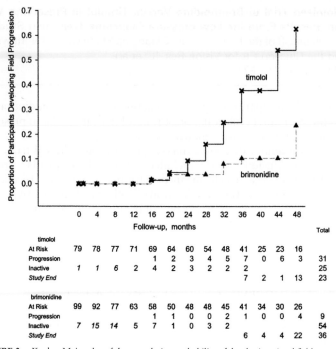

	0	4	8	12	16	20	24	28	32	36	40	44	48	Total
timolol														
At Risk	79	78	77	71	69	64	60	54	48	41	25	23	16	
Progression					1	2	3	4	5	7	0	6	3	31
Inactive	1	1	6	2	4	2	3	2	2	2				25
Study End										7	2	1	13	23
brimonidine														
At Risk	99	92	77	63	58	50	48	48	45	41	34	30	26	
Progression					1	1	0	0	2	1	0	0	4	9
Inactive	7	15	14	5	7	1	0	3	2					54
Study End										6	4	4	22	36

FIGURE 2.—Kaplan-Meier plot of the cumulative probability of developing visual field progression by Progressor analysis for the randomization groups in the Low-pressure Glaucoma Treatment Study. The numbers of active patients at risk and the number of patients developing visual field progression are presented at each 4-month period. Inactive (discontinued) patients and those reaching study end without field progression are withdrawn from the interval after their last completed visit. (Reprinted from Krupin T, on behalf of the low-pressure glaucoma study group. A randomized trial of brimonidine versus timolol in preserving visual function: results from the low-pressure glaucoma treatment study. *Am J Ophthalmol.* 2011;151:671-681, Copyright 2011, with permission from Elsevier.)

were observed in the remaining patients with regard to intraocular pressure reduction (Fig 3).

The brimonidine-treated patients experienced 3-fold less visual field progression than the timolol-treated eyes. This is a dramatic and profound result that was present with each of 3 different methods for visual field analysis.

The difference in outcomes does not seem related to underlying differences in the study groups or to the dropout rate in the brimonidine group. It seems possible that brimonidine had a neuroprotective effect beyond intraocular pressure reduction because similar pressure reduction in the timolol group did not result in the same level of protection against field loss. The only other obvious possibility is that timolol is detrimental to eyes with low-pressure glaucoma, which seems unlikely given the prior studies on this and similar groups. Although hemodynamic effects with timolol in low-pressure glaucoma have been feared, this group of patients did not have particularly low pressure (average about 16 mm Hg) or particular vasopathic risk factors.

Studies such as this are expensive and take many years. It is unlikely that another study of this caliber is done in the near future regarding brimonidine

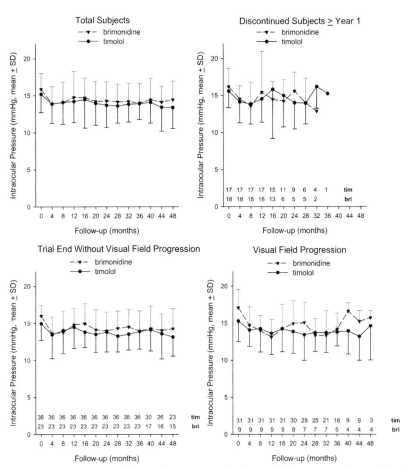

FIGURE 3.—Distribution of intraocular pressure at baseline and follow-up visits for timolol and brimonidine treatment groups of the Low-pressure Glaucoma Treatment Study. Intraocular pressure data is illustrated for all subjects (top left), discontinued subjects ≥ year 1 (top right), trial end without visual field progression (bottom left) and visual field progression (bottom right). Up error bars (standard deviation) for brimonidine treatment, down error bars for timolol treatment. Data below each figure represent the number of study patients at the follow-up months. (Reprinted from Krupin T, on behalf of the low-pressure glaucoma study group. A randomized trial of brimonidine vs timolol in preserving visual function: results from the low-pressure glaucoma treatment study. *Am J Ophthalmol.* 2011;151: 671-681, Copyright 2011, with permission from Elsevier.)

and timolol. The results of this prospective multicenter study should be considered when choosing therapy for low-pressure glaucoma.

J. S. Myers, MD

A Video Study of Drop Instillation in Both Glaucoma and Retina Patients with Visual Impairment

Hennessy AL, Katz J, Covert D, et al (Glaucoma Specialists, Baltimore, MD; Johns Hopkins Bloomberg School of Public Health, Baltimore, MD; Alcon Res Ltd, Fort Worth, TX; et al)
Am J Ophthalmol 152:982-988, 2011

Purpose.—To compare self-administration of drops in both visually impaired glaucoma subjects and retina subjects.

Design.—Prospective, observational study.

Methods.—*Setting*: Distinct glaucoma and retina practices.

Study Population: Subjects with glaucoma or retinal diseases with visual acuity of 20/60 or worse in 1 eye, significant field loss, or both.

Observation Procedures: Subjects were video recorded self-instilling a drop onto the worse eye.

Main Outcome Measure: Proper instillation of eye drop onto ocular surface.

Results.—We included 409 subjects (205 glaucoma, 204 retina). Differences between the groups included the following: glaucoma subjects included fewer females ($P = .05$), included fewer white persons ($P < .005$), had worse visual acuity ($P < .005$), had less self-reported arthritis ($P < .05$), were younger ($P < .005$), and had more previous exposure to drop use ($P < .005$). Glaucoma subjects had more bilateral impairment (60% vs 42%; $P < .0005$). Retina subjects instilled more drops (1.7 vs 1.4; $P = .02$) and more frequently touched the bottle to the eye (47% vs 33%; $P = .003$). Of subjects claiming not to miss the eye, nearly one third from each group ($P = .32$) actually missed. Approximately one third of each group could not get a drop onto the eye (30% retina vs 29% glaucoma; $P = .91$). Among subjects placing 1 drop onto the eye without touching the adnexae, there was a trend for glaucoma patients to perform better, although both groups did poorly (success, 39% glaucoma vs 31% retina; $P = .09$).

Conclusions.—Among visually impaired subjects, regardless of cause, drop administration was a problem. Both groups wasted drops, contaminated bottles, and had inaccurate perception of their abilities. This has implications for future therapeutic delivery systems.

▶ This prospective observational study examines the self-administration of eye drops in visually impaired patients with retinal disease and glaucoma. Ultimately, poor adherence to medication regimens, even if unintentional, may have adverse consequences for patients.

All patients in this study had Early Treatment Diabetic Retinopathy Study visual acuity of 20/60 or worse in at least 1 eye and/or demonstrated moderate or severe visual field damage by Hodapp-Parrish-Anderson criteria in 1 eye. The vast majority of patients with glaucoma had open-angle glaucoma, whereas a variety of retinal diseases were included. Age-related macular degeneration and diabetic retinopathy accounted for more than half of all retinal diseases in the study. Comorbid conditions such as cataract were allowed.

Subjects were given a sterile bottle of artificial tears and instructed to instill 1 drop into their worse-seeing eye using their dominant hand in a manner similar to their self-administration technique at home. Approximately 1 in 3 patients in both groups could not get a drop into the ocular surface. Subjects with retinal disease were statistically significantly more likely to instill more drops into the eye and to make more attempts and more frequently touched the tip of the bottle to the eye. One-third of patients in the glaucoma group and about half of patients in the retina group touched the tip of the bottle to the eye. Younger age (< 70 years old) seemed to be the biggest factor in determining a subject's ability to instill eye drops successfully.

In a questionnaire, about one-third of patients who reported they never missed their eye actually missed their eye during the videotaped administration. Although nearly 80% of subjects stated that they have no trouble taking eye drops, less than 30% were able to instill a drop on the eye. Of the subjects who denied touching the bottle tip to their eye, about 40% of patients with retinal disease and 25% of patients with glaucoma did touch the bottle to their eye.

The results of this study coincide well with previous important studies regarding patient adherence and persistency with medical management of glaucoma. In general, the success of patients in strictly following the instructions of their providers is dismal. Hopefully, the future holds promise for therapies that mitigate the burden of eye drop administration on patients. Already, slowly dissolving anti-inflammatory agents are injected into the vitreous and there is interest in glaucoma drugs that may be injected into the anterior segment.

J. S. Myers, MD

Increased iris thickness and association with primary angle closure glaucoma
Wang B-S, Narayanaswamy A, Amerasinghe N, et al (Singapore Eye Res Inst and Singapore Natl Eye Ctr; et al)
Br J Ophthalmol 95:46-50, 2011

Aims.—To investigate the relationship between quantitative iris parameters and angle closure disease.

Methods.—Participants with angle closure were recruited prospectively from glaucoma clinics. Anterior segment optical coherence tomography (AS-OCT) was performed under standardised dark conditions. Customised software was used on horizontal AS-OCT scans to measure iris thickness at 750 um (IT750) and 2000 um (IT2000) from the sclera spur, maximal iris thickness (ITM) and cross-sectional area of the iris (I-Area).

Results.—167 Angle closure (consisting of 50 primary angle-closure (PAC), 73 primary angle closure glaucoma (PACG) and 44 fellow eyes of acute PAC) and 1153 normal participants were examined. After adjusting for age, sex, pupil size and anterior chamber depth, mean IT750 (0.499 vs 0.451 mm, $p<0.001$), IT2000 (0.543 vs 0.479 mm, $p<0.001$), ITM (0.660 vs 0.602 mm, $p<0.001$) and I-Area (1.645 vs 1.570 mm^2, $p=0.014$) were significantly greater in angle closure (combined groups) versus normal eyes. Multivariate adjusted odd ratios (OR) of each parameter for the angle closure as compared with normal eyes were: IT750 OR1.7 (95% CI 1.1 to 2.7, p=0.032); IT2000 OR2.2 (95% CI 1.3 to 3.8, p=0.006) and ITM OR2.2 (95% CI 1.3 to 3.6, p=0.003), respectively, per 0.1 unit increase.

Conclusions.—Increased iris thickness is associated with angle closure (Fig 1, Table 2).

▶ This study is a follow-up to a previous study in which an independent association was found between narrow angles and iris curvature, cross-sectional area, and thickness. The previous study evaluated patients with only narrow angles, whereas this study focused on significant angle closure.

Patients were divided into 4 groups: primary angle closure, primary angle closure glaucoma (PACG), fellow eyes of acute primary angle closure, and normal controls. Primary angle closure was defined as presence of gonioscopically narrow angles with peripheral anterior synechiae and/or intraocular pressure > 21 mm Hg but without glaucomatous optic neuropathy or visual field loss. Primary angle closure glaucoma eyes were defined by a constellation of signs and symptoms. Past acute angle closure glaucoma may cause iris atrophy and thinning of the iris so the authors included only fellow eyes of patients with unilateral acute primary angle closure.

Anterior segment optical coherence tomography (OCT) scans were performed using Visante OCT (Carl Zeiss Meditec) under standardized dark conditions. Customized software was used to process the images. Using the scleral spur as the center of a circle with radius of 750 and 2000 μm, iris thickness was determined at the point of intersection of the circle and the anterior iris surface (Fig 1) to determine the IT750 and IT2000 parameters. The shortest

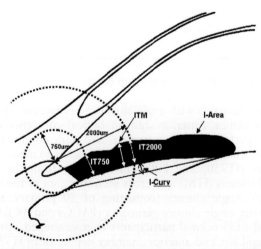

FIGURE 1.—A schematic diagram illustrates the automatic measurement of iris thickness (IT750, IT2000 and ITM), iris area (I-Area) and iris curvature (I-Curv). (Reprinted from Wang B-S, Narayanaswamy A, Amerasinghe N, et al. Increased iris thickness and association with primary angle closure glaucoma. *Br J Ophthalmol.* 2011;95:46-50, with permission from BMJ Publishing Group Ltd.)

TABLE 2.—Comparison of Iris Parameters in Angle Closure Eyes and Normal Eyes

Iris Measures	Mean (SD) in Angle Closure Eyes (n=167)	Mean (SD) in Normal Eyes (n=1153)	Mean Difference (95% CI)*	p Value
IT 750 (mm)	0.499 (0.14)	0.451 (0.10)	0.048 (0.024, 0.072)	<0.001
IT 2000 (mm)	0.543 (0.13)	0.479 (0.10)	0.063 (0.041, 0.085)	<0.001
ITM (mm)	0.660 (0.13)	0.602 (0.10)	0.058 (0.036, 0.080)	<0.001
I-Area (mm²)	1.645 (0.35)	1.570 (0.27)	0.075 (0.015, 0.135)	0.014
I-Curv (mm)	0.110 (0.27)	0.260 (0.12)	−0.328 (−0.361 to −0.294)	<0.001

IT750, iris thickness measured at 750 μm from the sclera spur; IT2000, iris thickness measured at 2000 μm from the sclera spur; I-Area, iris area; ITM, maximal iris thickness; I-Curv, iris curvature.
*Adjusted for age, sex, pupil size and anterior chamber depth.

distance from anterior to posterior surface at these points was used. The highest value of iris thickness along the entire iris was considered the maximal iris thickness (ITM), and cross-sectional area of the iris (I-Area) was calculated as the cumulative cross-sectional area of the full length of the iris. Finally, the iris curvature (I-Curv) parameter was determined by connecting the most central and peripheral points of the iris pigment epithelium and measuring the distance from this line to the iris at the point of greatest convexity.

The scleral spur may be difficult to identify on Visante OCT, and about 15% of patients from the angle closure groups and 25% of normals were excluded for undetectable scleral spur. Adjustments were made for age, sex, anterior chamber depth, and pupil size. The iris was statistically significantly thicker in angle closure patients than normal controls. This finding held for combined angle closure groups and all subgroups as well as for IT750, IT2000, and ITM (except for IT750 PACG vs normals). I-Curv was greater for normals than angle closure patients. I-Area yielded no statistically significant difference between angle closure patients and controls (Table 2).

This study indicates that iris thickness is independently associated with angle closure. Although it seems intuitive that a thicker iris may further crowd an already narrow angle, more evidence is needed to determine if the difference in iris thickness is enough to generate angle closure. The authors theorize that laser gonioplasty to thin the iris may be beneficial, but the risk/benefit analysis of this procedure requires consideration of other potential positives and negatives to determine its utility.

The authors acknowledge that limitations of this study include absence of lens thickness measurements, refraction, and axial length. Additionally, relatively small sample size limited the power of comparisons. Previous laser peripheral iridotomies and medications could have affected the iris measurements, as well.

S. J. Fudemberg, MD

Cerebrospinal fluid pressure in ocular hypertension

Ren R, Zhang X, Wang N, et al (Capital Med Univ, Beijing, China)
Acta Ophthalmol 89:e142-e148, 2011

Background.—To assess the lumbar cerebrospinal fluid pressure (CSF-P) in ocular hypertensive subjects with elevated intraocular pressure (IOP) but without development of glaucomatous optic nerve damage.

Methods.—The prospective interventional study included 17 patients with ocular hypertension and 71 subjects of a nonglaucomatous control group. All patients underwent a standardized ophthalmologic and neurological examination including measurement of lumbar CSF-P. In the ocular hypertensive group, the IOP was corrected for its dependence on central corneal thickness ($IOP_{corrected}$). The trans-lamina cribrosa pressure difference (Trans-LCPD) was calculated as $IOP_{corrected} - CSF\text{-}P$.

Results.—CSF-P was significantly ($p < 0.001$) higher in the ocular hypertensive group (16.0 ± 2.5 mmHg) than in the control group (12.9 ± 1.9 mmHg). CSF-P was significantly associated with $IOP_{corrected}$ ($p < 0.001$; $r = 0.82$). In multivariate analysis, CSF-P was significantly correlated with $IOP_{corrected}$ ($p < 0.001$) and marginally significantly with mean blood pressure ($p = 0.05$). Trans-LCPD was not associated significantly with blood pressure ($p = 0.69$).

Conclusion.—Some ocular hypertensive subjects with increased intraocular pressure measurements (after correction for their dependence on central corneal thickness) had an abnormally high lumbar cerebrospinal fluid pressure. Assuming that lumbar cerebrospinal fluid pressure correlated with orbital cerebrospinal fluid pressure, one may postulate that the elevated retro-lamina cribrosa pressure compensated for an increased

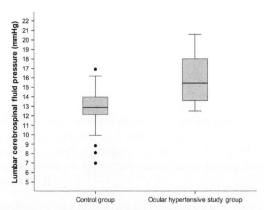

FIGURE 1.—Lumbar cerebrospinal fluid pressure in subjects with ocular hypertension and control subjects. Boxplots showing the distribution of cerebrospinal fluid pressure as measured by lumbar puncture in ocular hypertensive patients of the study group and subjects in the control group. The boxplots show the median, interquartile range, 95% percentile, outliers and extreme values. The difference between the groups was statistically significant ($p < 0.001$). (Reprinted from Ren R, Zhang X, Wang N, et al. Cerebrospinal fluid pressure in ocular hypertension. *Acta Ophthalmol*. 2011;89:e142-e148, with permission from Acta Ophthalmologica Scandinavica Foundation.)

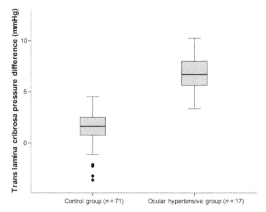

FIGURE 2.—Trans-lamina cribrosa pressure difference in subjects with ocular hypertension and control subjects. Boxplots showing distribution of the trans-lamina cribrosa pressure difference (intraocular pressure minus cerebrospinal fluid pressure) in ocular hypertensive patients and subjects in the control group. The difference between groups was statistically significant (p < 0.001). Boxplots show the median, interquartile range, 95% percentile, outliers and extreme values. (Reprinted from Ren R, Zhang X, Wang N, et al. Cerebrospinal fluid pressure in ocular hypertension. *Acta Ophthalmol.* 2011;89:e142-e148, with permission from Acta Ophthalmologica Scandinavica Foundation.)

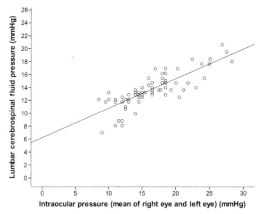

FIGURE 3.—Association between lumbar cerebrospinal fluid pressure measurements and intraocular pressure. Scatterplot showing distribution of cerebrospinal fluid pressure measurements (determined by lumbar puncture) and intraocular pressure in ocular hypertensive subjects of the study group and nonglaucomatous subjects of the control group. The correlation was statistically significant (p < 0.001; $r = 0.82$; equation of the regression line: cerebrospinal fluid pressure (mmHg) = 0.46 × intraocular pressure (mmHg) + 6.2 mmHg). (Reprinted from Ren R, Zhang X, Wang N, et al. Cerebrospinal fluid pressure in ocular hypertension. *Acta Ophthalmol.* 2011;89:e142-e148, with permission from Acta Ophthalmologica Scandinavica Foundation.)

intraocular pressure. The elevated retro-lamina cribrosa pressure may have led to a normal trans-laminar pressure difference in the eyes with elevated intraocular pressure, so that glaucomatous optic nerve damage did not develop. Intraocular pressure, cerebrospinal fluid pressure and arterial blood pressure were correlated with each other (Figs 1-3).

▶ The mechanical theory of glaucomatous optic neuropathy suggests that increased intraocular pressure may lead to duress on the ganglion cells. In recent years, research has suggested that patients with glaucoma may have lower intracranial pressure (ICP), exposing ganglion cells to an increased translaminar pressure gradient.

This study investigates ICP in ocular hypertensive patients—patients with high eye pressure but no signs of glaucomatous nerve damage. The results showed increasing eye pressure with increasing cerebrospinal fluid pressure, and higher ICP in the ocular hypertension (OHT) patients.

Shortcomings of this study include difference in the control group versus the OHT subjects: The controls were older and more were women, although neither of these differences is known to affect ICP or intraocular pressure. Also, controls were taken from a neurology clinic.

The translaminar pressure may be another factor helping to explain who gets glaucomatous optic neuropathy and who does not. More studies like this are needed to further clarify this exciting new concept.

J. S. Myers, MD

Anterior chamber angle imaging with optical coherence tomography
Leung CK-S, Weinreb RN (The Chinese Univ of Hong Kong, PR China; Univ of California, San Diego)
Eye 25:261-267, 2011

The technology of optical coherence tomography (OCT) has evolved rapidly from time-domain to spectral-domain and swept-source OCT over the recent years. OCT has become an important tool for assessment of the anterior chamber angle and detection of angle closure. Improvement in image resolution and scan speed of OCT has facilitated a more detailed and comprehensive analysis of the anterior chamber angle. It is now possible to examine Schwalbe's line and Schlemm's canal along with the scleral spur. High-speed imaging allows evaluation of the angle in 360°. With three-dimensional reconstruction, visualization of the iris profiles and the angle configurations is enhanced. This article summarizes the development and application of OCT for anterior chamber angle measurement, detection of angle closure, and investigation of the pathophysiology of primary angle closure.

▶ Gonioscopy is inherently subjective. In a perfect world, an objective measure of anterior chamber (AC) angle narrowing could be converted to a specific risk stratum for acute and chronic angle closure glaucoma. In this scenario, the decision to perform laser peripheral iridotomy would be based on better information than we currently use. Nonetheless, examination of the anterior chamber angle by gonioscopy provides extremely valuable information above and beyond an impression of angle narrowing.

In this article, the authors review optical coherence tomography (OCT) and its use in the anterior segment. OCT of the anterior segment has the potential to offer an accurate and precise objective measure of angle narrowing in a readily usable clinical format. Among the critical questions in applying the technique is: What should be measured to judge the angle? The authors summarize the evolution of OCT to current-generation, high-resolution machines that may identify particular angle structures and efforts to find a measurement that corresponds well with clinically significant AC angle narrowing.

Time-domain OCT was introduced in the early 1990s and has become an important tool for evaluation of macular and optic nerve diseases. The prototype OCT, OCT 1, and OCT 2000 did not generate sufficiently detailed images of the anterior segment. OCT 3, or Stratus OCT, scans at 400 A-scans per second with an axial resolution of about 10 µm. Although the configuration of the peripheral iris in relation to the scleral-corneal junction could be discerned, the scleral spur was not visible.

Two commercially available anterior-segment OCT systems, Visante OCT and SL-OCT, were introduced commercially between 2005 and 2006. The Visante has a faster scan speed and internal fixation target to adjust for the subject's refraction. Attempts were made to create a standard technique for measurement of the AC angle, but the advent of spectral-domain OCT permitted higher-resolution images of important structures.

In both time-domain and spectral-domain OCT, the interference pattern of light directed at a tissue of interest is compared with that from a reference mirror. In time-domain OCT, the mirror moves, and information is collected as a function of time, whereas in spectral-domain OCT, the mirror is stationary and the interference spectrum data are broken down by Fourier transform mathematics. Spectral domain is much faster with scan speeds of at least 20 000 A-scans per second. Ultimately, the next wave of innovation in OCT technology may be swept-source OCT, in which a tunable fast scanning laser source and photodetector enable scan speeds in the hundreds of thousands per second.

Spectral-domain OCT typically offers a view of angle configuration and the scleral spur but not the ciliary body. However, measurement reproducibility and repeatability data have not been reported. Current definitions of angle parameters assume the trabecular meshwork may be found about 500 to 750 µm from the scleral spur, but this assumption has not been validated. Perhaps instruments that better define the location and dimension of the trabecular meshwork will offer an improved way to detect angle closure.

In summary, anterior segment OCT offers tremendous potential for objectively determining angle narrowing. Further, more detailed understanding of AC angle structures and their relationship to one another with OCT measurements may contribute to our understanding.

J. S. Myers, MD

Sustained elevated intraocular pressures after intravitreal injection of bevacizumab, ranibizumab, and pegaptanib
Choi DY, Ortube MC, McCannel CA, et al (David Geffen School of Medicine at the Univ of California, Los Angeles)
Retina 31:1028-1035, 2011

Purpose.—To investigate elevated intraocular pressures (IOP) (defined by a measurement >25 mmHg at a follow-up visit) after an intravitreal injection of anti−vascular endothelial growth factor agents for age-related macular degeneration.

Methods.—Retrospective review of medical records.

Results.—A total of 127 patients (155 eyes) received an intravitreal injection of anti−vascular endothelial growth factor agents (bevacizumab, ranibizumab, or pegaptanib) ranging from 1 to 39 injections for more than a period of 30 to 1759 days. Among this population, 12 patients (14 eyes; 9.4%) developed elevated IOP >25 mmHg. Of these, 7 patients (5.5%) developed sustained elevated IOP (IOP >25 mmHg on 2 separate visits requiring glaucoma medication or surgery), of which 8 eyes required topical medications and 1 eye underwent glaucoma surgery. Mean IOP of injected eyes receiving intravitreal injection was 15.2 ± 2.4 mmHg, and the mean IOP was 14.9 ± 2.6 mmHg for noninjected eyes. Among eyes that had elevated IOPs, there was no association with injection frequency, number of injections, or anti−vascular endothelial growth factor agent used.

Conclusion.—Elevated IOP, sustained or unsustained, after intravitreal injection is not uncommon. No association with patient demographics or injection history was identified in the authors' study population (Fig 1).

▶ Transient intraocular pressure (IOP) elevation after intravitreal injection is expected. However, several case reports indicate that sustained IOP elevation may be a potential complication of intravitreal injections of vascular endothelial growth factor (VEGF) inhibitors. The MARINA and ANCHOR trials found no sustained increases in IOP with ranibizumab (Lucentis; Genetech, South San Francisco, California). The VISION and CORES trials also failed to show increases in IOP with pegaptanib (Macugen; Eyetech Pharmaceuticals/Pfizer, Inc., New York, New York) and bevacizumab (Avastin; Genetech).

This study is a retrospective review of patients who received anti-VEGF intravitreal injections between 2005 and 2010 for treatment of age-related macular degeneration (ARMD). Preexisting glaucoma diagnosis/treatment, diabetes, and retinal disorders besides ARMD were exclusion criteria. A total of 127 charts (254 eyes) were reviewed (Fig 1). Of these, 155 eyes received injections. Elevated IOP was defined as > 25 mm Hg, and 14 eyes met this threshold. Among eyes with elevated IOP, 9 were determined to have sustained IOP elevations. The majority of IOP measurements were made with Tono-Pen, which is subject to greater variability and less accuracy than Goldmann applanation tonometry. To mitigate the influence of this factor, the authors evaluated the variability of repeated Tono-Pen measurements for each eye across the entire cohort and confirmed that their threshold for elevated IOP was clearly outside the

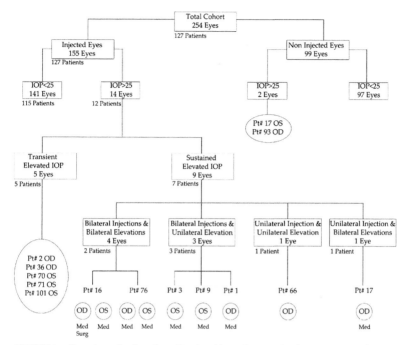

FIGURE 1.—Flow chart of entire cohort. (Reprinted from Choi DY, Ortube MC, McCannel CA, et al. Sustained elevated intraocular pressures after intravitreal injection of bevacizumab, ranibizumab, and pegaptanib. *Retina*. 2011;31:1028-1035, with permission from Ophthalmic Communications Society, Inc.)

normal range. They also examined IOP measurements for trends. No relationship was found between frequency of injections an eye received and progressive increase or decrease in IOP measurements during a 300-day interval. Fifty percent of patients received > 5 injections with a range of 1 to 39 injections.

Of the 9 eyes with sustained IOP elevations, 1 required trabeculectomy, and the rest were managed medically. The average number of injections to elevated IOP was 9.6 ± 7.7, but with a range of 1 to 24. Four eyes started to have sustained IOP elevation after ranibizumab, 3 after bevacizumab, and 2 after pegaptanib.

The incidence, prevalence, and etiology of sustained IOP increase after anti-VEGF injections are poorly understood. This study helps confirm anecdotal reports that sustained IOP increase may be a problem after intravitreal anti-VEGF injections. As the application of anti-VEGF agents extends beyond ARMD into treatment algorithms for other diseases, sustained IOP increase may become more widespread. For example, retinal vein occlusion and diabetes predispose patients to glaucoma more than ARMD; therefore, use of anti-VEGF agents in these conditions may yield more sustained IOP spikes.

A large prospective study is needed to consider this issue with rigorous and standardized follow-up. Unfortunately, information from patients followed up for ARMD, but not specifically for IOP elevations, is limited by factors, including but not limited to, variability in follow-up duration, absence of gonioscopic evaluations, and use of Tono-Pen IOP measurements. Also although ARMD patients with no other significant ocular conditions provide a relatively pure population in which to identify a causal link between intravitreal injections of anti-VEGF agents and IOP spike, other patient groups may be more commonly affected by sustained IOP spikes.

S. J. Fudemberg, MD

An Assessment of the Health and Economic Burdens of Glaucoma
Varma R, Lee PP, Goldberg I, et al (Univ of Southern California, Los Angeles, CA; Duke Eye Ctr, Durham, NC; Univ of Sydney, Australia; et al)
Am J Ophthalmol 152:515-522, 2011

Purpose.—To bring together information concerning the epidemiology and the economic and individual burdens of glaucoma.

Design.—Interpretive essay.

Methods.—Review and synthesis of selected literature published from 1991 through December 2010.

Results.—An estimated 3% of the global population over 40 years of age currently has glaucoma, the majority of whom are undiagnosed. Vision loss from glaucoma has a significant impact on health-related quality of life even in the early stages of disease. The overall burden increases as glaucomatous damage and vision loss progress. The economic burden of glaucoma is significant and increases as the disease worsens.

Conclusions.—Early identification and treatment of patients with glaucoma and those with ocular hypertension at high risk of developing vision loss are likely to reduce an individual's loss of health-related quality of life as well as the personal and societal economic burdens (Figs 2 and 5).

▶ This is an interpretive article aimed at synthesizing published information from 1991 to 2010 on the epidemiology as well as economic and individual burdens of glaucoma. Information regarding the extent of glaucoma throughout the world is staggering. Over 60 million people worldwide are estimated to have glaucoma. About 75% of these have primary open-angle glaucoma. The prevalence of glaucoma is expected to increase to almost 80 million people by the end of this decade. People of African descent and Latinos and Hispanics develop glaucoma at a rate 3 times that of white subjects. Asians represent nearly 90% of the population with primary angle-closure glaucoma.

The prevalence of glaucoma makes its economic impact significant. In the United States alone, roughly 2 million people have glaucoma and direct costs are around $3 billion per year. Direct costs include money spent for provider visits, medicines, and procedures related to glaucoma. Indirect costs, including lost productivity of patients and their caregivers, transportation, and nursing home care, likely add substantially to the direct costs. Not surprisingly, the financial implications are more profound as disease severity increases. One study indicated that direct costs per year increase 4-fold as the disease progresses from

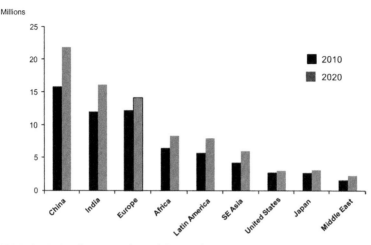

FIGURE 2.—Projected rise in prevalence of glaucoma between 2010 and 2020. Data from Quigley and Broman.[1] *Editor's Note*: Please refer to original journal article for full references. (Reprinted from Varma R, Lee PP, Goldberg I, et al. An assessment of the health and economic burdens of glaucoma. *Am J Ophthalmol.* 2011;152:515-522, Copyright 2011, with permission from Elsevier.)

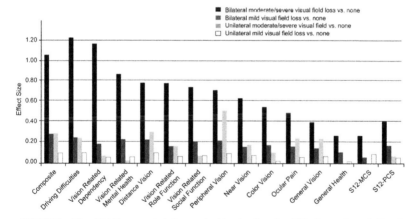

FIGURE 5.—Visual field loss negatively impacts health-related quality of life. Comparison of effect sizes (ES) between the no visual field loss (VFL) subgroup with subgroups with different severity levels of VFL. The level of VFL was stratified into 5 categories: no VFL (mean deviation [MD] > −2 decibels [dB] in both eyes), unilateral mild VFL (−6 dB < MD < −2 dB in the worse eye), unilateral moderate to severe VFL (MD < −6 dB in 1 eye, MD > −2 dB in the other eye), bilateral mild VFL (−6 dB < MD < −2 dB in both eyes; or −6 dB < MD < −2 dB in 1 eye, MD < −6 dB in the other eye), and bilateral moderate to severe VFL (MD < −6 dB in both eyes). The ES was calculated as the difference in the adjusted mean scores (between each of the severity levels of VFL and no VFL) divided by the standard deviation for the no-VFL group. Subscales are clustered in decreasing order of ES for the bilateral moderate to severe VFL vs none groups, for the 25-item National Eye Institute Visual Function Questionnaire (NEI-VFQ-25) vision-related subscales, and the Medical Outcomes Study 12-item Short-Form Health Survey (SF-12) general health subscale scores. ES below 0.20 represent no statistically significant effect. An ES of 0.20 to 0.49 is considered to be a small effect, 0.50 to 0.79 a medium effect, and 0.80 or more a large effect. Reprinted from McKean-Cowdin R et al.[27] Copyright © Elsevier; reprinted with permission. *Editor's Note*: Please refer to original journal article for full references. (Reprinted from Varma R, Lee PP, Goldberg I, et al. An assessment of the health and economic burdens of glaucoma. *Am J Ophthalmol.* 2011;152:515-522, Copyright 2011, with permission from Elsevier.)

early to end stages. Indirect costs also increase dramatically as severe disease limits function. Medications account for about half of all direct costs for glaucoma care.

The cost-effectiveness of glaucoma management depends on assumptions used in models designed to quantify treatment benefits. For example, treatment of ocular hypertensives was cost-effective when limited to patients with risk factors identified by the Ocular Hypertension Treatment Study, but treatment of all ocular hypertensives was not cost-effective.

Health-related quality of life may be severely reduced by glaucoma. Loss of independence through restrictions on driving, safely ambulating, and reading is magnified by the psychological burden of fear of blindness, social withdrawal, and depression. Glaucoma patients are more than 3 times more likely to have fallen within the prior year and more than 6 times more likely to have been involved in a motor vehicle collision over the prior 5 years.

This article highlights the real impact of glaucoma on patients and society. Capturing all of the direct and indirect costs of glaucoma in a quantifiable way is impossible. Therefore, even an excellent summary, such as this one, inherently underestimates the problem. Any disease treatment is a risk versus benefit analysis. The financial pressures affecting the modern health care system also may increasingly require a cost versus benefit analysis for disease treatment. A draft of the Agency for Healthcare Research and Quality's (AHRQ) review of the effectiveness of glaucoma screening sparked a strong rebuke from the American Academy of Ophthalmology and the American Glaucoma Society. The AHRQ draft called into question the utility and effectiveness of glaucoma screening. Regardless of debate about its methodology and conclusions, the AHRQ's effort demonstrates the importance of further understanding the total harm of glaucoma and improving our ability to detect as well as treat it. Future decisions about allocation of resources to prevent visual impairment from glaucoma are likely to depend on our understanding of the far-reaching impact of glaucoma.

J. S. Myers, MD

Use of Herbal Medicines and Nutritional Supplements in Ocular Disorders: An Evidence-Based Review
Wilkinson JT, Fraunfelder FW (Oregon Health & Science Univ, Portland)
Drugs 71:2421-2434, 2011

We sought to examine the evidence regarding the use of herbal medicines and nutritional supplements in age-related macular degeneration (AMD), cataracts, diabetic retinopathy and glaucoma, and to review the ocular adverse effects of herbal and nutritional agents of clinical importance to ophthalmologists. We performed a literature search of Ovid MEDLINE and selected websites including the American Academy of Ophthalmology (AAO), the Centers for Disease Control and Prevention (CDC), the National Institutes of Health (NIH) and the World Health Organization (WHO).

There is strong evidence supporting the use of antioxidants and zinc in patients with certain forms of intermediate and advanced AMD. However, there has been growing evidence regarding potential significant adverse effects associated with the AREDS (Age-Related Eye Disease Study) formula vitamins. Current data does not support the use of antioxidants or herbal medications in the prevention or treatment of cataracts, glaucoma or diabetic retinopathy.

It is important for providers to be aware of the benefits and the significant potential adverse effects that have been associated with nutritional supplements and herbal medications, and to properly inform their patients when making decisions about supplementation. Further rigorous evaluation of nutritional supplements and herbal medicines in the treatment of eye disease is needed to determine their safety and efficacy.

▶ In the United States alone, sales of dietary supplements were estimated at $27 billion in 2010. The use of complementary and alternative medicine (CAM) is becoming widespread. Between 1990 and 1997, use of herbal remedies increased nearly 4-fold. However, well-designed clinical trials for CAM therapies are often lacking. This article is an evidence-based review of the use of herbal medicines and nutritional supplements in ocular disorders, including glaucoma.

Many herbal remedies have been touted to provide ocular benefits (Table 1 in the original article) and many also carry the risk of adverse effects (Table 2 in the original article). Often, patients who use CAM do not report their use to their physicians. In a survey of over 1500 patients, about 14% reported past use of CAM therapy specifically for glaucoma. Of these patients, about 63% did not disclose the use of CAM therapy to their ophthalmologist and 41% believed their treatments were helping their glaucoma.

There are a number of vitamins thought to impact glaucoma. Vitamin C may transiently lower intraocular pressure (IOP) when given intravenously in acute angle closure glaucoma. However, the IOP-lowering effect of vitamin C administered orally, even in large doses, is inconsistent. Theoretically, intravenous doses of vitamin C may function purely as a hyperosmotic agent, like mannitol. The B vitamins have also been tried for glaucoma, although studies linking B vitamin deficiency and glaucoma are not conclusive. Vitamins A and E have been recommended for glaucoma, but a large epidemiological study evaluating nutritional supplements and glaucoma reported no strong association between risk of primary open angle glaucoma and use of antioxidants. Large doses of vitamin A have been associated with increased intracranial hypertension, and vitamin E supplementation has been linked with increased risk of heart failure.

Herbal remedies have also been tried for glaucoma. Marijuana has been shown to decrease IOP. The duration of the IOP-lowering effect is reported in the range of 3 to 4 hours, requiring frequent consumption to lower IOP consistently. Systemic toxicity and short half-life make marijuana a poor treatment option for glaucoma. It may also lower systemic blood pressure and could potentially decrease ocular perfusion. The American Glaucoma Society produced a position statement on the use of marijuana for glaucoma treatment that concluded, "although marijuana can lower the intraocular pressure (IOP), its side effects and short duration of action, coupled with a lack of evidence that its use alters the course of glaucoma, preclude recommending this drug in any form for the treatment of glaucoma at the present time."[1] Bilberry was reported to help in glaucoma and improve eyesight. It was also reported to increase ocular blood flow. Bilberry has not been reported to lower IOP. One report on ginkgo biloba indicated that it could improve preexisting visual field loss from glaucoma in normal tension patients. It is important to know that ginkgo biloba acts as a blood thinner by inhibiting platelet aggregation, which may increase the risk of serious adverse events from bleeding.

Ultimately, CAM therapies have not been clearly demonstrated to be beneficial in glaucoma treatment. Well-designed studies are needed to formally confirm or refute the use of popular CAM therapies for glaucoma. Even if CAM therapies prove useful in treating glaucoma, herbal and nutritional supplements are exempt from monitoring by the US Food and Drug Administration. These products may be sold with no burden to demonstrate efficacy and safety. Furthermore, wide variations in the concentration and purity of these products are possible because the industry is not tightly regulated.

J. S. Myers, MD

Reference

1. Jampel H. American glaucoma society position statement: marijuana and the treatment of glaucoma. *J Glaucoma.* 2010;19:75-76.

Incorporating life expectancy in glaucoma care
Wesselink C, Stoutenbeek R, Jansonius NM (Univ of Groningen, The Netherlands)
Eye 25:1575-1580, 2011

Aim.—To calculate for which combinations of age and perimetric disease stage glaucoma patients are unlikely to become visually impaired during their lifetime.

Methods.—We used residual life expectancy data (life expectancy adjusted for the age already reached) as provided by Statistics Netherlands and rates of progression as derived from published studies. We calculated the baseline mean deviation (MD) for which an individual would reach a MD of -20 dB at the end of life as a function of age and rate of progression. For situations in which the individual rate of progression is unknown, we used the 90th percentiles of rate of progression and residual life expectancy. For situations in which the individual rate of progression is known, we used the 95th percentile of the residual life expectancy.

Results.—An easily applicable graphical tool was developed that enables an accurate estimate of the probability of becoming visually impaired during lifetime, given age, current glaucomatous damage, and—if available—the individual rate of progression.

Conclusions.—This novel tool enables the clinician to incorporate life expectancy in glaucoma care in a well-founded manner and may serve as a starting point for personalized decision making (Fig 2).

▶ Most of glaucoma management is directed toward lowering intraocular pressure to prevent vision loss. However, the ultimate purpose of glaucoma care is to avoid functional vision loss, which is vision loss that actually affects an individual's ability to perform desired tasks. In general, glaucoma is a slowly progressive disease. In many patients, no functional impairment will occur even if some glaucoma progression occurs. Therefore, if the population of patients with almost no risk of functional impairment in their lifetime could be identified, the risks and costs of monitoring and treatment for these patients could be minimized. Life expectancy is fundamental to an analysis of the risk of functional impairment of vision.

The purpose of this article is to calculate which combinations of age and perimetric disease-stage glaucoma patients are unlikely to become visually impaired. The authors related statistics on the residual life expectancy (life expectancy adjusted for age already reached) to the rates of glaucoma progression from published studies. Residual life expectancy gives a chance of survival for a person of a given age. For example, according to the data used in this article, from Statistics Netherlands, a 70-year-old male has a 5% chance of dying by age 72 years. They also calculated a baseline mean deviation for each age at which a patient is unlikely to go blind in his or her lifetime. They assumed visual impairment to occur at −20 dB (chosen arbitrarily). The 90th percentile of the rate progression was assumed to be −2.5 dB per year for untreated glaucoma (based on 90th percentile from the Early Manifest Glaucoma Trial)[1] and −1 dB per year for treated glaucoma (based on 90th percentile from the Groningen Longitudinal Glaucoma Study).[2]

Graphing the baseline mean deviation versus age and plotting a line of progression for treated and untreated glaucoma, the authors created a tool by which one might gauge the risk of a visual impairment in an individual's lifetime (Fig 2).

This article draws attention to important issues for glaucoma patients and their eye care providers. The balance between overtreating and undertreating glaucoma is critically important. All available treatment options have real potential adverse effects. Undertreatment may result in blindness, and treatment exposes patients to the risks of side effects, procedure complications, and expense. Ultimately, complications of treatment may impair vision. Identifying patients unlikely to become visually impaired during their lifetime would help minimize the individual and societal impact of glaucoma treatment. However, a population analysis hinges on assumptions that limit its application in a clinical setting. A particular clinical setting or practice may suffer selection bias that skews the life expectancy data for this smaller subset of patients. Also, the assumptions about progression and relationship of mean deviation to visual impairment, while logical, are fundamentally just assumptions. In a broader perspective, the effort of a single practitioner to modify access to care for individual patients to achieve a societal benefit places both the patient and provider in jeopardy.

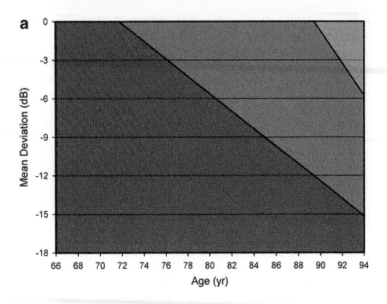

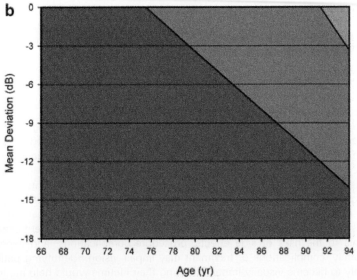

FIGURE 2.—Probability of becoming visually impaired before dying for the situation in which an individual rate of progression is unknown, for men (a) and women (b). If the combination of age and current mean deviation brings the patient in the red area, the probability of becoming visually impaired before dying exceeds 2.5%, even if treated. In the orange area, this probability is <2.5% if treated but >2.5% if untreated. In the green area, this probability is <2.5% even if untreated. Visually impaired was defined as a mean deviation of −20 dB. For interpretation of the references to color in this figure legend, the reader is referred to web version of this article. (Reprinted from Wesselink C, Stoutenbeek R, Jansonius NM. Incorporating life expectancy in glaucoma care. *Eye.* 2011;25:1575-1580, Copyright 2011, with permission from Macmillan Publishers Limited.)

Society as a whole may set standards of care based on rationing resources to save money, but it may be dangerous and disorganized for individual physicians to withhold care to save society money. In the absence of guidelines based on agreed standards of care, including withholding treatment for a condition like glaucoma as it worsens, it is unfair not to offer patients the choice to be treated and accept the risk of that treatment. Nonetheless, making an informed decision with a patient regarding the benefits and risks of treatment, including but not limited to its expense, is an essential part of glaucoma care.

J. S. Myers, MD

References

1. Leske MC, Heijl A, Hyman L, Bengtsson B. Early Manifest Glaucoma Trial: design and baseline data. *Ophthalmology.* 1999;106:2144-2153.
2. Wesselink C, Heeg GP, Jansonius NM. Glaucoma monitoring in a clinical setting: glaucoma progression analysis vs nonparametric progression analysis in the Groningen longitudinal Glaucoma Study. *Arch Ophthalmol.* 2009;127:270-274.

Biodegradable collagen matrix implant *vs* mitomycin-C as an adjuvant in trabeculectomy: a 24-month, randomized clinical trial
Cillino S, Di Pace F, Cillino G, et al (Univ of Palermo, Italy)
Eye 25:1598 1606, 2011

Aim.—To verify the safety and efficacy of Ologen (OLO) implant as adjuvant compared with low-dosage mitomycin-C (MMC) in trabeculectomy. *Methods.*—This was a prospective randomized clinical trial with a 24-month follow-up. Forty glaucoma patients (40 eyes) were assigned to trabeculectomy with MMC or OLO. Primary outcome includes target IOP at ≤ 21, ≤ 17, and ≤ 15 mm Hg; complete (target IOP without medications), and qualified success (target IOP regardless of medications). Secondary outcomes include bleb evaluation, according to Moorfields Bleb Grading System (MBGS); spectral domain optical coherence tomography (SD-OCT) examination; number of glaucoma medications; and frequency of postoperative adjunctive procedures and complications. *Results.*—The mean preoperative IOP was 26.5 (± 5.2) in MMC and 27.3 (± 6.0) in OLO eyes, without statistical significance. One-day postoperatively, the IOP dropped to 5.2 (± 3.5) and 9.2 (± 5.5) mm Hg, respectively ($P=0.009$). The IOP reduction was significant at end point in all groups ($P = 0.01$), with a mean IOP of 16.0 (± 2.9) and 16.5 (± 2.1) mm Hg in MMC and OLO, respectively. The rates and Kaplan—Meier curves did not differ for both complete and qualified success at any target IOP. The bleb height in OLO group was higher than MMC one ($P < 0.05$). SD-OCT analysis of successful/unsuccessful bleb in patients with or without complete success at IOP ≤ 17 mm Hg indicated a sensitivity of 83% and 73% and a specificity of 75% and 67%, respectively, for MMC and OLO groups. No adverse reaction to OLO was noted.

TABLE 3.—Success Rates (%) at the 24-Month Follow-up Study End Point in the Surgical Groups at Three Target IOP Levels

	MMC Group	OLO Group	P[a]
≤21 mm Hg			
Complete success	14 (70%)	15 (75%)	1.0
Qualified success	17 (85%)	18 (90%)	1.0
≤17 mm Hg			
Complete success	12 (60%)	11 (55%)	1.0
Qualified success	15 (75%)	15 (75%)	1.0
≤15 mm Hg			
Complete success	8 (40%)	10 (50%)	0.751
Qualified success	12 (60%)	14 (70%)	0.741

Abbreviations: MMC, mitomycin-C; OLO, Ologen.
[a]Fisher's exact test.

Conclusions.—Our results suggest that OLO implant could be a new, safe, and effective alternative to MMC, with similar long-term success rate (Table 3).

▶ This study is a prospective randomized clinical trial undertaken at Palermo University to verify the safety and efficacy of Ologen, a biodegradable collagen matrix implant, as an adjuvant to trabeculectomy with low-dose mitomycin-C. Theoretically, when Ologen is placed over the sclera flap, conjunctival fibroblasts and myofibroblasts should be forced to grow through the Ologen pores and secrete connective tissue in the form of a loose matrix. This matrix would reduce scar formation and wound contraction. The device should completely degrade within 90 to 180 days. A pilot study of Ologen failed to show any intraocular pressure (IOP)—lowering advantage and indicated a tendency to more complications. However, a randomized study comparing Ologen and trabeculectomy with mitomycin-C showed lower complete success, but also a lower bleb-associated complication rate compared with Ologen.

Forty consecutive white patients were included in this study. All patients had IOPs greater than 21 mm Hg or progressive visual field loss on maximum-tolerated medical therapy. Combined cataract extraction and trabeculectomy procedures were excluded. IOP was the primary outcome measure with 3 different target levels: 21, 17, or 15 mm Hg. Secondary outcome measures included bleb evaluation (using Moorfields bleb grading system), number of glaucoma medications, and frequency of postoperative adjunctive procedures and complications. All procedures were performed by 1 surgeon using a superior rectus bridle suture and limbus-incision/fornix-based conjunctival flap. Scleral flaps were 3 by 3.5 mm in size. Mitomycin-C was applied using a Weck-cell sponge of standard size soaked with 0.2 mg/mL mitomycin-C and left surrounding the sclera flap and on the sclera bed for 2 minutes. Flaps were secured using 2 loose 10-0 nylon stitches (one at each corner of the flap) for mitomycin-C cases and 1 loose stitch for Ologen cases. A cylindrical Ologen implant, about 2 mm in height and 6 mm in diameter, was centered on the sclera flap. Postoperative steroid regimen was topical dexamethasone drops 0.1% 5 times per day for 1 week, then 3 times per day for 6 weeks, then 2 times per day for 1 week. A protocol for more aggressive steroid therapy was in place and initiated based on clinical impression of bleb vasculature. IOP-lowering therapy was added for IOP greater than 21 mm Hg after topical steroid withdrawal.

The mean IOP reduction was statistically significant in both groups. No significant intergroup difference was present at any scheduled postoperative observation time. The percentage of IOP reduction from baseline was about 40% in both groups. Success rates are summarized in Table 3. Bleb height was higher in the Ologen group. Bleb needling for encapsulated bleb was performed 1 to 4 times in about one-third of patients in each group.

This study indicates that there may be a role for Ologen as an adjunct to trabeculectomy. Longer follow-up in a larger group of patients analyzed prospectively will help identify whether Ologen offers any real potential benefits or drawbacks in comparison with the traditional approach of trabeculectomy augmented by mitomycin-C. The delicate balance between trying to achieve lower IOP targets while managing the risk of creating dangerously avascular thin blebs will continue to demand the attention of glaucoma surgeons as long as shunting aqueous flow beneath the conjunctiva is a common technique. Exploring adjuvants to trabeculectomy is necessary, but it has been fraught with failure. In recent years, antivascular endothelial growth factor agents have also been tried in conjunction with trabeculectomy. Unfortunately, no clearly superior alternative to mitomycin-C has emerged.

J. S. Myers, MD

4 Cornea

Increased Risk of a Cancer Diagnosis after Herpes Zoster Ophthalmicus:
A Nationwide Population-Based Study
Ho J-D, Xirasagar S, Lin H-C (Taipei Med Univ Hosp, Taiwan; Univ of South
Carolina, Columbia; Taipei Med Univ, Taiwan)
Ophthalmology 118:1076-1081, 2011

Purpose.—Herpes zoster has been associated with immune suppression, as has an increased risk of cancer. This population-based follow-up study aimed to investigate the risk of a subsequent cancer diagnosis after herpes zoster ophthalmicus (HZO).

Design.—A retrospective cohort study.

Participants and Controls.—Retrospective claims data from the Taiwan National Health Insurance Research Database were analyzed. The study cohort comprised all patients with a diagnosis of HZO (International Classification of Diseases, 9th Revision, Clinical Modification code 053.2) in 2003 and 2004 (n=658). The comparison cohort consisted of randomly selected ambulatory care patients, 8 for every patient with HZO (n=5264) matched with the study group on age, gender, monthly income, and urbanization level of the patient's residence.

Methods.—The Kaplan—Meier method was used to compute 1-year cancer-free survival rate. Stratified Cox proportional hazard regressions were carried out to compute the adjusted 1-year cancer-free survival rate after adjusting for potential confounding factors.

Main Outcome Measures.—Subsequent claims for all study and comparison patients were captured over a 1-year follow-up period from their index ambulatory care visit to identify whether the patient received a cancer diagnosis during the follow-up period.

Results.—During 1-year follow-up, cancer was diagnosed in 4.86% of patients with HZO and 0.53% of patients in the comparison cohort. Patients with HZO had significantly lower 1-year cancer-free survival rates than the comparison cohort. After adjusting for patient age, gender, monthly income, and urbanization level, patients with HZO were found to have a 9.25-fold (95% confidence interval, 5.51—15.55) risk of a subsequent cancer diagnosis than the matched comparison cohort. No significant differences in cancer type were observed between the 2 cohorts.

TABLE 2.—Hazard Ratios of Malignancy Among the Sample Patients During the 1-Year Follow-up Period from the Index Ambulatory Care Visit (n=5922)

Presence of Malignancy	Total Sample n=5922 No.	%	Comparison n=5264 No.	%	Herpes Zoster Ophthalmicus n=658 No.	%
1-yr follow-up period						
Yes	60	1.01	28	0.53	32	4.86
No	5862	98.99	5236	99.47	626	95.14
HR* (95% CI)	—		1.00		9.25† (5.51−15.55)	

CI = confidence interval; HR = hazard ratio.
*Stratified Cox proportional regression stratified on patient's age, gender, monthly income, and urbanization level.
†$P<0.001$.

Conclusions.—Herpes zoster ophthalmicus may be a marker of increased risk of being diagnosed with cancer in the following year (Table 2).

▶ Each week we see new patients with herpes zoster ophthalmicus (HZO) and are faced with the question, either in our own mind or from the patient, "why did this happen?" and "what follow-up or testing should I recommend to look for underlying medical issues or malignancy?" The data to date have been conflicting regarding the risk of a cancer diagnosis following the new onset of HZO. This is a very large study of claims-based data from Taiwan, assessing the risk of cancer in 1 year following the diagnosis of HZO, compared with age-matched controls. The authors identify more than 650 patients with zoster and utilize a comparison cohort of more than 5000 age-matched controls. During the 1-year follow-up, 4.86% of patients with HZO received a cancer diagnosis, compared with 0.53% of control patients. The risk of a cancer diagnosis was 9 times higher in the group with zoster. Interestingly, this was more so in women (14.49 in women vs 7.23 in men). The types of cancer discovered were also of note. A previous population-based study out of Denmark found a high rate of hematologic cancers. That was not found here. While there was no difference in the 2 groups, gastrointestinal cancer was the most commonly discovered. This may be indicative of the genetic predisposition of the Asian population studied, a group in which stomach and esophageal cancers are much more common. It would be very interesting to repeat this study in other parts of the world where universal access, single-payer system is present. For now, I will continue to recommend to patients to have all health screenings up-to-date and have in mind that perhaps 1 in 20 of them will be diagnosed with cancer in the next year.

K. M. Hammersmith, MD

**Longer-Term Vision Outcomes and Complications with the Boston Type 1
Keratoprosthesis at the University of California, Davis**
Greiner MA, Li JY, Mannis MJ (Univ of California at Davis, Sacramento)
Ophthalmology 118:1543-1550, 2011

Purpose.—To evaluate retention of visual acuity and development of
complications after Boston type 1 keratoprosthesis implantation over a
longer follow-up period than previously reported.
Design.—Cohort study.
Participants.—Forty eyes of 35 patients who underwent Boston type 1
keratoprosthesis surgery at the University of California, Davis, between
2004 and 2010.
Methods.—Preoperative, intraoperative, and postoperative parameters
were collected and analyzed.
Main Outcome Measures.—Best-corrected visual acuity (BCVA) and
postoperative complications.
Results.—Preoperative visual acuity ranged from 20/150 to light perception and was ≤20/400 in 38 eyes (95%). Preoperative diagnoses included
failed corneal transplants (19 eyes, 47.5%), chemical injury (10 eyes, 25%),
and aniridia (5 eyes, 12.5%). Mean follow-up duration was 33.6 months
(range, 5−72 months). Of 36 eyes followed for ≥1 year, 32 eyes (89%)
achieved postoperative BCVA ≥20/200. Of eyes that achieved BCVA ≥20/
200, at last follow-up, 19 of 32 eyes (59%) followed for ≥1 year retained
BCVA ≥20/200; 16 of 27 eyes (59%) followed for ≥2 years retained
BCVA ≥20/200; 7 of 14 eyes (50%) followed for ≥3 years retained BCVA
≥20/200; and 2 of 7 eyes (29%) followed for ≥4 years retained BCVA
≥20/200. End-stage glaucoma most commonly caused vision loss (7 of 13
eyes, 54%) when BCVA ≥20/200 was not retained (follow-up ≥1 year).
Glaucoma was newly diagnosed in 11 eyes (27.5%); progression was
noted in 9 eyes (22.5%). Glaucoma drainage device erosion occurred in 9
eyes (22.5%). Retroprosthetic membrane formed in 22 eyes (55%), 5 eyes
(12.5%) developed endophthalmitis, 6 eyes (15%) developed corneal melt,
7 eyes (17.5%) underwent keratoprosthesis replacement, and 23 eyes
(57.5%) required major surgery to treat postoperative complications. The
initial keratoprosthesis was retained in 32 eyes (80%).
Conclusions.—Keratoprosthesis implantation remains a viable option
for salvaging vision. A significant number of patients lost vision over the
postoperative course. Glaucoma and complications related to glaucoma
surgery are significant challenges to maintaining good vision after keratoprosthesis surgery. Our study highlights the need for long-term follow-up
and a team approach to management, and points to a more guarded long-
term visual prognosis after surgery (Fig 2).

▶ One of my mentors always likened corneal surgery to the highlight film at the
end of the Olympics: moments of incredible jubilation mixed with devastating
defeats. There is no place that description is more apt than in the discussion of
keratoprosthesis surgery. The Boston keratoprosthesis offers the ability to quickly

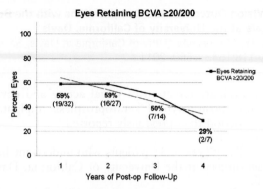

FIGURE 2.—Percentage of eyes that retained BCVA of 20/200 over time. After an initial plateau in the first and second postoperative years, a decreasing percentage of patients retain BCVA as the time from implantation increases. Progression to end-stage glaucoma was causal in the majority of cases. BCVA = best-corrected visual acuity. (Reprinted from Greiner MA, Li JY, Mannis MJ. Longer-term vision outcomes and complications with the Boston type 1 keratoprosthesis at the University of California, Davis. *Ophthalmology.* 2011;118:1543-1550, Copyright 2011, with permission from the American Academy of Ophthalmology.)

rehabilitate the patient's vision, usually very close to that eye's potential. This leads to those moments that we all hoped for as we entered ophthalmology, dramatic experiences of bringing someone out of blindness. However, as these patients now have increasingly longer follow-up, we find that later complications can destroy these early successes. This article describes such results, presenting visual results and complications with the Boston keratoprosthesis, with the mean follow-up of just under 3 years (33.6 months; range, 5-72 months). A retroprosthetic membrane was the most common complication (55%), but this is not usually sight threatening. The authors present that end-stage glaucoma was the most common cause of vision loss. They also describe 22.5% of patients with erosion around their glaucoma drainage device. We have seen this complication in increasing numbers over the past year, making the best management of these patients' glaucoma a continuing question. A disappointing 29% of patients followed up for more than 4 years retained vision better than 20/200 (Fig 2). The results presented here are, in the authors' own words, "sobering." Data such as these, and our own experience, reinforce our current practices when faced with the decision between repeat corneal transplant and keratoprosthesis. That is, whenever we feel that we can improve on prior attempts at corneal transplantation, we will favor repeating a traditional graft. We reserve keratoprosthesis surgery for those instances in which we don't feel that any modification of preoperative, postoperative, or intraoperative technique will result in a better outcome. We are thankful for the Boston keratoprosthesis but look forward to improvements in our ability to make this a longer-lasting outcome.

K. M. Hammersmith, MD

Split Cornea Transplantation for 2 Recipients – Review of the First 100 Consecutive Patients

Heindl LM, Riss S, Laaser K, et al (Friedrich-Alexander Univ Erlangen-Nürnberg, Germany)
Am J Ophthalmol 152:523-532, 2011

Purpose.—To evaluate the feasibility of split cornea transplantation for 2 recipients by combining deep anterior lamellar keratoplasty (DALK) and Descemet membrane endothelial keratoplasty (DMEK).

Design.—Interventional case series.

Methods.—Fifty consecutive eyes with anterior stromal disease suitable for DALK and 50 eyes with endothelial disease suitable for DMEK were scheduled for split cornea transplantation combining both procedures within 72 hours. Main outcome measures included success of using a single donor cornea for 2 recipients, best spectacle-corrected visual acuity (BSCVA), and complication rates within 6 months' follow-up.

Results.—A single donor cornea could be used for 2 recipients in 47 cases (94%). In 3 eyes (6%), the DALK procedure had to be converted to penetrating keratoplasty (PK) requiring a full-thickness corneal graft. Thereby, 47 donor corneas (47%) could be saved. Six months after surgery, mean BSCVA was 20/36 in the 47 eyes that underwent successful DALK, 20/50 in the 3 eyes that underwent conversion from DALK to PK, and 20/29 in the 50 eyes that underwent DMEK. Postoperative complications after DALK included Descemet folds in 5 eyes (11%) and epitheliopathy in 3 eyes (6%). After DMEK, partial graft detachment occurred in 26 eyes (52%) and was managed successfully with intracameral air reinjection. All corneas remained clear up to 6 months after surgery. No intraocular infections occurred.

Conclusion.—Split use of donor corneal tissue for combined DALK and DMEK procedures in 2 recipients within 3 subsequent days is a feasible approach to reduce donor shortage in corneal transplantation in the future.

▶ Availability of corneal tissue is a limiting factor in the treatment of corneal blindness around the world. During the transition to more lamellar corneal procedures in the last decade, the possibility that we can restore vision in 2 eyes from 1 cornea has been discussed. This article converts that possibility into a reality, following 50 corneas into nearly 100 eyes with excellent results. Descemet membrane endothelial keratoplasty still looks undesirable with a more than 50% rate of rebubbling. These procedures were performed more than 2 years ago, and the authors have published/presented additional data this year that show a significant reduction in the partial graft detachment. This is an encouraging article, especially in areas in which donor tissue is limited.

K. M. Hammersmith, MD

Herpes Zoster Ophthalmicus: Comparison of Disease in Patients 60 Years and Older Versus Younger than 60 Years
Ghaznawi N, Virdi A, Dayan A, et al (Thomas Jefferson Univ, Philadelphia, PA)
Ophthalmology 118:2242-2250, 2011

Objective.—To study the clinical course of herpes zoster ophthalmicus (HZO) and to compare the demographics, treatments, and outcomes in patients aged <60 years versus patients aged ≥60 years at the time of diagnosis.

Design.—Retrospective chart review of all 112 patients presenting for management of HZO from January 1, 2008 to December 31, 2008.

Participants.—A total of 112 patients (58 aged <60 years and 54 aged >60 years) at the time of HZO onset.

Interventions.—Anterior segment complications, treatments, and surgical procedures were documented at 3 months, 6 months, and 1 year, and then annually for the remainder of the follow-up period.

Main Outcome Measures.—Intraocular pressure, inflammation, steroid use, surgical procedures, anterior segment complications, post-herpetic neuralgia, and delayed herpes zoster pseudodendrites.

Results.—Equal numbers of patients were affected with HZO in the younger and older age groups (51.8%, n = 58 vs. 48.2%, n = 54, respectively, $P = 0.69$). The most common decade of HZO onset was between 50 and 59 years. Younger patients were more likely to be healthy compared with older patients ($P = 0.05$). Delayed herpes zoster pseudodendrites were more common in the younger patients (36.7% vs. 16.7%, $P = 0.03$). The mean number of flares per patient-years was significantly higher in the younger patients (z test, $P = 0.024$). Post-herpetic neuralgia, neurotrophic keratopathy, and secondary infectious keratitis were more frequent in the older patients ($P = 0.05$). Prevalence of corneal perforation, corneal thinning, cataract formation, and glaucoma was similar between the 2 groups. Most patients in both groups (84.2% of younger patients and 89.5% of older patients) were taking topical steroids 3 years after referral for HZO.

Conclusions.—Herpes zoster ophthalmicus affects individuals aged younger than and older than 60 years in similar numbers, with the most common decade of onset between age 50 and 59 years. Younger patients had more episodes of delayed pseudodendritiform keratitis and flares of inflammation compared with older patients, who had more problems related to neurotrophic keratopathy (Fig 1).

▶ The impetus for this study was the development of severe herpes zoster ophthalmicus (HZO) in one of the authors at the age of 58 years and the subsequent realization that many of our patients with chronic HZO were younger than 60 years, the recommended age for the varicella zoster vaccine. Thus, this study was undertaken to assess the age distribution in our practice of those with HZO and to compare the clinical characteristics and course in the 2 age groups. We found that half of the patients were younger than 60 years, with the most common decade of HZO onset between 50 and 60 years (Fig 1). Perhaps not

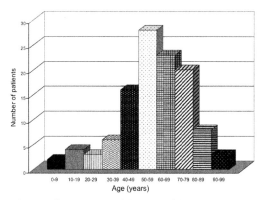

FIGURE 1.—Distribution of age at time of diagnosis of herpes zoster ophthalmicus by decade. (Reprinted from Ghaznawi N, Virdi A, Dayan A, et al, Herpes zoster ophthalmicus: comparison of disease in patients 60 years and older versus younger than 60 years. *Ophthalmology.* 2011;118:2242-2250, Copyright 2011, with permission from the American Academy of Ophthalmology.)

surprisingly, the younger patients were more likely to be healthy than the older patients. The mean number of flares per patient-years was statistically significantly higher in the younger group. Additionally, among those patients still followed up at 3 years, 85% of younger patients and 89.5% of older patients were still taking topical steroids. This signifies that this becomes a significant, chronic inflammatory condition in the younger as well as the older. Other studies have demonstrated that the vaccine response is actually more robust in the younger individuals. Certainly, a case is made to consider earlier vaccination, especially in those older than 50 years. The obstacles to this are availability of the vaccine and cost. Additionally, the primary caregivers' attitudes toward the vaccine, even in the approved age of greater than 60 years, are less than hoped for. We have added a question in our patient database about the use of the shingles vaccine. We have captured many patients in whom the vaccine is indicated and raised awareness within our own patients about the importance of vaccination. We look forward to more work in this area.

K. M. Hammersmith, MD

Randomized Comparison of Systemic Anti-Inflammatory Therapy Versus Fluocinolone Acetonide Implant for Intermediate, Posterior, and Panuveitis: The Multicenter Uveitis Steroid Treatment Trial

The Multicenter Uveitis Steroid Treatment (MUST) Trial Research Group (The Univ of Pennsylvania, Philadelphia, Univ of Wisconsin, Madison, Johns Hopkins Bloomberg School of Public Health, Baltimore, MD)
Ophthalmology 118:1916-1926, 2011

Objective.—To compare the relative effectiveness of systemic corticosteroids plus immunosuppression when indicated (systemic therapy) versus fluocinolone acetonide implant (implant therapy) for noninfectious intermediate, posterior, or panuveitis (uveitis).

Design.—Randomized controlled parallel superiority trial.

Participants.—Patients with active or recently active uveitis.

Methods.—Participants were randomized (allocation ratio 1:1) to systemic or implant therapy at 23 centers (3 countries). Implant-assigned participants with bilateral uveitis were assigned to have each eye that warranted study treatment implanted. Treatment-outcome associations were analyzed by assigned treatment for all eyes with uveitis.

Main Outcome Measures.—Masked examiners measured the primary outcome: change in best-corrected visual acuity from baseline. Secondary outcomes included patient-reported quality of life, ophthalmologist-graded uveitis activity, and local and systemic complications of uveitis or therapy. Reading Center graders and glaucoma specialists assessing ocular complications were masked. Participants, ophthalmologists, and coordinators were unmasked.

Results.—On evaluation of changes from baseline to 24 months among 255 patients randomized to implant and systemic therapy (479 eyes with uveitis), the implant and systemic therapy groups had an improvement in visual acuity of +6.0 and +3.2 letters ($P = 0.16$, 95% confidence interval on difference in improvement between groups, -1.2 to +6.7 letters, positive values favoring implant), an improvement in vision-related quality of life of +11.4 and +6.8 units ($P = 0.043$), a change in EuroQol-EQ5D health utility of +0.02 and -0.02 ($P = 0.060$), and residual active uveitis in 12% and 29% ($P = 0.001$), respectively. Over the 24 month period, implant-assigned eyes had a higher risk of cataract surgery (80%, hazard ratio [HR] = 3.3, $P < 0.0001$), treatment for elevated intraocular pressure (61%, HR = 4.2, $P < 0.0001$), and glaucoma (17%, HR = 4.2, $P = 0.0008$). Patients assigned to systemic therapy had more prescription-requiring infections than patients assigned to implant therapy (0.60 vs 0.36/person-year, $P = 0.034$), without notable long-term consequences; systemic adverse outcomes otherwise were unusual in both groups, with minimal differences between groups.

Conclusions.—In each treatment group, mean visual acuity improved over 24 months, with neither approach superior to a degree detectable with the study's power. Therefore, the specific advantages and disadvantages identified should dictate selection between the alternative treatments in consideration of individual patients' particular circumstances. Systemic therapy with aggressive use of corticosteroid-sparing immunosuppression was well tolerated, suggesting that this approach is reasonably safe for local and systemic inflammatory disorders (Table 4).

▶ This multicentered trial compares vision, vision-related quality of life, and complications in 2 groups treated for uveitis, 1 with the intravitreal fluocinolone acetonide implant and the other with systemic immunosuppression. The discussion of the exact immunosuppression is not included and was likely varied. The authors did discuss whether corticosteroids were initially used and other immunomodulators added when control was not met, when unable to taper to less than

TABLE 4.—Incidence of Ocular Complications of Uveitis or Its Treatment for the Two Treatment Groups, Among Eyes at Risk at Baseline*

	Implant Therapy		Systemic Therapy		Hazard Ratio	
	Number of Eyes at Risk	Cumulative % With Event by 2 Years (95% CI)‖	Number of Eyes at Risk	Cumulative % With Event by 2 Years (95% CI)	Implant/Systemic (95% CI)	P Value
IOP events						
IOP ≥30 mmHg	234	32.8 (27.1, 39.2)	229	6.3 (3.7, 10.3)	6.08 (3.32, 11.15)	<.0001
IOP ≥24 mmHg	234	53.1 (46.9, 59.7)	228	18.7 (14.2, 24.5)	3.59 (2.34, 5.50)	<.0001
IOP ≥10 mmHg increase from baseline	235	51.8 (45.5, 58.3)	230	15.5 (11.4, 20.9)	4.28 (2.78, 6.58)	<.0001
Glaucoma and IOP-lowering treatment						
Glaucoma	212	16.5 (12.1, 22.2)	202	4.0 (2.0, 7.8)	4.19 (1.82, 9.63)	0.0008
Use of any IOP-lowering therapy	201	61.1 (54.3, 67.8)	203	20.1 (15.1, 26.3)	4.16 (2.67, 6.47)	<.0001
IOP-lowering surgery	233	26.2 (21.0, 32.4)	226	3.7 (1.9, 7.2)	8.40 (3.39, 20.82)	<.0001
Cataract						
Incident cataract	54	90.7 (81.3, 96.6)	50	44.9 (32.3, 59.8)	4.12 (2.21, 7.67)	<.0001
Cataract surgery	140	80.4 (73.3, 86.6)	125	31.3 (23.9, 40.4)	3.33 (2.20, 5.04)	<.0001
Visual acuity worse than 20/40						
First visit with a reduced acuity	112	57.7 (48.2, 67.3)	117	35.6 (26.4, 44.8)	1.91 (1.26, 2.88)	0.0021
Reduced for two consecutive visits	112	31.2 (22.3, 40.1)	117	19.8 (12.2, 27.3)	1.68 (0.97, 2.90)	0.060
Visual acuity 20/200 or worse						
First visit with a reduced acuity	196	13.0 (8.2, 17.8)	193	9.9 (5.6, 14.1)	1.31 (0.68, 2.49)	0.41
Potential complications of implant surgery						
IOP >6 mmHg (hypotony)	228	8.4 (5.4, 12.8)	218	6.1 (3.6, 10.2)	1.46 (0.60, 3.54)	0.41
Vitreous hemorrhage	236	15.7 (11.6, 21.0)	230	4.9 (2.7, 8.6)	3.57 (1.60, 7.96)	0.0019
Endophthalmitis	237	1.3 (0.4, 4.0)	230	0	Not estimable	
Rhegmatogenous retinal detachment	236	2.1 (0.9, 5.0)	230	0.44 (0.1, 3.1)	4.91 (0.57, 42.56)	0.15
Implant extrusion	204	0	231	0	Not estimable	

Hazard ratios are adjusted for bilateral disease and uveitis stratum.
CI = confidence interval; IOP = intraocular pressure.
*Eyes with prevalent complications or missing data at enrollment were excluded from the risk set; the Table only assesses first events, not multiple events.

10 mg/day of prednisone, or in "specific high-risk uveitis syndromes." Both groups showed improvement in mean visual acuity, with neither significantly better. Control of overall inflammation was slightly better in the implant group at all times. However, the very high rate of ocular morbidity related to the implant cannot be minimized. Eighty percent of patients developed a need for cataract surgery, and 60% were treated for high intraocular pressure. Perhaps most concerning, 17% developed true glaucoma. The systemically treated patients fared much better in the eye but did have more infections requiring prescription than those with implants. Overall, the systemic therapy was well tolerated and appears victorious.

K. M. Hammersmith, MD

Corticosteroids for Bacterial Keratitis: The Steroids for Corneal Ulcers Trial (SCUT)
Srinivasan M, for the Steroids for Corneal Ulcers Trial Group (Aravind Eye Care System, Madurai, India; et al)
Arch Ophthalmol 130:143-150, 2012

Objective.—To determine whether there is a benefit in clinical outcomes with the use of topical corticosteroids as adjunctive therapy in the treatment of bacterial corneal ulcers.

Methods.—Randomized, placebo-controlled, double-masked, multi-center clinical trial comparing prednisolone sodium phosphate, 1.0%, to placebo as adjunctive therapy for the treatment of bacterial corneal ulcers. Eligible patients had a culture-positive bacterial corneal ulcer and received topical moxifloxacin for at least 48 hours before randomization.

Main Outcome Measures.—The primary outcome was best spectacle-corrected visual acuity (BSCVA) at 3 months from enrollment. Secondary outcomes included infiltrate/scar size, reepithelialization, and corneal perforation.

Results.—Between September 1, 2006, and February 22, 2010, 1769 patients were screened for the trial and 500 patients were enrolled. No significant difference was observed in the 3-month BSCVA (-0.009 logarithm of the minimum angle of resolution [logMAR]; 95% CI, -0.085 to 0.068; $P = .82$), infiltrate/scar size ($P = .40$), time to reepithelialization ($P = .44$), or corneal perforation ($P > .99$). A significant effect of corticosteroids was observed in subgroups of baseline BSCVA ($P = .03$) and ulcer location ($P = .04$). At 3 months, patients with vision of counting fingers or worse at baseline had 0.17 logMAR better visual acuity with corticosteroids (95% CI, -0.31 to -0.02; $P = .03$) compared with placebo, and patients with ulcers that were completely central at baseline had 0.20 logMAR better visual acuity with corticosteroids (-0.37 to -0.04; $P = .02$).

Conclusions.—We found no overall difference in 3-month BSCVA and no safety concerns with adjunctive corticosteroid therapy for bacterial corneal ulcers.

Application to Clinical Practice.—Adjunctive topical corticosteroid use does not improve 3-month vision in patients with bacterial corneal ulcers.

Trial Registration.—clinicaltrials.gov Identifier: NCT00324168.

▶ One of the most debated controversies in cornea and external disease—the use of topical steroids as adjunctive therapy—is assessed in this large, well-designed randomized controlled trial. The authors compare 500 patients with bacterial corneal ulcers, half of whom had prednisolone sodium phosphate added to their antibiotic regimen after 2 days of intensive therapy and the other half of whom had placebo. The authors found no overall difference in the 3-month best spectacle-corrected visual acuity and no safety concerns with adjunctive corticosteroid therapy. These findings are interesting but do little to distinguish the "correct" way to treat these patients. For those who are not "fans" of steroids, there is now evidence that the use of them is not necessary and will not result in better visual acuity. For those who use a heavier hand with steroids, there were no more perforations, only scant evidence of delayed epithelial healing, and really no significant adverse events to deter their use. So, a little finding for everyone. The most surprising finding was the fact that the largest ulcers with the worst presenting vision were actually the only group in whom steroid use was significantly beneficial. This has certainly affected our thought process as we approach these severe infections. The patients in the study are mostly from Aravind Eye Hospital in Madurai, India, where the etiology of bacterial keratitis was most commonly trauma and the pathogens distinct from our practice. In fact, only 8 of the 500 patients were contact lens wearers. The eyes seen there have significant infection, as is evidenced by the fact that nearly 25% of patients seen during the study period were not eligible for the study because of impending perforation. It is interesting to note that the steroid-treated group had a larger number of *Nocardia* patients, who fare poorly on steroids. If there had been fewer, or an equal number of *Nocardia* patients, perhaps steroid use would have been more beneficial. Thus, it is hard to extrapolate perfectly how these data should be used, but it certainly supports further study to help answer these questions.

K. M. Hammersmith, MD

Descemet's Stripping Endothelial Keratoplasty Under Failed Penetrating Keratoplasty: Visual Rehabilitation and Graft Survival Rate
Anshu A, Price MO, Price FW Jr (Cornea Res Foundation of America, Indianapolis, IN; Price Vision Group, Indianapolis, IN)
Ophthalmology 118:2155-2160, 2011

Purpose.—To evaluate graft survival, risk factors for failure, complications, and visual rehabilitation in patients who underwent Descemet's stripping endothelial keratoplasty (DSEK) under a failed penetrating keratoplasty (PK).
Design.—Retrospective interventional case series.
Participants.—Sixty eyes (60 patients) treated at Price Vision Group, Indianapolis, Indiana.
Methods.—Graft diameters ranged from 8 to 9 mm and were ~1 mm larger than the previous PK. The Descemet's membrane was not stripped

in the majority (54, 84%). The graft was inserted using forceps or a Busin funnel glide (Moria, Anthony, France). The probability of graft survival was calculated by Kaplan—Meier survival analysis.

Main Outcome Measures.—Graft survival, best-corrected visual acuity (BCVA), and complications.

Results.—The mean recipient age was 68 years (range, 17—95 years). Forty eyes had 1 previous failed PK, 14 eyes had 2 previous failed PKs, and 6 eyes had 3 previous failed PKs. Thirty-one eyes (52%) had preexisting glaucoma, and 16 eyes (27%) had prior glaucoma surgery (trabeculectomy in 4, shunt procedure in 12). Fifty-five grafts were performed for visual rehabilitation, and 5 grafts were performed for pain relief. Median follow-up was 2.3 years (range, 2 months to 6 years). Median preoperative BCVA was 1.23 logarithm of the minimum angle of resolution (logMAR) (range, 0.2—3, Snellen 20/340), and median postoperative visual improvement was 0.6 logMAR (6 lines), range −0.3 to +2.7. Four eyes had graft detachment (6.6%), 7 eyes (10.5%) had endothelial rejection, and 10 eyes (16.6%) had graft failure (primary failure in 2, secondary failure in 8). The overall secondary graft survival rates were 98%, 90%, 81%, and 74% at 1, 2, 3, and 4 years, respectively. Prior glaucoma shunt was the principal risk factor for graft failure. The graft survival rates were 100%, 96%, 96%, and 96% in eyes without a prior shunt versus 93%, 74%, 44%, and 22% with a prior shunt at 1, 2, 3, and 4 years, respectively (P=0.0005; relative risk = 20). Peripheral anterior synechiae (P=0.14), neovascularization (P=0.88), endothelial rejection (P=0.59), and number of prior PKs (P=0.13) were not independent risk factors for graft failure.

Conclusions.—Endothelial keratoplasty under a previous failed PK is a useful alternative to a repeat standard PK, particularly in eyes with an acceptable topography and refractive outcome before failure.

▶ Over its evolution of the past decade, Descemet's stripping endothelial keratoplasty (DSEK) has been shown to have clear advantages over penetrating keratoplasty (PK). The authors present exciting data regarding the results of DSEK after failed PK. They present the results of 60 patients who underwent DSEK following failed PK and noted good graft survival of 98%, 90%, 81%, and 74% at 1, 2, 3, and 4 years. They found previous glaucoma shunt was a main risk factor for failure and noted excellent survival rates (100% at 1 year, 96% at 4 years) in eyes without a previous tube. Eyes with previous tubes were noted to be 20 times more likely to fail, and prior glaucoma shunt surgery was the only statistically significant risk factor for failure. Known risk factors for PK failure, including peripheral anterior synechiae, corneal neovascularization, more than 1 previous PK, and preexisting glaucoma were not independent risk factors of failure in this study.

The authors described a few modifications of the DSEK procedure specifically for these cases. They noted oversizing endothelial grafts by 1 mm to ensure that the endothelial graft overlapped the PK graft-host junction and leaving recipient Descemet's membrane intact when possible. The larger graft ensured higher endothelial cell counts, and avoiding removal of Descemet's may decrease the risk of PK wound dehiscence. We have not adopted these modifications and remove endothelium as well as same size or undersize our endothelial graft because of concerns regarding endothelial graft fit at the graft-host junction; we have had good results overall.

These results are highly encouraging for DSEK after PK and should be considered in patients with reasonable topography and refraction before graft failure, especially those without previous tube shunts.

P. K. Nagra, MD

Comparison of Fibrin Glue versus Suture for Conjunctival Autografting in Pterygium Surgery: A Meta-Analysis
Pan H-W, Zhong J-X, Jing C-X (First Affiliated Hosp of Jinan Univ, Guangzhou, China; Jinan Univ, Guangzhou, Japan)
Ophthalmology 118:1049-1054, 2011

Purpose.—To evaluate the safety and clinical efficacy of fibrin glue in pterygium surgery with conjunctival autografting.

Design.—The use of fibrin glue has been introduced in the treatment of pterygium. However, its role versus traditional suturing is still a matter of debate. We performed a meta-analysis to compare the safety and clinical efficacy of fibrin glue with suture for conjunctival autograft attachment in pterygium surgery.

Participants.—A total of 342 participants with 366 eyes in 7 studies were analyzed.

Methods.—We searched Medline, EMBASE, Web of Science, Cochrane Central Register of Controlled Trials, and Google Scholar for relevant randomized controlled trials (RCTs).

Main Outcome Measures.—The methodological quality of all the included trials was assessed with the Jadad score. The meta-analysis was performed with the fixed-effects model for complication rate and recurrence rate, and random-effects model for operating time.

Results.—Fibrin glue was associated with a significantly decreased operating time (weighted mean difference -17.61 minutes, 95% confidence interval [CI], -26.03 to -9.18, $P < 0.0001$) and was more effective in reducing the recurrence rate (Peto odds ratio [OR] 0.33, 95% CI, 0.15-0.71, $P = 0.004$) compared with suture. There were no significant differences in the complication rate (Peto OR 1.82, 95% CI, 0.63-5.27, $P = 0.27$) between the 2 groups.

Conclusions.—Our meta-analysis supports the superiority of fibrin glue to suture in pterygium surgery with conjunctival autografting in that the use of fibrin glue can significantly reduce the recurrence rate without increasing the risk of complications. Ophthalmologists should consider the use of fibrin glue in pterygium surgery.

▶ With the evolution of new surgical methods and techniques, there is always a question of whether the latest modification truly adds any benefit to the procedure overall.

This meta-analysis involving 7 studies aimed at answering that question, comparing the efficacy and safety of sutures versus fibrin glue in pterygium surgery. Benefits of fibrin glue are widely known, including less discomfort, faster operating room time, and ease of use; this study assessed these issues to show a statistically significant advantage of fibrin glue over sutures. Longer operating room times were associated with sutures, and this was suggested to be associated with increased operating room costs (although comparison between the cost of the glue and sutures was not mentioned). Complication rates between the 2 techniques were similar, although graft dehiscence was noted more frequently in the fibrin glue group. All the complications in both groups, including dehiscences, hemorrhage, granuloma, and conjunctival cyst were managed successfully without visual acuity loss.

One of the most frustrating aspects of pterygium excision, for both surgeons and patients alike, is the risk of recurrence. This meta-analysis found that fibrin glue was associated with a significantly decreased risk of recurrence compared to sutures. This finding was felt to be related in part to fibrin glue's anti-inflammatory properties, compared with sutures pro-inflammatory properties.

The authors' recommended surgeons consider using fibrin glue over sutures, given its lower risk of recurrence, shorter operating times, and decreased patient discomfort compared with sutures. Although the safety profile of glue appears similar to sutures in this study, the authors acknowledged the risk, albeit low, of transmission of infectious disease, although no cases have yet been reported.

Overall, this study provides further compelling evidence of the benefit of fibrin glue and may change practices among surgeons.

P. K. Nagra, MD

Corneal Arcus is a Sign of Cardiovascular Disease, Even in Low-Risk Persons
Ang M, Wong W, Park J, et al (Singapore Eye Res Inst, Republic of Singapore; et al)
Am J Ophthalmol 152:864-871, 2011

Purpose.—To examine the association of corneal arcus to cardiovascular disease (CVD) in an adult, ethnic Indian population.

Design.—Population-based cross-sectional study.

Methods.—Population-based study of ethnic South Asian Indians 40 to 80 years of age in Singapore from June 2007 through March 2009. We obtained a 75.5% response rate (3397/4497). All participants underwent standardized interview and systemic and ocular examinations, followed by nonfasting blood sampling. Corneal arcus was detected using a standardized slit-lamp examination. The main outcome measure was CVD, defined from a self-reported history of previous myocardial infarction, angina, or stroke.

Results.—Corneal arcus, found in 1701 (50.1%) of 3397 participants, was associated with older age (odds ratio [OR], 3.07; 95% CI, 2.78 to 3.40; P < .001), male gender (OR, 2.17; 95% CI, 1.81 to 2.62; P < .001), higher levels of total cholesterol (OR, 1.14; 95% CI, 1.05 to 1.24; $P = .002$), hypertension (OR, 1.14; 95% CI, 1.05 to 1.24; $P = .013$), and cigarette smoking (OR, 1.59; 95% CI, 1.25 to 2.03; $P < .001$). Corneal arcus was associated with CVD (OR, 1.31; 95% CI, 1.02 to 1.7; $P = .0038$) independent of the above-named cardiovascular risk factors. Participants with low-risk Framingham scores were more likely to be associated with CVD if they had corneal arcus (men: OR, 2.02; 95% CI, 1.20 to 3.40; $P = .008$; women: OR, 2.78; 95% CI, 1.36 to 3.01; $P < .001$). Corneal arcus was associated with CVD independent of the Framingham score (men: Akaike information criterion, 1524.39 for Framingham Score and corneal arcus vs 1527.38 for Framingham Score alone; women: 1000.14 vs 1003.54, respectively).

Conclusions.—Corneal arcus is associated with CVD, independent of risk factors in ethnic Indian adults, even in those at low risk for vascular disease.

▶ In examination of the eye, there are a number of situations in which ocular findings may be harbingers of systemic disease. Corneal arcus, for example, is common and benign among elderly patients; in younger patients, however, it may be associated with familial hyperlipidemia or hypercholesterolemia.

The authors of this study performed a large population-based evaluation of the association of cardiovascular disease and arcus in an adult, ethnic Indian population. Based on interviews, systemic and ophthalmic examinations, and blood work, they found arcus was associated with older age, male gender, high cholesterol, hypertension, and cigarette smoking. In addition, they found arcus was an independent risk factor for cardiovascular disease. Further, they found that the presence of arcus, when added to a Framingham score, gave additional information regarding the risk of cardiovascular disease.

This study assessed cardiovascular risk in patients with arcus in a single ethnic population, Asian Indians living in Singapore. It is not clear how these findings may compare to other Asian or ethnic populations, and further studies are certainly warranted to see whether comparable results may be found.

Overall, the independent association of arcus with cardiovascular disease in the Asian Indian population is an important finding and may justify referral to internists or cardiologist for additional, and potentially lifesaving, evaluation and treatment.

P. K. Nagra, MD

Repeat Penetrating Corneal Transplantation in Patients with Keratoconus
Kelly T-L, Coster DJ, Williams KA (Flinders Univ, Adelaide, Australia)
Ophthalmology 118:1538-1542, 2011

Purpose.—To determine factors influencing penetrating corneal graft survival in patients receiving repeat grafts in the same eye after a failed first graft for keratoconus.

Design.—Large cohort study from a national register of corneal grafts, in which data were recorded prospectively and analyzed retrospectively. Follow-up extended to 23 years.

Participants.—Follow-up was available for 229 regrafts performed in 177 eyes of 173 patients. Regrafts were performed more than once in 16 eyes.

Methods.—Corneal graft survival was analyzed using Kaplan–Meier survival plots and Cox proportional hazards regression, clustered by patient.

Main Outcome Measures.—Graft survival.

Results.—Graft survival was significantly worse (*P*<0.001) for second (n = 176) and third or greater grafts (n = 20), compared with first grafts for keratoconus (n = 4871). Kaplan–Meier survivals at 1, 5, and 15 years postgrafting were 88%, 69%, and 46% for second grafts, and 65%, 49%, and 33% for third and subsequent grafts, respectively (*P*<0.001). Risk factors associated with graft failure of repeat grafts in multivariate analysis were the geographic location of surgery ("center"; *P* = 0.04), failure of the previous graft within 10 years of surgery (*P* = 0.02), recipient age at graft ≥60 years (*P* = 0.04), occurrence of rejection episodes (*P* = 0.007), and corneal neovascularization postoperatively (*P* = 0.007).

TABLE 2.—Multivariate Risk Factors for Graft Failure in Regrafts after a First Penetrating Graft Performed for Keratoconus—Final Cox Model (n = 191)

Risk Factor	Hazard Ratio (95% CI)*	*P* Value
Geographic location		0.04
Center 1	1.0	
Center 2	0.86 (0.09, 8.62)	
Center 3	4.17 (1.16, 15.0)	
Center 4	5.84 (1.59, 21.5)	
Center 5	5.42 (1.40, 21.0)	
Survival time of previous graft, yrs		0.02
<10	1.0	
≥10	0.25 (0.08, 0.78)	
Rejection episodes in repeat graft		0.007
None	1.0	
≥1	2.12 (1.23, 3.66)	
Vascularization postgrafting		0.007
No	1.0	
Yes	2.86 (1.33, 6.18)	
Recipient age at grafting, yrs		0.04
<60	1.0	
≥60	1.87 (1.02, 3.43)	
Variables examined but removed from the final Cox model		
Reason for failure of previous graft		
Reasons 1–4†	0.36 (0.04, 3.00) to 1.09 (0.53, 2.24)	0.81
Occurrence rejection in previous graft	1.56 (0.55, 4.47)	0.41
Each additional previous graft	1.07 (0.45, 2.54)	0.88
Vascularization at grafting	1.22 (0.61, 2.44)	0.57
Inflammation at grafting	1.55 (0.85, 2.83)	0.15

CI = % confidence interval.
*Global *P* values reported for risk factors with multiple categories.
†Including endothelial cell failure, unspecified graft failure, astigmatism, and other specified reason.

Conclusions.—Repeat corneal grafts in eyes originally grafted for keratoconus showed better survival when the previous graft had survived ≥10 years, surgery was performed at a favorable location, the recipient was <60 years old at grafting, and graft rejection and neovascularization were circumvented (Table 2).

▶ Keratoconus patients are known to have a high success rate following corneal transplantation, which is important because this is a common indication for corneal transplantation, as well as a condition affecting younger, otherwise healthy patients with decades of life ahead of them. Inevitably, however, we do see patients with a history of keratoconus requiring repeat corneal grafting, which makes the results of this study important and applicable to most corneal surgeons' practices.

As detailed in Table 2, the authors found several significant variables increasing the risk of failure in regrafts, specifically graft survival of initial transplant less than 10 years, rejection, vascularization, and patient age. Interestingly, the authors noted that 14% of the regrafts were for primary graft failure, which seems high and perhaps not comparable to our practice in the United States; these patients were excluded from the study. In addition, a difference in graft survival based on center location of the graft was also noted, which again, may or may not be translatable to experiences outside Australia.

Although the authors recognized the weaknesses of their retrospective study, they demonstrated the importance of inflammation as a major risk factor for failure of repeat grafts in patients with a history of keratoconus. As they stated, initial transplant survival in keratoconus "was not indefinite," and we all encounter the need to regraft these patients. The results of this study may help in understanding which patients have a higher risk of failure in regrafts, which can aid in our counseling of these patients preoperatively and alter our postoperative treatment regimen.

P. K. Nagra, MD

Clinical outcomes and prognostic factors associated with acanthamoeba keratitis
Chew HF, Yildiz EH, Hammersmith KM, et al (Thomas Jefferson Univ, Philadelphia, PA)
Cornea 30:435-441, 2011

Purpose.—To describe the clinical characteristics, time of presentation, risk factors, treatment, outcomes, and prognostic factors on a recent series of Acanthamoeba keratitis (AK) treated at our institution.

Methods.—Retrospective case series of 59 patients diagnosed with AK from January 1, 2004 to December 31, 2008. Of these 59 patients, 51 had complete follow-up data and were analyzed using univariate and multivariate logistic regression analyses performed with "failure" defined as requiring a penetrating keratoplasty (PKP) and/or having (1) best-corrected visual acuity (BCVA) <20/100 or (2) BCVA <20/25 at the last follow-up. A single multivariate model incorporating age, sex, steroid use before diagnosis, time to diagnosis, initial visual acuity (VA), stromal involvement, and diagnostic method was performed.

Results.—Symptom onset was greatest in the summer and lowest in the winter. With failure defined as requiring PKP and/or final BCVA <20/100, univariate analysis suggests that age >50 years, female sex, initial VA <20/50, stromal involvement, and patients with a confirmed tissue diagnosis had a significant risk for failure; however, none of these variables were significant using multivariate analysis. Univariate analysis, with failure defined as requiring PKP and/or final BCVA <20/25, showed stromal involvement and initial VA <20/50 were significant for failure-only initial VA <20/50 was significant using multivariate analysis.

Conclusions.—Symptom onset for AK is greatest in the summer. Patients with confirmed tissue diagnosis and female patients may have a higher risk for failure, but a larger prospective population-based study is required to confirm this. Failure is likely associated with patients who present with stromal involvement and patients presenting with an initial BCVA worse than 20/50.

▶ Over the last decade, we have seen an increase in Acanthamoeba keratitis in our clinics. However, as it remains an uncommon diagnosis, our understanding of risk factors and management has been slower to progress. This study details characteristics associated with this infection. The authors present 51 patients with this condition who they treated (59 patients were diagnosed with acanthamoeba during the 4-year period, 8 of whom did not have complete follow-up). They found symptom onset was greatest during the summer, and certain risk factors were associated with a poorer outcome (20/200 or worse final visual acuity [VA] or requiring penetrating keratoplasty) such as older age (> 50 years), female sex, confirmed tissue diagnosis, initial VA worse than 20/50, and stromal involvement, although these factors were significant on univariate analysis only, not multivariate. Initial VA worse than 20/50 was significant on multivariate analysis when the definition for failure was changed to final VA worse than 20/25 or requiring corneal transplantation. The authors also identified complications, noting that uveitic glaucoma occurred in 20% of patients, superinfection in 16%, and rapid cataract formation in 24%. As the authors acknowledge, a definite weakness of this article was using final VA as an endpoint, with variable posttreatment time periods.

Given the apparent increase in Acanthamoeba keratitis (Fig 1 in the original article illustrates the increase noted at Wills Eye Institute over a 13-year period), this article helps increase our understanding of this condition and potential prognostic risk factors for treatment failure or success.

P. K. Nagra, MD

Corneal collagen crosslinking for keratoconus and corneal ectasia: One-year results
Hersh PS, Greenstein SA, Fry KL (Cornea and Laser Eye Inst—Hersh Vision Group, Teaneck, NJ)
J Cataract Refract Surg 37:149-160, 2011

Purpose.—To evaluate 1-year outcomes of corneal collagen crosslinking (CXL) for treatment of keratoconus and corneal ectasia.
Setting.—Cornea and refractive surgery subspecialty practice.
Design.—Prospective randomized controlled clinical trial.
Methods.—Collagen crosslinking was performed in eyes with keratoconus or ectasia. The treatment group received standard CXL and the sham control group received riboflavin alone. Principal outcomes included uncorrected (UDVA) and corrected (CDVA) distance visual acuities, refraction, astigmatism, and topography-derived outcomes of maximum and average keratometry (K) value.
Results.—The UDVA improved significantly from 0.84 logMAR ± 0.34 (SD) (20/137) to 0.77 ± 0.37 logMAR (20/117) ($P = .04$) and the CDVA, from 0.35 ± 0.24 logMAR (20/45) to 0.23 ± 0.21 logMAR (20/34) ($P<.001$). Fifteen patients (21.1%) gained and 1 patient lost (1.4%) 2 or more Snellen lines of CDVA. The maximum K value decreased from baseline by 1.7 ± 3.9 diopters (D) ($P<.001$), 2.0 ± 4.4 D ($P = .002$), and 1.0 ± 2.5 D ($P = .08$) in the entire cohort, keratoconus subgroup, and ectasia subgroup, respectively. The maximum K value decreased by 2.0 D or more in 22 patients (31.0%) and increased by 2.0 D or more in 3 patients (4.2%).
Conclusions.—Collagen crosslinking was effective in improving UDVA, CDVA, the maximum K value, and the average K value. Keratoconus patients had more improvement in topographic measurements than patients with ectasia. Both CDVA and maximum K value worsened between baseline and 1 month, followed by improvement between 1, 3, and 6 months and stabilization thereafter.

▶ Collagen crosslinking has become an important treatment for early keratoconus throughout most of the world. However, while US Food and Drug Administration (FDA) approval is pending in the United States (although Avedro did receive FDA approval for its riboflavin drop, VibeX, in September 2011, approval for the ultraviolet A light source is still pending), most of us in this country have been limited to reading studies by our European, Canadian, and Asian counterparts for understanding the role of this treatment.

In this study, Hersh and his colleagues present the results of their arm of the prospective, multicenter FDA-guided trial looking at crosslinking in the treatment of keratoconus and ectasia in this country. They had a total of 71 eyes (49 keratoconus and 22 post—laser-assisted in situ keratomileusis [LASIK]ectasia), and noted a mean improvement in uncorrected visual acuity of 1 Snellen line in 1 year, with 21.1% of patients gaining more than 2 Snellen lines, and 1.4% losing 2 Snellen line best-corrected distance acuity (this 1 patient with loss of vision had post-LASIK ectasia, the etiology of visual loss was not clear). Regarding topography, maximum keratometry readings decreased by 1.7 diopters (D) (2.0 D in the keratoconus patients and 1.0 D in ectasia patients). The results suggested that keratoconus patients may have a better response compared with ectasia patients, which they hypothesize may be related to issues associated with the LASIK flap or pathophysiologic differences between keratoconus and post-LASIK ectasia.

This study supports much of the data already published looking at collagen crosslinking for keratoconus. A small improvement in visual acuity, keratometry readings may be noted, and perhaps more importantly, stability in the cornea over time. As the authors suggest, further studies would be helpful to distinguish efficacy of this treatment between keratoconus and post-LASIK ectasia. In addition, as our experience with this procedure grows, further defining patient criteria for enrollment (ie, less steep keratometry values, early diagnosis, defined criteria for progression), may aid in further stratification of those who may have the best response to this treatment.

P. K. Nagra, MD

Factors Influencing Outcomes of the Treatment of Allograft Corneal Rejection

Perera C, Jhanji V, Vajpayee RB (Monash Univ, Melbourne, Australia; The Chinese Univ of Hong Kong; Univ of Melbourne, East Melbourne, Australia)
Am J Ophthalmol 152:358-363, 2011

Purpose.—To identify patient characteristics influencing treatment outcomes of allograft corneal rejection.

Design.—Retrospective case file review.

Methods.—Files containing details of first episode of corneal allograft rejections in patients who underwent penetrating keratoplasty at the Royal Victorian Eye and Ear Hospital, Melbourne, Australia from 1991 to 2006 were reviewed. Cases were divided into 2 groups based on the response to treatment for graft rejection: treatment responders and failures. Main parameters evaluated were demographic characteristics, preoperative clinical profile, donor characteristics, surgical technique, presentation, and treatment of rejection episode.

Results.—A total of 235 cases of graft rejection were identified, of which 195 cases (83%) were successfully treated and 40 (17%) failed to respond. Age ($P = .08$) and gender ($P = .61$) were comparable in both groups. On univariate analysis, primary diagnosis of keratoconus ($P = .04$) and phakic lens status at the time of surgery ($P = .02$) were more common in treatment responders whereas aphakic bullous keratopathy ($P \leq .01$), history of glaucoma ($P < .01$), aphakia ($P < .01$), and previous grafts ($P < .01$) were more common among treatment failures. Multivariate analysis revealed that preoperative corneal neovascularization (adjusted odds ratio [aOR] 3.6, 95% CI: 1.3-9.7, $P = .01$), a larger (>9 mm) donor size (aOR 5.7, 95% CI: 1.3-24.9, $P = .02$), and corneal edema at presentation (aOR 4.7, 95%

TABLE 1.—Preoperative Clinical Characteristics of Patients With Corneal Allograft Rejection in Treatment Responder and Treatment Failure Groups

	All (n=235)	Treatment Responders (n=195)	Treatment Failures (n=40)	P Value
Gender				
Male	55%	57%	53%	.61
Female	45%	43%	47%	
Age (years)				
(Mean ± SD)	60 ± 19	60 ± 19	64 ± 22	.08
Indication for graft				
PBK	32%	30%	38%	.46
Keratoconus	19%	21%	8%	**.04**
Corneal ydstrophy	17%	19%	13%	.49
Herpetic keratitis	13%	13%	12%	1.0
Postinfectious keratitis scar	6%	7%	5%	1.0
Post-traumatic scar	6%	5%	7%	.71
ABK	6%	4%	17%	**<.01**
Other	1%	1%	0%	1.0
Previous grafts				
None	83%	85%	73%	**<.01**
1	10%	9%	12%	
2	4%	4%	5%	
3 or more	3%	2%	10%	
Past ocular history				
Glaucoma	19%	15%	38%	**<.01**
HSV	10%	10%	10%	1.0
Diabetes	8%	8%	5%	.75
Prior retinal surgery	6%	5%	13%	.07
Lens status				
Phakic	52%	56%	35%	**.02**
Pseudophakic	38%	38%	40%	.86
Aphakic	10%	6%	25%	**<.01**
Presence of preoperative clinical signs				
Corneal edema	64%	76%	62%	.07
Corneal neovascularization				
−0 quadrant	75%	81%	47%	**<.01**
−1 quadrant	6%	6%	8%	
−≥2 quadrants	19%	13%	45%	
Intraocular pressure mm Hg (mean ± SD)	15 ± 5	15 ± 5	16 ± 5	.50

ABK = aphakic bullous keratopathy; HSV = herpes simplex virus; PBK = pseudophakic bullous keratopathy; SD = standard deviation.
Bold font indicates statistically significant P values (<.05).

CI: 1.7-13.2, $P < .01$), were independently associated with failure of treatment of graft rejection.

Conclusions.—Treatment failure in cases of corneal allograft rejection is more likely to occur among patients with corneal neovascularization, large donor graft buttons, and corneal edema at presentation (Table 1).

▶ The onset of allograft corneal rejection remains a source of weakness in our management of patients following corneal transplantation. This study thoroughly reviewed characteristics separating treatment responders and failures in graft rejection. Overall, among the 235 cases of rejection identified, 83% were noted to respond to treatment successfully, while 17% were treatment failures.

As shown in Table 1, the authors found that patients with keratoconus were more likely to respond to treatment, whereas aphakia, glaucoma, previous grafts, and corneal neovascularization were associated with failure. The study also showed that graft size larger than 9 mm and corneal edema on presentation were also associated with an increased risk of graft failure.

Given the retrospective nature of the study, one major limitation was that there was no standardized treatment. In fact, the results suggested that the use of fluorometholone acetate drops was associated with decreased graft failure; most likely, those patients treated with fluorometholone had more mild forms of rejection (SEIs vs endothelial rejection with corneal edema) and therefore were more likely to respond. Another major limitation of this retrospective study was the authors' inability to quantify the length of time between onset of symptoms and presentation because of inconsistent notations in medical records; these data would be very interesting, specifically to see how strong a correlation there is between delayed presentation and failure.

In general, the authors present a very useful study in which they identify risks associated with an increased risk of graft failure. As these data suggest, certain patient characteristics are high risks for failure to treatment of allograft rejection; perhaps more aggressive treatment with close follow-up may be warranted for high-risk patients.

P. K. Nagra, MD

Antibiotic Resistance in Microbial Keratitis: Ten-Year Experience of Corneal Scrapes in the United Kingdom
Shalchi Z, Gurbaxani A, Baker M, et al (William Harvey Hosp, Ashford, Kent, UK)
Ophthalmology 118:2161-2165, 2011

Purpose.—To determine the scale of antibiotic resistance in microbial keratitis in East Kent, United Kingdom.

Design.—Retrospective, observational case series.

Participants.—Corneal scrapes over a 10-year period to December 2008 were identified using the local microbiology database, which provided culture results and antibiotic sensitivity-resistance profiles.

Testing.—Isolate sensitivity to chloramphenicol, cefuroxime, gentamicin, and ciprofloxacin was determined by microdilution using the Microscan System (Siemens Diagnostics, Dearfield, IL).

Main Outcome Measures.—Isolates were graded as sensitive, intermediate, or resistant to the tested antibiotics, with minimal inhibitory concentrations interpreted against breakpoints from the Clinical and Laboratory Standards Institute.

Results.—There were 476 scrapes from 440 patients (female, 57.6%; mean age, 53.5 years). All samples were cultured. Culture was positive in 163 samples (34.2%), growing 172 organisms. Bacterial keratitis accounted for 162 isolates (94.2%), of which 99 (61.1%) were gram-negative. There was a general increase in the number of gram-negative isolates with time

(P=0.003). In vitro testing showed widespread gram-negative resistance to chloramphenicol (74.1%), with reducing sensitivity over the study period (P=0.004). There was 97.3% sensitivity to combination gentamicin and cefuroxime, and 94.4% sensitivity to ciprofloxacin. Ciprofloxacin resistance was found in 8 (17.0%) of 47 gram-positive isolates tested, with no trend toward increasing resistance.

Conclusions.—This study has documented the highest levels of gram-negative keratitis in any open retrospective survey to date and highlights a trend of increasing gram-negative infection. We have demonstrated reducing chloramphenicol sensitivity, with high sensitivity to combination gentamicin and cefuroxime, as well as ciprofloxacin. Gram-positive fluoroquinolone resistance was higher than previously reported in the United Kingdom, but showed no evidence of increasing resistance. Second-generation fluoroquinolone monotherapy remains the recommended empirical treatment in microbial keratitis in the United Kingdom, and a change to fourth-generation compounds is not advised. Continued testing is essential to monitor for increasing resistance (Table 1).

▶ In the Cornea Service at Wills Eye Institute, we see several corneal ulcers on a weekly basis. Many of these ulcers are cultured and started empirically on broad-spectrum fortified antibiotics, typically when the ulcers are large, central, and suspicious for and/or have a history of treatment failure on monotherapy. Fourth-generation fluoroquinolone may be instituted if these ulcers are smaller and peripheral in location; rarely do we start patients on second-generation fluoroquinolones empirically, as may be common practice in the United Kingdom.

I read with great interest this article regarding antibiotic resistance in the United Kingdom. The authors noted that 476 cultures were performed over a 10-year period, of which 163 samples were positive (34.2%). As Table 1 illustrates, the authors found that a majority of these culture-positive results were gram-negative isolates (61.1%), and they noted this trend appeared to be increasing. *Pseudomonas aeruginosa* was the most common organism, identified in 49.4% of positive

TABLE 1.—Bacterial Keratitis by Gram-Positive and Gram-Negative Species

	No. of Positive Cultures	% of Total Bacterial Organisms
Gram-positive isolates	63	38.9
Staphylococcus aureus	24	14.8
Coagulase-negative *Staphylococcus*	13	8.0
Streptococcus pneumoniae	9	5.6
Propionibacterium acnes	3	1.9
Bacillus spp.	3	1.9
Other	11	6.8
Gram-negative isolates	99	61.1
Pseudomonas aeruginosa	80	49.4
Serratia spp.	5	3.1
Klebsiella oxytoca	3	1.9
Moraxella spp.	3	1.9
Enterobacter spp.	2	1.2
Other	6	3.7
Total	162	100

scrapings. Gentamicin has a low resistance rate of 2.2%, with 3 resistant *Staphylococcus* organisms. Cefuroxime, on the other hand, had a high gram-negative resistance rate (94.6%) with moderate gram-positive resistance (25.6%). Ciprofloxacin also had a low resistance rate of 5.6%, all 8 of which were *Staphylococcus* infections (5 were methicillin-resistant *Staphylococcus aureus*).

Based on these findings, the patient population amongst these patients with keratitis was likely skewed toward contact lens wearers with fewer trauma cases, perhaps more similar to a suburban private practice than an urban tertiary eye care center. Because of occasional difficulty obtaining fortified antibiotics and ease of monotherapy, it is encouraging to know that most organisms were sensitive to ciprofloxacin. However, as fourth-generation fluoroquinolones are more commonly used as monotherapy in the United States with differing resistance patterns noted, how these results translate to our US experience is questionable. There are other limitations of this article, including small sample size and low culture yield (34.2%). However, the trend toward increasing gram-negative infections was noteworthy, and I look forward to additional data confirming or rejecting this apparent trend.

P. K. Nagra, MD

Clinical and Microbiological Characteristics of Fungal Keratitis in the United States, 2001–2007: A Multicenter Study

Keay LJ, Gower EW, Iovieno A, et al (Univ of Sydney, Australia; Johns Hopkins Univ, Baltimore, MD; CIR Laboratory of Ophthalmology, Rome, Italy; et al)
Ophthalmology 118:920-926, 2011

Objective.—To study the epidemiology, clinical observations, and microbiologic characteristics of fungal keratitis at tertiary eye care centers in the United States.

Design.—Retrospective multicenter case series.

Participants.—Fungal keratitis cases presenting to participating tertiary eye care centers.

Methods.—Charts were reviewed for all fungal keratitis cases confirmed by culture, histology, or confocal microscopy between January 1, 2001, and December 31, 2007, at 11 tertiary clinical sites in the United States.

Main Outcome Measures.—Frequency of potential predisposing factors and associations between these factors and fungal species.

Results.—A total of 733 cases of fungal keratitis were identified. Most cases were confirmed by culture from corneal scraping (n = 693) or biopsies (n = 19); 16 cases were diagnosed by microscopic examination of corneal scraping alone; and 5 cases were diagnosed by confocal microscopy alone. Some 268 of 733 cases (37%) were associated with refractive contact lens wear, 180 of 733 cases (25%) were associated with ocular trauma, and 209 of 733 cases (29%) were associated with ocular surface disease. No predisposing factor was identified in 76 cases (10%). Filamentous fungi were identified in 141 of 180 ocular trauma cases (78%) and in 231 of 268 refractive contact lens-associated cases (86%). Yeast was the causative organism

TABLE 1.—Patient Demographics and Rate of Surgical Intervention by Primary Presenting Factor

	Refractive Contact Lens Wear*	Ocular Trauma†	Ocular Surface Disease‡	No Identified Risk Factor at Presentation
Total cases	268	180	209	76
Age (mean ± SD)	38.9±16.5	46.2±16.5	60.3±18.5	49.8±19.8
Female No. (%)	169 (63.1)	40 (22.2)	106 (50.7)	28 (36.8)
Multiple risk factors No. (%)	41 (15.3)	13 (7.2)	72 (34.4)	0 (0)
Surgical intervention required No. (%)	45 (16.8)	33 (18.3)	93 (44.4)	21 (27.6)

SD = standard deviation.
*Limited to patients in whom contact lenses were used for correction of simple refractive error.
†Corneal foreign body injury or major ocular trauma.
‡Includes therapeutic contact lens wearers, postsurgical cases, chronic steroid or antibiotic use and ocular surface disease, or systemic disease.

in 111 of 209 cases (53%) associated with ocular surface disease. Yeast accounted for few cases of fungal keratitis associated with refractive contact-lens wear (20 cases), therapeutic contact-lens wear (11 cases), or ocular trauma (21 cases). Surgical intervention was undertaken in 26% of cases and was most frequently performed for fungal keratitis associated with ocular surface disease (44%). Surgical intervention was more likely in cases associated with filamentous fungi ($P = 0.03$). Among contact lens wearers, delay in diagnosis of 2 or more weeks increased the likelihood of surgery (age-adjusted odds ratio = 2.2; 95% confidence interval, 1.2–4.2).

Conclusions.—Trauma, contact lens wear, and ocular surface disease predispose patients to developing fungal keratitis. Filamentous fungi are most frequently the causative organism for fungal keratitis associated with trauma or contact lens wear, whereas yeast is most frequently the causative organism in patients with ocular surface disease. Delay in diagnosis increases the likelihood of surgical intervention for contact lens-associated fungal keratitis (Table 1).

▶ Fungal keratitis is one of the more challenging infections to manage, from initial diagnosis through final treatment and visual rehabilitation. This large, multicenter study provides an overview of the epidemiology of fungal keratitis in the United States. Unlike many studies assessing the epidemiology coming from tropical developing countries where the most common risk factor for fungal keratitis is ocular trauma, the authors of this study noted refractive contact lens wear was the predominant risk factor, found in 37% of patients compared with 25% of cases associated with ocular trauma. As Table 1 displays, female age was more commonly associated with refractive contact lens-related ulcers, patients with ocular trauma were predominantly men, and patients with ocular surface disease were older (although this was not statistically significant) and more likely to require surgical intervention. Yeast was the most common organism following corneal transplantation and in cases associated with ocular surface disease, whereas filamentous fungi were more common in refractive contact lens cases and ocular trauma. As has been previously noted, this study also confirmed the preponderance of fungal infections, especially filamentous fungi, in warmer climates, particularly outside the period of ulcers related to exposure to ReNu MoistureLoc.

The study provides noteworthy details regarding the epidemiology of fungal keratitis. I look forward to additional studies by these authors, especially one assessing antifungal treatments and specific surgical interventions.

P. K. Nagra, MD

5 Retina

Safety of Vitrectomy for Floaters
Tan HS, Mura M, Lesnik Oberstein SY, et al (Univ of Amsterdam, The Netherlands)
Am J Ophthalmol 151:995-998, 2011

Purpose.—To assess the risks of vitrectomy for the removal of primary and secondary vitreous opacities.

Design.—Retrospective, nonrandomized, interventional case series.

Methods.—We reviewed the results of 116 consecutive cases of vitrectomy for vitreous floaters. Eighty-six cases were primary and 30 cases were secondary floaters. Main outcome measures were the incidence of iatrogenic retinal breaks and postoperative rhegmatogenous retinal detachments.

Results.—We found iatrogenic retinal breaks in 16.4% of operations. There was no statistically significant difference in risk between cases of primary and secondary floaters. Intraoperative posterior vitreous detachment induction was found to increase significantly the risk of breaks. Retinal detachment occurred in 3 cases (2.5%), all after operations for primary floaters. One case of complicated retinal detachment ended with a low visual acuity of hand movements. Cataract occurred in 50% of phakic cases. Transient postoperative hypotony was found after 5.2% of our operations, and transient postoperative high intraocular pressure was encountered in 7.8%. An intraoperative choroidal hemorrhage occurred in 1 case, which resolved spontaneously. The mean visual acuity improved from 0.20 to 0.13 logarithm of the minimal angle of resolution units.

Conclusions.—The risk profile of vitrectomy for floaters is comparable with that of vitrectomy for other elective indications. Retinal breaks are a common finding during surgery and treatment of these breaks is crucial for the prevention of postoperative retinal detachment. Patients considering surgery for floaters should be informed specifically about the risks involved.

▶ Although floaters are an extremely common and generally minor nuisance rather than significant visual problem for most patients, there is a small subset of patients who are extremely disturbed by vitreous opacities. For these individuals, there is a strong desire for relief, even though the Snellen measurement may be 20/20. With refinements in vitrectomy techniques, visual results are more predictable, and complication rates have been reduced. This retrospective study found very high patient satisfaction after vitrectomy. Most patients had no other predisposing pathology, although a few had prior inflammation or retinal detachment.

Despite the favorable results for the large majority, side effects and complications must be emphasized before elective surgery. The authors report a cataract progression rate of 50%, but with longer follow-up, it is likely that this number will be much higher. The retinal detachment rate of 2% to 3% with permanent severe vision loss in 1 patient despite appropriate measures to prevent this worrisome result is the critical factor to bear in mind. Furthermore, although there were no cases of endophthalmitis or severe hemorrhage, with enough cases, these complications will inevitably occur as well. Vitrectomy for floaters can be a highly beneficial treatment for a severely affected patient, but case selection and informed consent are critical aspects of management.

J. F. Vander, MD

Vitreoretinal Interface and Foveal Deformation in Asymptomatic Fellow Eyes of Patients with Unilateral Macular Holes

Kumagai K, Hangai M, Larson E, et al (Shinjo Ophthalmologic Inst, Miyazaki, Japan; Kyoto Univ, Japan; Miyazaki Prefectural Nursing Univ, Japan)
Ophthalmology 118:1638-1644, 2011

Purpose.—To compare the vitreoretinal interface of the asymptomatic fellow eyes of patients with unilateral macular holes (MHs) with that of the asymptomatic fellow eyes of patients with other retinal diseases and with that of healthy eyes.

Design.—Retrospective, observational cross-sectional study.

Participants.—This study included 137 healthy volunteers and 929 eyes of 929 patients with various unilateral retinal diseases.

Methods.—We reviewed medical charts, fundus photographs, and spectral-domain optical coherence tomographic (SD OCT) images. The incidence of the features of the vitreoretinal interface and foveal structures in the SD OCT images were compared among the asymptomatic fellow eyes of patients with unilateral MHs (n = 242), age-related macular degeneration (n = 129), epiretinal membrane (n = 185), macular pseudohole (n = 48), rhegmatogenous retinal detachment (n = 68), retinal vein occlusion (n = 257), and 1 of the eyes of healthy individuals (n = 137).

Main Outcome Measures.—Findings of slit-lamp biomicroscopy and SD OCT B-scan images.

Results.—The SD OCT B-scan images showed different types of foveal deformations associated with vitreofoveal adhesions in eyes without a posterior vitreous detachment (PVD) in the macular area. The incidence of the foveal deformations associated with vitreofoveal adhesions was significantly higher ($P<0.0001$) in the fellow eyes of the unilateral MH group (17%) than that in the other groups (0%−2%), except for the macular pseudohole group (8%). The SD OCT B-scan images also showed residual foveal deformations in eyes with a macular PVD. The incidence of a residual foveal deformation in eyes with a macular PVD was significantly higher ($P<0.0001$) in the MH group (32%) than that in any other group (0%−9%).

Conclusions.—The higher incidence of foveal deformations in the fellow eyes of patients with unilateral MHs with and without vitreofoveal adhesions suggests that patients in whom MHs develop have abnormally strong vitreofoveal adhesions sufficient to cause foveal deformation.

▶ This retrospective study does not provide us with new information that will transform the care of patients with macular hole and related entities caused by an abnormal vitreoretinal interface, at least not yet. We have long appreciated that the fellow eye of a patient with a macular hole has an elevated risk of a similar problem in the fellow eye. Previous series have described the nature of the vitreomacular interface of the fellow eye using high-resolution optical coherence tomography. This report reaffirms the higher frequency of abnormal findings by comparing with alternative types of macular disease not typically associated with vitreomacular interface issues. Currently, this information is interesting and may help when counseling patients with a macular hole. Intervention to alter the course for the fellow eye at this point isn't an option because this would consist of prophylactic vitrectomy. We are getting closer to an exciting alternative, however, that could have a major impact for these patients. There is increasing evidence that intravitreal injection of microplasmin may precipitate induction of vitreofoveal separation. If this evidence holds up in terms of efficacy and safety, we may be able to greatly reduce the development of fellow eye macular hole. If so, then an excellent understanding of the various details of analyzing the vitreomacular interface will be critical for case selection.

J. F. Vander, MD

Comparison of Pars Plana Vitrectomy With and Without Scleral Buckle for the Repair of Primary Rhegmatogenous Retinal Detachment
Kinori M, Moisseiev E, Shoshany N, et al (The Goldschleger Eye Inst, Tel Hashomer, Israel; Tel Aviv Med Ctr, Israel; Tel Aviv Univ, Israel)
Am J Ophthalmol 152:291-297, 2011

Purpose.—To compare pars plana vitrectomy (PPV) with combined PPV and scleral buckle (SB) for the repair of noncomplex primary rhegmatogenous retinal detachment (RRD).

Design.—Retrospective, nonrandomized, interventional case series.

Methods.—We reviewed 181 consecutive cases of vitrectomy for primary RRD at 2 major medical centers in Israel. The follow-up was at least 3 months. There were 96 eyes in the PPV group and 85 eyes in the PPV plus SB group. Main outcome measures were single-surgery anatomic success (SSAS) and final visual acuity (VA).

Results.—SSAS was achieved in 81.3% and 87.1% in the PPV and PPV plus SB groups, respectively ($P = .29$). Final anatomic success rate was 98.9% and 98.8%, respectively ($P = .61$). Final VA was 0.41 (20/51) in the PPV group and 0.53 (20/68) in the PPV plus SB group ($P = .13$). The final VA was significantly better than the preoperative VA in both groups

($P < .0001$). In detachments caused by inferior tears, SSAS rates were 80.9% and 81.5% in the PPV and PPV plus SB groups, respectively ($P = .74$). In phakic eyes, SSAS rates were 92% and 87.5%, respectively, and in pseudophakic eyes, SSAS rates were 77.5% and 86.7%, respectively, in the PPV and PPV plus SB groups ($P = .29$).

Conclusions.—The reattachment rate and the final VA were similar in both groups. The addition of SB did not improve the results and was associated with slightly lower VA than with PPV alone. Tear location or lens status had no significant effect on success rates. It is likely that in eyes undergoing PPV for primary RRD, addition of a SB is not warranted.

▶ There are now numerous studies assessing the merits of adding a scleral buckle (SBP) to the performance of pars plana vitrectomy (PPV) versus PPV alone for managing primary retinal detachment. Comparing surgical papers tends to be difficult in that confirming consistency of preoperative factors and intraoperative techniques is generally difficult. Thus, prior reports on this subject have found wide ranges of single-surgery success ranging from just over 50% to 97% for what are allegedly similar pools of patients treated with similar techniques. In addition, sufficient numbers of patients to ensure a reasonable power to detect important differences are often hard to achieve. In this report, the group treated with PPV and SBP had a 6% higher single-surgery success rate than PPV alone, but this did not come close to statistical significance. Considering that this was a nonrandomized study, it is possible that surgeons tended to recommend the more extensive procedure for patients with clinical features that put them at somewhat higher risk for failure. In fact, the 6% differential might have been higher if patients had been randomized and assessed prospectively. It is reassuring that final anatomic and visual results were excellent for both groups, and it is likely that individual surgeon ability matters more than which of the 2 techniques is used. Definitive evidence-based support for assertions of equivalence between the 2 strategies is lacking thus far.

J. F. Vander, MD

Sustained Benefits from Ranibizumab for Macular Edema Following Branch Retinal Vein Occlusion: 12-Month Outcomes of a Phase III Study
Brown DM, Campochiaro PA, Bhisitkul RB, et al (Retinal Consultants of Houston, TX; Johns Hopkins School of Medicine, Baltimore, MD; Univ of California San Francisco; et al)
Ophthalmology 118:1594-1602, 2011

Purpose.—Assess 12-month efficacy and safety of intraocular injections of 0.3 mg or 0.5 mg ranibizumab in patients with macular edema after branch retinal vein occlusion (BRVO).

Design.—Prospective, randomized, sham injection-controlled, double-masked, multicenter trial.

Participants.—A total of 397 patients with macular edema after BRVO.

Methods.—Eligible patients were randomized 1:1:1 to 6 monthly injections of 0.3 mg or 0.5 mg ranibizumab or sham injections. After 6 months, all patients with study eye best-corrected visual acuity (BCVA) ≤20/40 or central subfield thickness ≥250 μm were to receive ranibizumab. Patients could receive rescue laser treatment once during the treatment period and once during the observation period if criteria were met.

Main Outcome Measures.—The main efficacy outcome reported is mean change from baseline BCVA letter score at month 12. Additional visual and anatomic parameters were assessed.

Results.—Mean (95% confidence interval) change from baseline BCVA letter score at month 12 was 16.4 (14.5—18.4) and 18.3 (15.8—20.9) in the 0.3 mg and 0.5 mg groups, respectively, and 12.1 (9.6—14.6) in the sham/0.5 mg group ($P < 0.01$, each ranibizumab group vs. sham/0.5 mg). The percentage of patients who gained ≥15 letters from baseline BCVA at month 12 was 56.0% and 60.3% in the 0.3 mg and 0.5 mg groups, respectively, and 43.9% in the sham/0.5 mg group. On average, there was a marked reduction in central foveal thickness (CFT) after the first as-needed injection of 0.5 mg ranibizumab in the sham/0.5 mg group, which was sustained through month 12. No new ocular or nonocular safety events were identified.

Conclusions.—At month 12, treatment with ranibizumab as needed during months 6—11 maintained, on average, the benefits achieved by 6 monthly ranibizumab injections in patients with macular edema after BRVO, with low rates of ocular and nonocular safety events. In the sham/0.5 mg group, treatment with ranibizumab as needed for 6 months resulted in rapid reduction in CFT to a similar level as that in the 0.3 mg ranibizumab treatment group and an improvement in BCVA, but not to the extent of that in the 2 ranibizumab groups. Intraocular injections of ranibizumab provide an effective treatment for macular edema after BRVO.

▶ This report details the follow-up data from the BRAVO (Branch Retinal Vein Occlusion: Evaluation of Efficacy and Safety) trial, which demonstrated the effectiveness of repeated intravitreal injection of ranibizumab for macular edema associated with branch retinal vein occlusion (BRVO) after 6 months. This report demonstrates that ongoing injections will be needed for most patients, although possibly not with the same frequency during the subsequent 6 months. We do not know if scheduled monthly injections would be superior, nor do we know how many injections and for how long after the 12-month point. Patients who had been treated with sham injections do respond when given injections 6 months after presentation, but their response is not as extensive when compared with those injected initially. Prolonged delay of treatment after presentation would seem to be unwise. Grid laser photocoagulation has been shown to be superior to observation for many patients with BRVO and macular edema. Ideally, we can devise a strategy that combines the initial dramatic effects of injections with the sustained effects of laser. This would improve vision and minimize the burden of treatment. This study, unfortunately, does not provide guidance on this subject.

J. F. Vander, MD

Central and Hemicentral Retinal Vein Occlusion: Role of Anti–Platelet Aggregation Agents and Anticoagulants

Hayreh SS, Podhajsky PA, Zimmerman MB (Univ of Iowa)
Ophthalmology 118:1603-1611, 2011

Objective.—To investigate systematically the role of anti–platelet aggregating drugs or anticoagulants in central retinal vein occlusion (CRVO) and hemi-CRVO.

Design.—Cohort study.

Participants.—Six hundred eighty-six consecutive patients with CRVO (567 patients, 585 eyes) and nonischemic hemi-CRVO (119 patients, 122 eyes).

Methods.—At first visit, all patients had a detailed ophthalmic and medical history (including the use of anti–platelet aggregating drugs or anticoagulants), and comprehensive ophthalmic and retinal evaluation. Visual evaluation was carried out by recording visual acuity, using the Snellen visual acuity chart, and visual fields with a Goldmann perimeter. The same ophthalmic evaluation was performed at each follow-up visit. At the initial visit, CRVO and hemi-CRVO were classified as nonischemic and ischemic.

Main Outcome Measures.—Visual acuity, visual fields, and severity of retinal hemorrhages.

Results.—All 3 types of CRVO, showed a significantly greater severity of retinal hemorrhages among aspirin users than nonusers (P<0.001). Initial visual acuity and visual fields were significantly worse in aspirin users than nonusers in nonischemic CRVO and hemi-CRVO, but did not differ for ischemic CRVO. Among patients with nonischemic CRVO who initially had 20/60 or better visual acuity, there was a significant association of aspirin use with visual acuity deterioration. The odds ratio of visual acuity deterioration, adjusting for age, diabetes, ischemic heart disease, and hypertension, for aspirin users relative to nonusers was 2.24 (95% confidence interval [CI], 1.14–4.41; $P = 0.020$). Of those whose macular edema resolved, overall cumulative visual acuity outcome also suggested a higher percentage with deterioration among aspirin users, odds ratio for deterioration of 3.62 (95% CI, 0.97–13.54; $P = 0.05$) for aspirin users relative to nonusers. For the nonischemic CRVO patients with 20/70 or worse visual acuity at the initial visit, after resolution of macular edema, improvement in visual acuity was less likely in the aspirin users than in nonusers (odds ratio, 0.18; 95% CI, 0.04–0.72; $P = 0.016$).

Conclusions.—Findings of this study indicate that, for patients with CRVO and hemi-CRVO, the use of aspirin, other anti–platelet aggregating agents, or anticoagulants was associated with a worse visual outcome and no apparent benefit.

▶ Dr Hayreh has contributed an enormous amount to our understanding of retinal vascular occlusive disease over several decades in large part because of his meticulous attention to detail and a consistent, thorough evaluation and follow-up protocol. This provides excellent natural history data, in particular. This retrospective analysis of a large series of vein occlusion patients allows us to say with confidence that for those unfortunate individuals who developed occlusions in an era when there was no effective treatment, the use of aspirin or other anticoagulants at the time of presentation did not improve the prognosis and might have made it worse. Additional conclusions are made, however, that are more problematic. There is no way to know how patients using these medications would have done had the drug been stopped nor can we know what the consequences of initiation of drug upon presentation might have been. Furthermore, there are additional considerations such as possible prevention of thrombotic events in the fellow eye or systemically. A rationale is offered in favor of retinal vein occlusion not being a risk factor for thrombotic disease elsewhere, but there is a significant rate of bilateral involvement in other series and many researchers would disagree with the hypotheses offered in this report. Perhaps more importantly with the advent of meaningful and effective treatment for vein occlusions with anti-VEGF injections, it is possible that anticoagulants will behave quite differently in treated patients. Whether aspirin should be discontinued or initiated in a patient with a fresh vein occlusion remains a question without a definitive answer.

J. F. Vander, MD

Sustained Benefits from Ranibizumab for Macular Edema following Central Retinal Vein Occlusion: Twelve-Month Outcomes of a Phase III Study

Campochiaro PA, Brown DM, Awh CC, et al (The Johns Hopkins School of Medicine, Baltimore, MD; Retinal Consultants of Houston, TX; Tennessee Retina, Nashville; et al)

Ophthalmology 118:2041-2049, 2011

Purpose.—Assess the 12-month efficacy and safety of intraocular injections of 0.3 mg or 0.5 mg ranibizumab in patients with macular edema after central retinal vein occlusion (CRVO).

Design.—Prospective, randomized, sham injection-controlled, double-masked, multicenter clinical trial.

Participants.—We included 392 patients with macular edema after CRVO.

Methods.—Eligible patients were randomized 1:1:1 to receive 6 monthly intraocular injections of 0.3 mg or 0.5 mg of ranibizumab or sham injections. After 6 months, all patients with BCVA ≤20/40 or central subfield thickness ≥250 μm could receive ranibizumab.

Main Outcome Measures.—Mean change from baseline best-corrected visual acuity (BCVA) letter score at month 12, additional parameters of visual function, central foveal thickness (CFT), and other anatomic changes were assessed.

Results.—Mean (95% confidence interval) change from baseline BCVA letter score at month 12 was 13.9 (11.2−16.5) and 13.9 (11.5−16.4) in the 0.3 mg and 0.5 mg groups, respectively, and 7.3 (4.5–10.0) in the sham/0.5 mg group (*P*<0.001 for each ranibizumab group vs. sham/0.5 mg). The percentage of patients who gained ≥15 letters from baseline BCVA at month 12 was 47.0% and 50.8% in the 0.3 mg and 0.5 mg groups, respectively, and 33.1% in the sham/0.5 mg group. On average, there was a marked reduction in CFT after the first as-needed injection of 0.5 mg ranibizumab in the sham/0.5 mg group to the level of the ranibizumab groups, which was sustained through month 12. No new ocular or nonocular safety events were identified.

Conclusions.—On average, treatment with ranibizumab as needed during months 6 through 11 maintained the visual and anatomic benefits achieved by 6 monthly ranibizumab injections in patients with macular edema after CRVO, with low rates of ocular and nonocular safety events. After sham injections for 6 months, treatment with ranibizumab as needed for 6 months resulted in rapid reduction in CFT in the sham/0.5 mg group to a level similar to that in the 2 ranibizumab treatment groups and an improvement in BCVA, but not to the same level as that in the 2 ranibizumab groups. Intraocular injections of ranibizumab provide an effective treatment for macular edema after CRVO.

▶ This is a follow-up report of the CRUISE study, which had demonstrated the value of intravitreal ranibizumab for the treatment of macular edema associated with central retinal vein occlusion (CRVO). The initial randomized data showed the benefits of monthly injections versus sham injections for what has previously been a condition without proven treatment options. This follow-up report adds a few key pieces to the puzzle of managing CRVO. First, about two-thirds of patients receiving injections for 6 months are still dependent on ranibizumab injections for maintenance of a dry macula and best possible vision as evidenced by the rate of recurrence of edema when injections were withheld at month 6. Whether continuing with monthly injections beyond this point or treating on an as-needed basis is superior is unknown at this time. Second, when treatment is withheld for 6 months and then initiated, the patients will respond but not as fully as patients treated at presentation. This suggests that there is no rationale to withhold treatment initially, at least not for several months. Whether any delay is acceptable is also unknown. We are still learning about the ideal strategy for treating CRVO, but at least now we have a treatment that is generally effective even though it requires ongoing care for at least 12 months.

J. F. Vander, MD

The Effect of Adjunctive Intravitreal Bevacizumab for Preventing Postvitrectomy Hemorrhage in Proliferative Diabetic Retinopathy

Ahn J, Woo SJ, Chung H, et al (Seoul Natl Univ College of Medicine, Korea)
Ophthalmology 118:2218-2226, 2011

Objective.—To assess the effects of preoperative and intraoperative intravitreal bevacizumab (IVB) injection on the incidence of postoperative vitreous hemorrhage (VH) after vitrectomy for proliferative diabetic retinopathy (PDR).

Design.—Prospective, randomized, clinical trial.

Participants.—One hundred seven eyes of 91 patients undergoing pars plana vitrectomy (PPV) for the management of PDR-related complications were enrolled.

Methods.—One hundred seven cases were assigned randomly to either group 1 (intravitreal 1.25 mg/0.05 ml bevacizumab injection 1 to 14 days before PPV), group 2 (intravitreal 1.25 mg/0.05 ml bevacizumab injection at the end of PPV), or group 3 (no IVB injection).

Main Outcome Measures.—The primary outcome was the incidence of early ($\leq$4 weeks) and late (>4 weeks) recurrent VH. Secondary outcome measures were the initial time of vitreous clearing (ITVC) and best-corrected visual acuity (BCVA) at 6 months after surgery.

Results.—The incidences of early recurrent VH were 22.2%, 10.8%, and 32.4% in groups 1, 2, and 3, respectively ($P = 0.087$). A subgroup pairwise analysis showed significantly decreased early VH incidence in group 2 compared with that of group 3 ($P = 0.026$). The incidences of late recurrent VH were 11.1%, 16.2%, and 14.7% in groups 1, 2, and 3, respectively ($P = 0.813$). The ITVC in groups 1, 2, and 3 were 26.4 ± 42.5 days, 10.3 ± 8.2 days, and 25.2 ± 26.1 days, respectively. The ITVC was significantly shorter in group 2 compared with that in groups 1 and 3 ($P = 0.045$ and $P = 0.015$, respectively). The BCVA at 6 months after surgery did not differ significantly among the 3 groups ($P = 0.418$).

Conclusions.—This study found no substantial evidence to support the adjunctive use of preoperative IVB to reduce postoperative recurrence of VH in vitrectomy for PDR. For select cases in which adjunctive IVB use is considered, intraoperative administration seems to be the better option for reducing postoperative VH.

▶ Postvitrectomy vitreous hemorrhage in patients with proliferative diabetic retinopathy tends to be self-limited, and in the vitrectomized eye, even a substantial amount of blood will usually clear spontaneously, especially if meticulous attention to vitreous removal, relief of retinal traction, and panretinal photocoagulation are performed. Therefore, it is not surprising that this study did not identify any meaningful long-term benefit to the adjunctive use of intravitreal bevacizumab either days before or at the conclusion of vitrectomy. More important than the use of drugs is the adequacy of the procedure performed. This study did not, however, address the surgeon's ability to effectively perform the procedure. Although it is difficult to quantify and stratify the preoperative attributes that make certain vitrectomy procedures in the diabetic patient more challenging, in general, highly vascularized extraretinal proliferation and the extent of membranes and traction have great bearing on the success of the case. Intravitreal bevacizumab will produce a substantial reduction in vascularity of epiretinal membranes within days and may greatly facilitate the performance of surgery, reducing the rates of intraoperative breaks and other complications. Fear of inducing acute retinal traction is also a legitimate concern. This study demonstrates that routine use of this drug may not be needed but does not rule out the benefits of use for selected patients.

J. F. Vander, MD

A Randomized Pilot Study of Low-Fluence Photodynamic Therapy Versus Intravitreal Ranibizumab for Chronic Central Serous Chorioretinopathy
Bae SH, Heo JW, Kim C, et al (Seoul Natl Univ, Korea; Seoul Natl Univ Hosp, Korea; et al)
Am J Ophthalmol 152:784-792, 2011

Purpose.—To report 6-month outcomes of a prospective, randomized study comparing the efficacy and safety between low-fluence photodynamic therapy (PDT) and intravitreal injections of ranibizumab in the treatment of chronic central serous chorioretinopathy.

Design.—Prospective, randomized, single-center pilot study.

Methods.—Sixteen eyes with chronic central serous chorioretinopathy were randomized to receive either low-fluence PDT or intravitreal injections of ranibizumab: 8 eyes in the low-fluence PDT group and 8 in the ranibizumab group. Rescue treatment was considered if subretinal fluid was sustained after completion of primary treatment: low-fluence PDT for the ranibizumab group and ranibizumab injection for the low-fluence PDT group. Main outcome measures were excess foveal thickness, resolution of subretinal fluid, choroidal perfusion on indocyanine green angiography, and best-corrected visual acuity.

Results.—At 3 months, the mean excess foveal thickness was reduced from 74.1 ± 56.0 μm to −35.4 ± 44.5 μm in the low-fluence PDT group ($P = .017$) and from 26.3 ± 50.6 μm to −23.1 ± 56.5 μm in the ranibizumab group ($P = .058$). After a single session of PDT, 6 eyes (75%) in the low-fluence PDT group achieved complete resolution of subretinal fluid and reduction of choroidal hyperpermeability, whereas 2 (25%) eyes in the ranibizumab group achieved this after consecutive ranibizumab injections. Four eyes (50%) in the ranibizumab group underwent additional low-fluence PDT and accomplished complete resolution. At 3 months, significant improvement of best-corrected visual acuity was not demonstrated in the low-fluence PDT group ($P = .075$), whereas it was observed in the ranibizumab group ($P = .012$). However, the tendency toward improvement of best-corrected visual acuity was not maintained.

Conclusions.—In terms of anatomic outcomes, the effect of ranibizumab injections was not promising compared with that of low-fluence PDT.

▶ Central serous chorioretinopathy (CSCR) has traditionally been considered a relatively benign condition with a majority of patients experiencing spontaneous recovery. Although this is true for many affected individuals, there is a sizable percentage of patients who are not as fortunate. Considering that these patients are typically relatively young, active, and leading a high-visual-demand lifestyle, the consequences can be substantial. The treatment of exudative macular diseases has been transformed in the past decade, first by the introduction of photodynamic therapy (PDT) and more recently by the widespread use of intravitreal vascular endothelial growth factor (VEGF) inhibitors. For most patients with a "wet macula," there is now good reason to expect preservation of vision and often improvement. Unfortunately for the chronic CSCR patient, neither of these treatments is likely a panacea for what ails them. PDT (and thermal laser for that matter) can help to reduce subretinal fluid but may not help improve final visual results to any great degree. VEGF inhibition, as this pilot study reports, seems to do little, if anything, for the CSCR patient in terms of reducing fluid or providing sustained visual recovery. The most meaningful conclusion one can draw from this report is that we still do not have effective treatment for CSCR.

J. F. Vander, MD

Efficacy of Intravenous Tissue-Type Plasminogen Activator in Central Retinal Artery Occlusion: Report From a Randomized, Controlled Trial

Chen CS, Lee AW, Campbell B, et al (Flinders Med Centre and Univ, Australia; Royal Melbourne Hosp, Parkville, Australia; et al)
Stroke 42:2229-2234, 2011

Background and Purpose.—Central retinal artery occlusion is caused by a platelet-fibrin thrombus or embolic occlusion and is a stroke of the eye. Observational studies suggest that thrombolytics may restore ocular perfusion and visual function. We hypothesized that intravenous tissue-type plasminogen activator (tPA) administered within 24 hours of symptom onset might restore ocular perfusion and visual function.

Methods.—A placebo-controlled, randomized trial of intravenous tPA versus intravenous saline was performed in patients with clinically defined central retinal artery occlusion within 24 hours of symptom onset. tPA was administered at a total dose of 0.9 mg/kg, with 10% given as a 1-minute bolus and the remainder over 1 hour. An improvement of visual acuity of 3 lines or more was considered significant.

Results.—Twenty-five percent (2 of 8) of the tPA group experienced the primary outcome at 1 week after tPA versus none of the placebo group. One patient had an intracranial hemorrhage. The visual acuity improvement of these 2 patients was not sustained at 6 months. In both patients, tPA was administered within 6 hours of symptom onset.

Conclusions.—Although essentially a negative study, it does add to the evidence base of reperfusion in central retinal artery occlusion by showing that the time window for intervention is likely to be <6 hours. Reocclusion is a potential problem and may require adjuvant anticoagulation. Future studies should concentrate on determining the efficacy of thrombolytics in the <6-hour time window.

Clinical Trial Registration.—URL: http://www.anzctr.org.au. Unique identifier: 83102.

▶ Central retinal artery occlusion (CRAO) is an infrequent cause of vision loss but generally quite devastating when it occurs. There is no proven effective therapy, and, after the publication of this report, that remains the case. This is a small study because of the difficulty with recruitment and the discontinuation due to a single severe adverse event (intracranial bleed) and no apparent sustained therapeutic effect. It is noteworthy that this does not disprove the hypothesis that timely use of intravenous thrombolytic medication may increase visual recovery in acute CRAO. Two of the 8 patients in the treatment group had relatively short duration of symptoms, and both had a significant visual improvement. This effect was not sustained, but, because the protocol did not call for ongoing anticoagulation after the initial treatment, it is likely that reocclusion occurred. If patients with a short duration of symptoms (< 6 hours) were treated with thrombolysis and then followed up with anticoagulation, the effect might have been more positive. It is important to recall that 1 of 8 patients had a life-threatening complication. This treatment is not the standard of care, but, in an unusual circumstance such as acute CRAO in a monocular patient with a few hours of vision loss, it might be worth considering.

J. F. Vander, MD

Cataract Surgery in Ranibizumab-Treated Patients With Neovascular Age-Related Macular Degeneration From the Phase 3 ANCHOR and MARINA Trials
Rosenfeld PJ, on behalf of the MARINA and ANCHOR Study Groups (Univ of Miami Miller School of Medicine, FL; et al)
Am J Ophthalmol 152:793-798, 2011

Purpose.—To investigate whether cataract surgery was beneficial in patients with neovascular age-related macular degeneration (AMD) receiving monthly ranibizumab injections in the ANCHOR (Anti-VEGF Antibody for the Treatment of Predominantly Classic Choroidal Neovascularization in AMD) and MARINA (Minimally Classic/Occult Trial of the Anti-VEGF Antibody Ranibizumab in the Treatment of Neovascular AMD) phase 3 trials.

Design.—Retrospective analysis.

Methods.—0Patients were identified who underwent cataract surgery during the 2 pivotal trials. For this analysis, the best-corrected visual acuity

(VA) just prior to cataract surgery was referred to as the redefined baseline VA. For the period after cataract surgery, endpoints included change in VA, time to first postsurgery injection, and total number of injections. Monthly follow-up visits after surgery were defined at 30-day intervals ± 15 days.

Results.—Three subgroups were identified: study eyes of ranibizumab-treated patients (758 eyes [23 undergoing surgery]), fellow eyes of ranibizumab-treated patients (758 eyes [28 undergoing surgery]), and eyes of non-ranibizumab patients (762 [16 undergoing surgery]). Three months postsurgery, the VA of ranibizumab-treated eyes improved by a mean of 10.4 (± 3.4) letters compared to the redefined baseline (n = 20; 95% confidence interval +3.3 letters to +17.5 letters). The mean VA change from redefined baseline VA was not significantly different between the 3 groups at any of the evaluated time points postsurgery ($P > .44$ for all comparisons between each pair of the 3 groups at 1, 2, 3, and 4 months following surgery).

Conclusions.—In the phase 3 trials, cataract surgery appeared to be safe and beneficial for all eyes with AMD, including ranibizumab-treated eyes with neovascular AMD. An average VA improvement of more than 2 lines was typically observed.

▶ The Anchor and Marina Trials were vitally important studies serving to guide the rapid evolution of treatment for wet age-related macular degeneration (ARMD) into the current era of serial injections with anti—vascular endothelial growth factor medications for virtually all forms of macular degeneration. This study extracts a fairly small subgroup of patients from the larger randomized study populations and attempts to assess an endpoint not considered in the original study design. It is quite tempting to draw on the wealth of data established in high quality randomized trials and put it to additional valuable purpose. This approach is fraught with danger, however, and it is difficult to reach conclusions possessing any degree of statistical confidence in this setting. Cataracts and wet ARMD often coexist, and the issue addressed herein is of great clinical relevance. It is reassuring to learn that in this study population, the patients with treated ARMD who underwent cataract surgery seemed to do as well as the control populations. Lacking high-quality, prospective data, this type of report is the best we have thus far, and it seems reasonable to consider cataract surgery for patients with similar features to those reported. We still need more information about questions such as whether there is any added risk, when in the injection cycle is the ideal time for surgery, and what features make surgery more or less successful, among many others.

J. F. Vander, MD

Randomized Comparison of Systemic Anti-inflammatory Therapy Versus Fluocinolone Acetonide Implant for Intermediate, Posterior, and Panuveitis: The Multicenter Uveitis Steroid Treatment Trial

The Multicenter Uveitis Steroid Treatment (MUST) Trial Research Group (The Univ of Pennsylvania, Philadelphia; Univ of Wisconsin, Madison; Johns Hopkins Bloomberg School of Public Health, Baltimore, MD)

Ophthalmology 118:1916-1926, 2011

Objective.—To compare the relative effectiveness of systemic corticosteroids plus immunosuppression when indicated (systemic therapy) versus fluocinolone acetonide implant (implant therapy) for noninfectious intermediate, posterior, or panuveitis (uveitis).

Design.—Randomized controlled parallel superiority trial.

Participants.—Patients with active or recently active uveitis.

Methods.—Participants were randomized (allocation ratio 1:1) to systemic or implant therapy at 23 centers (3 countries). Implant-assigned participants with bilateral uveitis were assigned to have each eye that warranted study treatment implanted. Treatment-outcome associations were analyzed by assigned treatment for all eyes with uveitis.

Main Outcome Measures.—Masked examiners measured the primary outcome: change in best-corrected visual acuity from baseline. Secondary outcomes included patient-reported quality of life, ophthalmologist-graded uveitis activity, and local and systemic complications of uveitis or therapy. Reading Center graders and glaucoma specialists assessing ocular complications were masked. Participants, ophthalmologists, and coordinators were unmasked.

Results.—On evaluation of changes from baseline to 24 months among 255 patients randomized to implant and systemic therapy (479 eyes with uveitis), the implant and systemic therapy groups had an improvement in visual acuity of +6.0 and +3.2 letters ($P = 0.16$, 95% confidence interval on difference in improvement between groups, -1.2 to +6.7 letters, positive values favoring implant), an improvement in vision-related quality of life of +11.4 and +6.8 units ($P = 0.043$), a change in EuroQol-EQ5D health utility of +0.02 and -0.02 ($P = 0.060$), and residual active uveitis in 12% and 29% ($P = 0.001$), respectively. Over the 24 month period, implant-assigned eyes had a higher risk of cataract surgery (80%, hazard ratio [HR] = 3.3, $P < 0.0001$), treatment for elevated intraocular pressure (61%, HR = 4.2, $P < 0.0001$), and glaucoma (17%, HR = 4.2, $P = 0.0008$). Patients assigned to systemic therapy had more prescription-requiring infections than patients assigned to implant therapy (0.60 vs 0.36/person-year, $P = 0.034$), without notable long-term consequences; systemic adverse outcomes otherwise were unusual in both groups, with minimal differences between groups.

Conclusions.—In each treatment group, mean visual acuity improved over 24 months, with neither approach superior to a degree detectable with the study's power. Therefore, the specific advantages and disadvantages identified should dictate selection between the alternative treatments in consideration of individual patients' particular circumstances. Systemic therapy with aggressive use of corticosteroid-sparing immunosuppression was well tolerated, suggesting that this approach is reasonably safe for local and systemic inflammatory disorders.

▶ Noninfectious uveitis may be mild and self-limiting at one extreme to severe, refractory and potentially blinding at the other. Often patients with more severe bilateral disease will have systemic evidence of inflammatory disease requiring significant systemic immunosuppression. For individuals with severe bilateral uveitis but without evidence for nonocular inflammation, a critical decision is whether to treat locally or systemically. This randomized trial assesses this question with 2 years' worth of careful follow-up. In terms of visual acuity results, there is not a substantial difference. Patients undergoing surgical placement of a long-term sustained release fluocinolone acetonide intravitreal implant had good control of intraocular inflammation, but virtually all required cataract surgery, and 25% required glaucoma surgery. These numbers are high, and presumably the number of patients requiring glaucoma procedures will increase with time, especially if additional treatment with corticosteroids is required beyond 24 months. In contrast, steroid sparing systemic immunosuppression produces fewer ocular issues but, not surprisingly, increases the likelihood of systemic infections, or at least prescribed treatment for systemic infection. Serious systemic adverse events were not more frequent in the systemic immunosuppression group. The apparent answer to which method is preferable is, "it depends." Given that many uveitis patients already have some degree of cataract and likely have been exposed to corticosteroids, use of implants seems reasonable if such a patient is not known to be a steroid pressure responder. Otherwise, systemic immunosuppression with careful monitoring for systemic side effects is a reasonable, possibly preferable strategy.

J. F. Vander, MD

Medicare Costs for Neovascular Age-Related Macular Degeneration, 1994–2007
Day S, Acquah K, Lee PP, et al (Duke Eye Ctr, Durham, NC; Duke Univ, Durham, NC)
Am J Ophthalmol 152:1014-1020, 2011

Purpose.—To assess changes in Medicare payments for neovascular age-related macular degeneration (AMD) since introduction of anti–vascular endothelial growth factor (VEGF) therapies.
Design.—Retrospective, longitudinal cohort study.
Methods.—Using the Medicare 5% sample, beneficiaries with new diagnoses of neovascular AMD in 1994 (N = 2497), 2000 (N = 3927), and 2006 (N = 6041) were identified using International Classification of Diseases (ICD-9-CM). The total first-year health care and eye care costs were calculated for each beneficiary. Propensity score matching was used to match individuals in the 2000 and 2006 cohorts with the 1994 cohort on age, sex, race, Charlson Comorbidity Index, and low vision/blindness.

Results.—The number of beneficiaries newly diagnosed with neovascular AMD more than doubled between the 1994 and 2006 cohorts. Overall yearly Part B payments per beneficiary increased significantly from $3567 for the 1994 to $5991 for the 2006 cohort (*P* < .01) in constant 2008 dollars. Payments for eye care alone doubled from $1504 for the 1994 cohort to $3263 for the 2006 cohort (*P* < .01). Most of the increase in payments for eye care in 2006 reflected payments for anti-VEGF injections, which were $1609 over 1 year. Mean annual numbers of visits and imaging studies also increased significantly between the 1994 and 2006 cohort. Results were similar in the matched sample.

Conclusions.—The introduction of anti-VEGF intravitreal injections has offered remarkable clinical benefits for patients with neovascular AMD, but these benefits have come at the cost of an increased financial burden of providing care for these patients.

▶ There is not a significant medical advance described in this article, and yet it is of considerable importance as a matter of public health and public policy. With the development and high acceptance of treatment using injectable medications for neovascular age-related macular degeneration (ARMD) has come a major change in the economics of eye care for the elderly population. Expenditures more than doubled between 1994 and 2006, and this does not include the period of the largest increase in usage of ranibizumab, which followed shortly thereafter. Numbers for 2008 and later are undoubtedly even higher. As indications for usage have broadened and newer drugs, such as aflibercept, which is comparably priced to ranibizumab and was just approved by the U.S. Food and Drug Administration, come to market, the potential for even higher costs is substantial. One fortuitous circumstance that will likely help to restrain cost increases is the availability of bevacizumab, as this report describes. As recently shown in a nationwide randomized trial (the CATT Trial), this much lower cost alternative seems to be roughly equally effective for many patients with wet ARMD and helps to provide downward pressure in the marketplace. Although not mentioned in this article, which only looks at Medicare data, many private insurers are reducing or eliminating support for the use of the more expensive drugs in favor of the lower-cost option. Whether CMS will follow suit is unknown at this time.

J. F. Vander, MD

Incidence of Retinal Pigment Epithelial Tears after Intravitreal Ranibizumab Injection for Neovascular Age-Related Macular Degeneration
Cunningham ET Jr, Feiner L, Chung C, et al (Stanford Univ School of Medicine, CA; Retina Associates of New Jersey, Teaneck; Genentech, Inc, South San Francisco, CA)
Ophthalmology 118:2447-2452, 2011

Objective.—To explore the association between treatment for neovascular age-related macular degeneration (AMD) and incidence and timing of retinal pigment epithelium (RPE) tears in ranibizumab-treated patients versus control treatment.

Design.—Results from 3 phase III clinical trials (*A*Nti-VEGF antibody for the treatment of predominantly classic *CHO*Roidal neovascularization in age-related macular degeneration [ANCHOR], *M*inimally classic/occult trial of the *A*nti-VEGF antibody *R*anibizumab *I*n the treatment of *N*eovascular *A*ge-related macular degeneration [MARINA], and A *P*hase IIIb, Multicenter, Randomized, Double-Masked, Sham *I*njection-Controlled Study of the *E*fficacy and Safety of *R*anibizumab in Subjects with Subfoveal Choroidal Neovascularization [CNV] with or without Classic CNV Secondary to Age-Related Macular Degeneration [PIER]) were retrospectively reviewed to identify patients who developed RPE tears during the study period, detected on fluorescein angiography performed at prespecified intervals.

Participants.—Patients with baseline and post-baseline angiographic assessments.

Methods.—Patients received intravitreal ranibizumab (0.3 or 0.5 mg) or control treatment (verteporfin photodynamic therapy [PDT] in ANCHOR and sham intravitreal injections in ANCHOR, MARINA, and PIER).

Main Outcome Measures.—Incidence and timing of RPE tears during the treatment period.

Results.—Data from 1298 patients were analyzed. No statistically significant differences in RPE tear incidence were observed. The pooled rate of RPE tears was 1.8% with 0.5 mg ranibizumab, 3.0% with 0.3 mg ranibizumab, and 1.6% in the control group. Most (76%; 16/21) RPE tears in ranibizumab-treated patients were identified within 3 months of initiating treatment, whereas the majority (80%; 4/5) of late-onset RPE tears occurred in control patients. In patients who developed RPE tears, better visual acuity (VA) outcomes were observed in those treated with ranibizumab versus control treatment.

Conclusions.—As studied in these trials, no statistically significant differences in the incidence of RPE tears within a 2-year treatment period were observed in patients who received ranibizumab (0.5 or 0.3 mg) versus control treatment, although most RPE tears with ranibizumab occurred within 3 months of initiating treatment. Mean VA was better in patients who developed RPE tears while receiving ranibizumab than in those who received control treatment, suggesting a potential benefit of continued ranibizumab therapy in patients with neovascular AMD who developed RPE tears.

▶ The introduction of anti–vascular endothelial growth factor (VEGF) medications into our armamentarium for treatment of wet age-related macular degeneration (AMD) has transformed a once ominous diagnosis into a manageable problem associated with a reasonable prognosis, albeit with the burden of ongoing injections. Most patients do well with preserved or improved vision. One uncommon but important group of patients who do not fare so well are those who develop a retinal pigment epithelium (RPE) tear or rip. Although the rate of RPE tears in wet AMD is only 2% to 6%, for patients with an associated pigment epithelial detachment (PED), the number is 25% or higher. The risk is highest for large PEDs. Although it is reassuring that the overall rate of RPE tears is not different in the treated group versus untreated or photodynamic therapy controls, there is an important difference between the 2 groups. The ranibizumab-treated groups tend to have their tear form early in the course of treatment. The report indicates 3 months, but that is likely because the first fluorescein angiogram was done 3 months after enrollment. It is possible (and in my experience likely) that a large percentage of these tears occurred after the first injection. Presumably rips occur with contracture of the choroidal neovascularization (CNV) associated with the PED. The most dramatic change in the CNV based on angiography and optical coherence tomography tends to be shortly after the first injection. Although patients with moderate to severe vision loss before the tear may not notice a dramatic change, patients with fairly good vision will describe a sudden and sometimes quite marked visual loss at the time of the tear. Patients with a large PED and good vision are therefore a setup for trouble. They are at risk for developing an RPE tear and for having severe vision loss associated with a tear should it occur, not infrequently after the first injection. This is not a happy circumstance. Great caution and extra counseling of such patients are required before treatment. For patients with a very large PED and little overlying intraretinal and subretinal fluid, observation may be the preferred option even with angiographic evidence of CNV.

J. F. Vander, MD

Comparison of Hemorrhagic Complications of Warfarin and Clopidogrel Bisulfate in 25-Gauge Vitrectomy versus a Control Group

Mason JO III, Gupta SR, Compton CJ, et al (Retina Consultants of Alabama, Birmingham; Univ of Alabama at Birmingham School of Medicine)
Ophthalmology 118:543-547, 2011

Purpose.—To estimate the risk of hemorrhagic complications associated with 25-gauge pars plana vitrectomy (PPV) when warfarin (Coumadin; Bristol-Myers Squibb, New York, NY) or clopidogrel (Plavix; Bristol-Myers Squibb) are continued throughout the surgical period, as compared with a control group.

Design.—A single-center, retrospective, cohort study of 289 consecutive patients receiving either warfarin therapy or clopidogrel therapy or neither of those therapies who underwent 25-gauge PPV.

Participants.—Included were 61 patients (64 eyes; 64 PPV procedures) in the warfarin group and 118 (125 eyes; 136 PPV procedures) in the clopidogrel group. Warfarin patients were subdivided into 4 groups by international normalized ratio (INR). A control group included 110 patients (110 eyes; 110 PPV procedures) who were not receiving warfarin or clopidogrel.

Methods.—Retrospective chart review for which the criteria included: 25-gauge PPV, minimum age of 19 years, warfarin or clopidogrel use, and, if taking warfarin, an INR obtained within 5 days of surgery.

Main Outcome Measures.—Incidence of intraoperative and postoperative hemorrhagic complications.

Results.—The most common indications for anticoagulation therapy included: atrial fibrillation (38%), valvular heart disease (17%), and thromboembolic disease (16%). The most common indications for antiplatelet therapy included: cardiac stent (49%), coronary artery bypass grafting (24%), and history of transient ischemic attack (16%). No patient experienced anesthesia-related hemorrhagic complications resulting from peribulbar or retrobulbar block. Transient vitreous hemorrhage occurred in 1 (1.6%) of 64 PPV procedures in the warfarin group ($P = .6531$), 5 (3.7%) of 136 PPV procedures in the clopidogrel group ($P = 1.0$), and 4 (3.6%) of 110 PPV procedures in the control group. No choroidal or retrobulbar hemorrhages occurred in any patient.

Conclusions.—The rate of 25-gauge PPV hemorrhagic complications in patients who underwent systemic anticoagulation or who were receiving platelet inhibitor therapy is extremely low. Given the risks associated with stopping these therapies, the authors recommend that patients continue their current therapeutic regimen without cessation.

▶ As the authors of this report point out, it is increasingly common to encounter patients requiring pars plana vitrectomy who are using 1 or more oral anticoagulants, thereby making this study clinically relevant. The authors used a 25-gauge technique, but it is reasonable to extrapolate to other incision techniques because the pars plana incisions are not the likely sources of bleeding during vitrectomy. The pars plana is relatively avascular. The anesthetic injection technique and intraoperative intraocular bleeding from highly vascularized tissue such as proliferative retinopathy or the choroid are more likely to be problematic. Although it is reassuring that the authors did not find a significant increase in hemorrhagic risk with continued anticoagulant use at the time of surgery, it is important to recognize the limitations that the authors acknowledge. Given the incidence of these complications, the study is underpowered and is retrospective. Furthermore, given the potentially catastrophic consequences of uncontrolled bleeding, it makes sense to take all reasonable precautions despite the encouraging results reported. Rather than use a retrobulbar injection for anesthesia, a small conjunctival incision after topical anesthetic placement will allow for a blunt tipped sub-Tenon's injection of anesthetic, which should reduce the risk of retrobulbar bleeding. Also, if patients can have the anticoagulant temporarily suspended after consultation with their internist or cardiologist, this may provide additional safety. A single rigid approach that ignores the patient's particular risk factors does not seem justified by the level of evidence provided herein.

J. F. Vander, MD

Dexamethasone Intravitreal Implant for Noninfectious Intermediate or Posterior Uveitis

Lowder C, for the Ozurdex HURON Study Group (Cole Eye Inst, Cleveland, OH; et al)

Arch Ophthalmol 129:545-553, 2011

Objective.—To evaluate the safety and efficacy of 2 doses of dexamethasone intravitreal implant (DEX implant) for treatment of noninfectious intermediate or posterior uveitis.

Methods.—In this 26-week trial, eyes with noninfectious intermediate or posterior uveitis were randomized to a single treatment with a 0.7-mg DEX implant (n=77), 0.35-mg DEX implant (n=76), or sham procedure (n=76).

Main Outcome Measure.—The main outcome measure was the proportion of eyes with a vitreous haze score of 0 at week 8.

Results.—The proportion of eyes with a vitreous haze score of 0 at week 8 was 47% with the 0.7-mg DEX implant, 36% with the 0.35-mg DEX implant, and 12% with the sham ($P<.001$); this benefit persisted through week 26. A gain of 15 or more letters from baseline best-corrected visual acuity was seen in significantly more eyes in the DEX implant groups than the sham group at all study visits. The percentage of eyes with intraocular pressure of 25 mm Hg or more peaked at 7.1% for the 0.7-mg DEX implant, 8.7% for the 0.35-mg DEX implant, and 4.2% for the sham ($P>.05$ at any visit). The incidence of cataract reported in the phakic eyes was 9 of 62 (15%) with the 0.7-mg DEX implant, 6 of 51 (12%) with the 0.35-mg DEX implant, and 4 of 55 (7%) with the sham ($P>.05$).

Conclusions.—In patients with noninfectious intermediate or posterior uveitis, a single DEX implant significantly improved intraocular inflammation and visual acuity persisting for 6 months.

Application to Clinical Practice.—Dexamethasone intravitreal implant may be used safely and effectively for treatment of intermediate and posterior uveitis.

Trial Registration.—clinicaltrials.gov Identifier: NCT00333814.

▶ Corticosteroids, given in adequate doses, are effective at reducing intraocular inflammation and the secondary effects of the inflammation in patients with intermediate and posterior uveitis. This is the primary conclusion of this report, and it is unremarkable if left at that. It is also well known that, if given in sufficient doses, patients treated with corticosteroids will develop cataracts and, in a significant minority, glaucoma, if followed over adequate periods of time. In this regard, this study is lacking in that with only 26 weeks of follow-up, we can not comment on these important safety aspects. Perhaps most problematic is the group of patients not assessed in this trial. Given current treatment strategies, the most relevant control group to compare with the Ozurdex sustained-release device would be recipients of standard intravitreal injection of either dexamethasone or triamcinolone. Using a 30-gauge needle, it is possible to quickly, nearly painlessly, and cheaply inject high levels of drug in the office and repeating every 2 to 3 months if needed. In contrast, the Ozurdex device requires a 22-gauge injector and is considerably more expensive. Admittedly, it has the theoretical advantage of flattening out the peaks and valleys of drug level in the vitreous, but the number of patients requiring rescue treatment toward the end of the 6-month trial suggests that the period of sustained efficacy may not be that much longer than the standard injection will provide. While the concept of a sustained-release mechanism for drug administration is appealing, thus far the added value when considering the cost and logistics of administration may not justify widespread application of this device. Furthermore, until we find an alternative to corticosteroids, we will continue to wrestle with their side effects, regardless of how they are delivered.

J. F. Vander, MD

Ranibizumab and Bevacizumab for Neovascular Age-Related Macular Degeneration

The CATT Research Group (Cleveland Clinic Cole Eye Inst, OH; Univ of Pennsylvania, Philadelphia; et al)

N Engl J Med 364:1897-1908, 2011

Background.—Clinical trials have established the efficacy of ranibizumab for the treatment of neovascular age-related macular degeneration (AMD). In addition, bevacizumab is used off-label to treat AMD, despite the absence of similar supporting data.

Methods.—In a multicenter, single-blind, noninferiority trial, we randomly assigned 1208 patients with neovascular AMD to receive intravitreal injections of ranibizumab or bevacizumab on either a monthly schedule or as needed with monthly evaluation. The primary outcome was the mean change in visual acuity at 1 year, with a noninferiority limit of 5 letters on the eye chart.

Results.—Bevacizumab administered monthly was equivalent to ranibizumab administered monthly, with 8.0 and 8.5 letters gained, respectively. Bevacizumab administered as needed was equivalent to ranibizumab as needed, with 5.9 and 6.8 letters gained, respectively. Ranibizumab as needed was equivalent to monthly ranibizumab, although the comparison between bevacizumab as needed and monthly bevacizumab was inconclusive. The mean decrease in central retinal thickness was greater in the ranibizumab-monthly group (196 μm) than in the other groups (152 to 168 μm, $P=0.03$ by analysis of variance). Rates of death, myocardial infarction, and stroke were similar for patients receiving either bevacizumab or ranibizumab ($P>0.20$). The proportion of patients with serious systemic adverse events (primarily hospitalizations) was higher with bevacizumab than with ranibizumab (24.1% vs. 19.0%; risk ratio, 1.29; 95% confidence interval, 1.01 to 1.66), with excess events broadly distributed in disease categories not identified in previous studies as areas of concern.

Conclusions.—At 1 year, bevacizumab and ranibizumab had equivalent effects on visual acuity when administered according to the same schedule.

Ranibizumab given as needed with monthly evaluation had effects on vision that were equivalent to those of ranibizumab administered monthly. Differences in rates of serious adverse events require further study. (Funded by the National Eye Institute; ClinicalTrials.gov number, NCT00593450.).

▶ This is a tremendously important article. Neovascular age-related macular degeneration (AMD) is a major public health issue, and, with 2 medications widely used for treatment, a head-to-head comparison in the form of a well-conceived, well-controlled randomized clinical trial provides the highest level of evidence to guide treatment strategies going forward. It is important to note that the 2 drugs were compared using each with 2 distinct treatment strategies. As with virtually every other study reported to date, patients with neovascular AMD treated using monthly injections tend to do better both in terms of anatomic endpoints as well as visual acuity results when compared with any less frequent injection protocol. Whether a "treat when wet" or gradually lengthened treatment interval ("treat and extend") might be a reasonable compromise (reducing the costs, risks, and burden of treatment without sacrificing much in terms of long-term visual results) is not yet firmly established. Similarly, although bevacizumab and ranibizumab appear to be roughly equivalent in terms of effectiveness and safety over the course of 1 year, there are still some unanswered questions. Specific subtypes of AMD (eg, vascularized pigment epithelial detachment) tend to respond less completely to treatment. There might be an advantage in using one or the other drug in selected resistant cases that did not show up in this study. Furthermore, the data are only for 1 year, and given the trend toward a difference in foveal thickness noted in these data, we should eagerly look forward to 2-year data and beyond.

J. F. Vander, MD

Primary Endpoint Results of a Phase II Study of Vascular Endothelial Growth Factor Trap-Eye in Wet Age-related Macular Degeneration
Brown DM, for the CLEAR-IT 2 Investigators (The Methodist Hosp, Houston, TX; et al)
Ophthalmology 118:1089-1097, 2011

Objective.—To evaluate the biologic effects and safety of vascular endothelial growth factor (VEGF) Trap-Eye during a 12-week fixed-dosing period in patients with neovascular (wet) age-related macular degeneration (AMD).

Design.—Multicenter, prospective, randomized, double-masked clinical trial with initial 12-week fixed dosing period. Data were analyzed to week 16.

Participants.—We included 159 patients with subfoveal choroidal neovascularization secondary to wet AMD.

Methods.—Patients were randomized 1:1:1:1:1 to VEGF Trap-Eye during the fixed-dosing phase (day 1 to week 12): 0.5 or 2 mg every 4 weeks (0.5 mg q4wk, 2 mg q4wk) on day 1 and at weeks 4, 8, and 12;

or 0.5, 2, or 4 mg every 12 weeks (0.5 mg q12wk, 2 mg q12wk, or 4 mg q12wk) on day 1 and at week 12.

Main Outcome Measures.—The primary endpoint was change from baseline in central retinal/lesion thickness (CR/LT) at week 12; secondary outcomes included change in best-corrected visual acuity (BCVA), proportion of patients with a gain of ≥15 letters, proportion of patients with a loss of >15 letters, and safety.

Results.—At week 12, treatment with VEGF Trap-Eye resulted in a significant mean decrease in CR/LT of 119 μm from baseline in all groups combined ($P<0.0001$). The reduction in CR/LT with the 2 mg q4wk and 0.5mg q4wk regimens was significantly greater than each of the quarterly dosing regimens. The BCVA increased significantly by a mean of 5.7 letters at 12 weeks in the combined group ($P<0.0001$), with the greatest mean gain of >8 letters in the monthly dosing groups. At 8 weeks, BCVA improvements were similar with 2 mg q4wk and 2 mg q12wk dosing. After the last required dose at week 12, CR/LT and visual acuity were maintained or further improved at week 16 in all treatment groups. Ocular adverse events were mild and consistent with safety profiles reported for other intraocular anti-VEGF treatments.

Conclusions.—Repeated monthly intravitreal dosing of VEGF Trap-Eye over 12 weeks demonstrated significant reductions in retinal thickness and improvements in visual acuity, and was well-tolerated in patients with neovascular AMD.

▶ This published report demonstrates 2 important facts. First, the vascular endothelial growth factor (VEGF) Trap compound is a promising alternative to ranibizumab and bevacizumab in the management of exudative macular degeneration. As with earlier studies looking at currently available anti-VEGF medications, patients receiving more medication, whether higher doses or more frequent treatment, tended to do better in terms of macular thickness and visual acuity. The ideal dosing regimen is not yet clear, although it is likely that dosing schedules may need to be customized for individual patients. The second fact is that when following rapidly evolving fields such as the treatment of wet age-related macular degeneration, there is a substantial lag between the peer-reviewed published literature and the forefront of current information. The authors of this Phase 2 report acknowledge the release of the data from the Phase 3 trials that followed this study. It is highly likely that before the end of 2011, this drug will have received Food and Drug Administration approval and may be clinically available just months after the printing of this Phase 2 report. Stay tuned.

J. F. Vander, MD

Dietary ω-3 Fatty Acid and Fish Intake and Incident Age-Related Macular Degeneration in Women
Christen WG, Schaumberg DA, Glynn RJ, et al (Brigham and Women's Hosp and Harvard Med School, Boston, MA)
Arch Ophthalmol 129:921-929, 2011

Objective.—To examine whether intake of ω-3 fatty acids and fish affects incidence of age-related macular degeneration (AMD) in women.

Design.—A detailed food-frequency questionnaire was administered at baseline among 39 876 female health professionals (mean [SD] age: 54.6 [7.0] years). A total of 38 022 women completed the questionnaire and were free of a diagnosis of AMD. The main outcome measure was incident AMD responsible for a reduction in best-corrected visual acuity to 20/30 or worse based on self-report confirmed by medical record review.

Results.—A total of 235 cases of AMD, most characterized by some combination of drusen and retinal pigment epithelial changes, were confirmed during an average of 10 years of follow-up. Women in the highest tertile of intake for docosahexaenoic acid, compared with those in the lowest, had a multivariate-adjusted relative risk of AMD of 0.62 (95% confidence interval, 0.44-0.87). For eicosapentaenoic acid, women in the highest tertile of intake had a relative risk of 0.66 (95% confidence interval, 0.48-0.92). Consistent with the findings for docosahexaenoic acid and eicosapentaenoic acid, women who consumed 1 or more servings of fish per week, compared with those who consumed less than 1 serving per month, had a relative risk of AMD of 0.58 (95% confidence interval, 0.38-0.87).

Conclusion.—These prospective data from a large cohort of female health professionals without a diagnosis of AMD at baseline indicate that regular consumption of docosahexaenoic acid and eicosapentaenoic acid and fish was associated with a significantly decreased risk of incident AMD and may be of benefit in primary prevention of AMD.

▶ The role of diet and nutritional supplementation in the development and progression of age-related macular degeneration (AMD) is a topic of great interest to many. Given the scope of the public health problem caused by AMD and the lack of effective treatment for the large majority of people affected by AMD (ie, the dry form), this is understandable. It has been many years since the AREDS trial gave us powerful evidence showing the substantial benefits of nutraceuticals in reducing progression of AMD, and we will not have the opportunity to assess data from the follow-up AREDS 2 trial until at least 2013. In the interim, many studies have been published trying to assess the role of diet and supplements by looking at associations in large populations. This report describes a particularly large and well-organized prospective cohort study and finds a convincing link between relatively frequent fish consumption and a reduced rate of AMD development over an average of 10 years' follow-up in women. This finding is fairly consistent with expectations and the majority of studies on the subject. What is surprising is that some large and, apparently well-done, studies have not come to this conclusion. It is not clear why such a strong association would not consistently appear in virtually all large trials on this subject. Most researchers expect the new AREDS 2 formula with inclusion of the long-chain fatty acids to be strongly beneficial, but the answer is still not in.

J. F. Vander, MD

Fluocinolone Acetonide Intravitreal Implant for Diabetic Macular Edema: A 3-Year Multicenter, Randomized, Controlled Clinical Trial
Pearson PA, Comstock TL, Ip M, et al (Univ of Kentucky, Lexington; Bausch & Lomb, Inc, Rochester, NY; Univ of Wisconsin Med School, Madison; et al)
Ophthalmology 118:1580-1587, 2011

Purpose.—We studied the 3-year efficacy and safety results of a 4-year study evaluating fluocinolone acetonide (FA) intravitreal implants in eyes with persistent or recurrent diabetic macular edema (DME).

Design.—Prospective, evaluator-masked, controlled, multicenter clinical trial.

Participants.—We included 196 eyes with refractory DME.

Methods.—Patients were randomized 2:1 to receive 0.59-mg FA implant (n = 127) or standard of care (SOC additional laser or observation; n = 69). The implant was inserted through a pars plana incision. Visits were scheduled on day 2, weeks 1, 3, 6, 12, and 26, and thereafter every 13 weeks through 3 years postimplantation.

Main Outcome Measures.—The primary efficacy outcome was ≥15-letter improvement in visual acuity (VA) at 6 months. Secondary outcomes included resolution of macular retinal thickening and Diabetic Retinopathy Severity Score (DRSS). Safety measures included incidence of adverse events (AEs).

Results.—Overall, VA improved ≥3 lines in 16.8% of implanted eyes at 6 months ($P=0.0012$; SOC, 1.4%); in 16.4% at 1 year ($P=0.1191$; SOC, 8.1%); in 31.8% at 2 years ($P=0.0016$; SOC, 9.3%); and in 31.1% at 3 years ($P=0.1566$; SOC, 20.0%). The number of implanted eyes with no evidence of retinal thickening at the center of the macula was higher than SOC eyes at 6 months ($P<0.0001$), 1 year ($P<0.0001$; 72% vs 22%), 2 years ($P=0.016$), and 3 years ($P=0.861$). A higher rate of improvement and lower rate of decline in DRSS occurred in the implanted group versus the SOC group at 6 months ($P=0.0006$), 1 year ($P=0.0016$), 2 years ($P=0.012$), and 3 years ($P=0.0207$). Intraocular pressure (IOP) ≥30 mm Hg was recorded in 61.4% of implanted eyes (SOC, 5.8%) at any time and 33.8% required surgery for ocular hypertension by 4 years. Of implanted phakic eyes, 91% (SOC, 20%) had cataract extraction by 4 years.

Conclusions.—The FA intravitreal implant met the primary and secondary outcomes, with significantly improved VA and DRSS and reduced DME. The most common AEs included cataract progression and elevated

IOP. The 0.59-mg FA intravitreal implant may be an effective treatment for eyes with persistent or recurrent DME.

▶ Corticosteroids delivered to the retina reduce edema associated with diabetic macular leakage. It has been 10 years since it was first reported that a striking but, unfortunately, temporary reduction in edema can be achieved with the intravitreal injection of triamcinolone acetonide. Since then, a variety of steroids and a variety of delivery methods have been investigated trying to find a safe and effective longer-term solution to this common problem. Certain recurrent themes have been discovered by these efforts, including this report. When active drug is in the vitreous, the edema generally resolves. The greater the amount and potency of the steroid, the greater the effect on the macula. At least one-third of patients have a substantial rise in intraocular pressure, which may require surgical intervention, and nearly all phakic patients will develop a cataract. While focal laser generally works very gradually and frequently requires repeated treatment, the early benefits of steroid treatment over laser are not sustained with longer-term follow-up. Pharmacologic treatment is an appealing strategy, as is a sustained release approach. The problem is that corticosteroids are not likely the best choice for this purpose. Recent evidence demonstrates the efficacy of anti—vascular endothelial growth factor agents injected into the vitreous with a superior safety profile. It is not clear whether a sustained release vehicle for delivery of this drug class will be possible. In the meantime, it appears that corticosteroids are not the preferred method for treating diabetic macular edema regardless of delivery strategy.

J. F. Vander, MD

Economic Considerations of Macular Edema Therapies
Smiddy WE (Univ of Miami Miller School of Medicine, FL)
Ophthalmology 118:1827-1833, 2011

Purpose.—To relate costs and treatment benefits for diabetic macular edema (DME), branch retinal vein occlusion (BRVO), and central retinal vein occlusion (CRVO).

Design.—A model of resource use, outcomes, and cost-effectiveness and utility.

Participants.—None.

Methods.—Results from published clinical trials (index studies) of laser, intravitreal corticosteroids, intravitreal anti-vascular endothelial growth factor (VEGF) agents, and vitrectomy trials were used to ascertain visual benefit and clinical protocols. Calculations followed from the costs of 1 year of treatment for each treatment modality and the visual benefits as ascertained.

Main Outcome Measures.—Visual acuity (VA) saved, cost of therapy, cost per line saved, cost per line-year saved, and costs per quality-adjusted life years (QALYs).

Results.—The lines saved for DME (0.26—2.02), BRVO (0.74—4.92), and CRVO (1.2—3.75) yielded calculations of costs/line of saved VA for DME

($1329—$11,609), BRVO ($494—$13,039), and CRVO ($704—$7611); costs/line-year for DME ($60—$561), BRVO ($25—$754), and CRVO ($45—$473); and costs/QALY ($824 to $25,566).

Conclusions.—Relative costs and benefits should be considered in perspective when applying and developing treatment strategies.

▶ Ten years ago, a report like this would likely never have seen the light of day. The author has not done any original research regarding the effects of treatment in any medical sense, and yet the information found in this article is far more likely to have an impact on how we practice in 5 or 10 years than virtually any scientific report one is likely to read. The reason is simple. The development of new, effective medications for managing the wide array of exudative macular diseases has revolutionized the practice of retina. Many more patients are being treated and treated more often than was the case 10 years ago. Anatomic and visual results are impressive. Although the burden of treatment can be substantial, the proof that patients value the results is plain to see; they keep coming back for more! Some treatments are more expensive than others, as the author outlines nicely, and whether the added value of certain treatments justifies the added costs is unclear. When there is no connection between the choice of treatment and the costs, patients are likely to make different choices than when there is a direct impact to the patient in economic terms. The role we as physicians and our patients play in making these choices now is likely to be of diminishing importance in the years to come, as governmental and insurance imperatives drive the evolution of our health care system. How much is one more Snellen line worth?

J. F. Vander, MD

6 Oculoplastic Surgery

Changes to Upper Eyelid Orbital Fat from Use of Topical Bimatoprost, Travoprost, and Latanoprost

Park J, Cho HK, Moon J-I (The Catholic Univ of Korea, Seoul)
Jpn J Ophthalmol 55:22-27, 2011

Purpose.—To confirm the possible mechanism by which topical prostaglandin antiglaucoma drugs cause a deep superior sulcus.

Methods.—Among patients who used bimatoprost (Lumigan), latanoprost (Xalatan), or travoprost (Travatan) and who developed a deep upper lid sulcus, 18 eyes of 11 patients (mean age, 58.2 ± 8.9 years) were studied. Seven patients were binocular users of one of the eye drops and four were monocular users. Preaponeurotic orbital fat was obtained, and the mean adipocyte density compared.

Results.—In the four monocular users, mean adipocyte density of treated eyes was 1758.21 ± 158.15 cells/mm^2, and that of untreated eyes was 1258.73 ± 127.54 cells/mm^2. This difference was statistically significant ($P = 0.04$), suggesting that the adipocytes were atrophied in the treated eyes. The mean adipocyte density of the bimatoprost group was 2073.35 ± 184.89 cells/mm^2, that of the travoprost group was 1623.46 ± 218.99 cells/mm^2, and that of the latanoprost group was 1468.20 ± 113.44 cells/mm^2. The densities of the bimatoprost and travoprost groups, but not of the latanoprost group ($P = 0.75$), were significantly different from that of the untreated group ($P < 0.001$).

Conclusions.—Fat atrophy can be considered a mechanism of upper eyelid sulcus deepening in patients using topical prostaglandin analogs (Table 1).

▶ This is a small study that attempts to show pathologic evidence for why topical prostaglandin analogues cause a deeper superior sulcus in some patients. The study took fat samples from the upper lids of patients on topical bimatoprost, travoprost, and latanoprost who had developed a deepened superior sulcus. Samples were also from untreated eyes.

The results revealed a higher density of adipocytes in the treated eyes compared with controls. As adipocytes atrophy, their cell density goes up. This atrophy was most marked in the bimatoprost users followed by travoprost, and the least difference was seen in the latanoprost users. The difference between these groups and the nonusers was statistically significant with bimatoprost and travoprost but not with latanoprost. Those results seem to go along with clinical observations that

153

TABLE 1.—Characteristics of the Patients

	Treated Group Bimatoprost (Lumigan)	Travoprost (Travatan)	Latanoprost (Xalatan)	Untreated Group
Number of eyes	5	5	8	4
Number of patients (binocular users/monocular users)	3 (2/1)	3 (2/1)	5 (3/2)	
Mean age (years), mean ± SD	58.6 ± 10.3	61.3 ± 9.8	57.9 ± 7.5	59.3 ± 6.4
Sex (M:F)	1:2	2:1	3:2	2:2
Duration of eye-drop usage (years), mean ± SD*	2.4 ± 0.8	4.8 ± 2.3	5.9 ± 3.6	—
Cosopt co-use (eyes)	—	—	2	—
Cosopt & Alphgan P co-use (eyes)	3	4	3	—

Age and sex did not differ significantly among the groups (age, $P = 0.76$; sex, $P = 0.35$).
*$P = 0.02$.

bimatoprost and travoprost are the most likely to cause a deepening of the superior sulcus and latanoprost is less likely to cause it.

It must be remembered this is a very small study, so the statistical strength is not high. Also, the development of a deeper superior sulcus compared with visual loss from glaucoma is a small cosmetic issue. However, the knowledge that this can happen, why it happens, and that it is often reversible makes for better patient care and a better-informed patient.

R. B. Penne, MD

Ocular Surface Morbidity in Eyes with Senile Sunken Upper Eyelids
Liang L, Sheha H, Fu Y, et al (Sun Yat-sen Univ, Guangzhou, China; Ocular Surface Ctr, Miami, FL)
Ophthalmology 118:2487-2492, 2011

Purpose.—To report ocular surface findings in eyes manifesting senile sunken upper eyelids.

Design.—Cross-sectional comparative case series.

Participants.—A study group of 38 eyes of 38 patients with sunken upper eyelids was compared with a control group of 26 age- and gender-matched patients without sunken upper eyelids.

Methods.—Patient records were retrieved and compared between the 2 groups and among different severities of sunken upper lids.

Main Outcome Measures.—Ocular surface deficits were measured by symptoms, eyelid blinking and closure, Bell's phenomenon, apposition of lids and puncta to the globe, conjunctiva inflammation and chalasis, corneal epithelial breakdown by fluorescein and Rose Bengal staining, and the fluorescein clearance test.

Results.—Ocular irritation or pain was less common, but tearing and mucous buildup were more common in the study group than the control group, and it tended to be worse in the morning. Incomplete blinking, incomplete closure, abnormal Bell's phenomenon, lid/punctum ectropion, and delayed tear clearance were more frequently detected in the study group than the control group and were more evident in severely affected eyes. Incomplete blinking was significantly correlated with incomplete closure, whereas abnormal Bell's phenomenon was significantly correlated with early morning symptoms. Conjunctivochalasis was less common in the study group than the control group. Corneal epithelial breakdown was more common in the study group than the control group, and was more severe in severely affected eyes.

Conclusions.—Sunken upper eyelids are associated with ocular surface morbidity characterized by corneal epithelial breakdown because of an array of ocular surface deficits leading to exposure and desiccation, not only during the day but also in the night. Recognition of this potential risk factor will help to understand pathogenesis and formulate effective therapies in complex ocular surface diseases (Fig 1).

▶ This is a chart review of patients with a sunken upper eyelid compared with age-matched controls with specific attention to the ocular surface. The theory is that patients with sunken upper eyelids have changes in their eyelid and orbital anatomy so that they will have more ocular surface problems. The results did

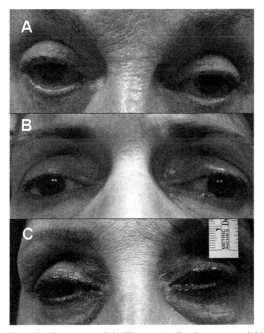

FIGURE 1.—Grading of sunken upper eyelids. The severity of sunken upper eyelid is graded according to the presence of an enlarged invaginated skin space between the brow bone and the upper eyelid as (A) "mild," a space of ≥1 mm mostly in the nasal aspect, (B) "moderate," a space of >3 mm mostly in the nasal but not the entire superior sulcus, or (C) "severe," a space of >3 mm involving the entire superior sulcus. (Reprinted from Liang L, Sheha H, Fu Y, et al. Ocular surface morbidity in eyes with senile sunken upper eyelids. *Ophthalmology.* 2011;118:2487-2492, Copyright 2011, with permission from the American Academy of Ophthalmology.)

156 / Ophthalmology

show a statistically significant increase in corneal surface problems in the patient with a sunken upper eyelid.

The term *senile sunken upper eyelid* has been called many different things. It is a loss of orbital volume that results in this defect and also causes changes in the relationship between the eyelid and the corneal surface and even how the eyelids work to protect and lubricate the eye. The classic appearance of this deepened upper eyelid does not always go along with corneal problems. However, I have seen a few patients like those in the study with significant corneal surface problems, and they have been very difficult to treat.

This is another thing to think about when people have significant corneal surface problems that do not respond to the usual treatment. The difficulty is we don't have any standard treatment for the orbital volume deficiency to easily solve this. The thought would be to place an orbital implant of some type in the orbit to increase the volume. I have never done that for this problem, but from the anatomic approach it should help. Further study of potential treatments and their effectiveness is the next step.

R. B. Penne, MD

Selenium and the Course of Mild Graves' Orbitopathy
Marcocci C, for the European Group on Graves' Orbitopathy (Univ of Pisa, Italy; et al)
N Engl J Med 364:1920-1931, 2011

Background.—Oxygen free radicals and cytokines play a pathogenic role in Graves' orbitopathy.

Methods.—We carried out a randomized, double-blind, placebo-controlled trial to determine the effect of selenium (an antioxidant agent) or pentoxifylline (an antiinflammatory agent) in 159 patients with mild Graves' orbitopathy. The patients were given selenium (100 μg twice daily), pentoxifylline (600 mg twice daily), or placebo (twice daily) orally for 6 months and were then followed for 6 months after treatment was withdrawn. Primary outcomes at 6 months were evaluated by means of an overall ophthalmic assessment, conducted by an ophthalmologist who was unaware of the treatment assignments, and a Graves' orbitopathy–specific quality-of-life questionnaire, completed by the patient. Secondary outcomes were evaluated with the use of a Clinical Activity Score and a diplopia score.

Results.—At the 6-month evaluation, treatment with selenium, but not with pentoxifylline, was associated with an improved quality of life (P<0.001) and less eye involvement (P=0.01) and slowed the progression of Graves' orbitopathy (P=0.01), as compared with placebo. The Clinical Activity Score decreased in all groups, but the change was significantly greater in the selenium-treated patients. Exploratory evaluations at 12 months confirmed the results seen at 6 months. Two patients assigned to placebo and one assigned to pentoxifylline required immunosuppressive therapy for deterioration in their condition. No adverse events were evident

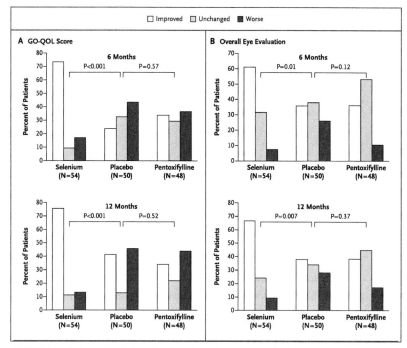

FIGURE 2.—Primary End Points. Panel A shows the changes reflected in the score on the Graves' orbitopathy—specific quality-of-life questionnaire (GO-QOL) at 6 months and 12 months. This questionnaire measures limitations in visual functioning (as a consequence of diplopia, decreased visual acuity, or both) and in psychosocial functioning (as a consequence of a changed appearance). Panel B shows the changes at 6 months and 12 months in overall results of the eye evaluation performed by an ophthalmologist who was unaware of the treatment assignments. The quality of life and overall eye evaluations were considered to be improved, unchanged, or worsened according to predefined criteria. Differences in proportions were tested with the use of the contingency 3×2 chi-square test. (Reprinted from Marcocci C, for the European Group on Graves' Orbitopathy. Selenium and the course of mild Graves' orbitopathy. *N Engl J Med*. 2011;364:1920-1931, Copyright 2011 Massachusetts Medical Society. All rights reserved.)

with selenium, whereas pentoxifylline was associated with frequent gastro-intestinal problems.

Conclusions.—Selenium administration significantly improved quality of life, reduced ocular involvement, and slowed progression of the disease in patients with mild Graves' orbitopathy. (Funded by the University of Pisa and the Italian Ministry for Education, University and Research; EUGOGO Netherlands Trial Register number, NTR524.) (Fig 2).

▶ This is a very interesting article using selenium to treat Graves' orbitopathy (GO). The study is well designed. It is a randomized, double-blind, placebo-controlled trial with 3 arms. Patients were given selenium, pentoxifylline (an anti-inflammatory agent), or placebo twice a day for 6 months and then followed for an additional 6 months. All patients had mild GO. They were examined at baseline, 3, 6, and 12 months after initiation of the study. Evaluation was done by an ophthalmologist, and the patient completed a Graves' orbitopathy-specific quality-of-life questionnaire.

The results showed the patients taking selenium had improved quality of life, reduced ocular involvement, and slowed progression of the disease compared with the other 2 groups. These effects were maintained 6 months after completion of the treatment (Fig 2).

This is remarkable work that requires further study; it suggests that the use of a simple chemical element, selenium, an antioxidant, may improve GO. Multiple follow-up questions to be answered from this study include: whether these patients could have been selenium-deficient, (selenium levels were not checked); whether selenium would have any effect in more advanced GO; and whether selenium should be continued beyond 6 months?

At the very least, I think this suggests that patients with mild GO should be on selenium for at least 6 months. The dose is low (100 μg twice a day) and appears safe; there were no adverse effects in the study. Selenium toxicity is possible, but it is thought that up to 800 μg per day is safe. Whether this proves to be a useful treatment only time will tell, but for now, it is one small thing to help patients with GO when we often have limited options.

R. B. Penne, MD

Oral Propranolol for Treatment of Periocular Infantile Hemangiomas
Missoi TG, Lueder GT, Gilbertson K, et al (Univ of Missouri—Columbia; Washington Univ in St Louis, MO)
Arch Ophthalmol 129:899-903, 2011

Objective.—To evaluate the efficacy and adverse effects of oral propranolol for treatment of periocular infantile hemangioma.

Methods.—Participants were treated with oral propranolol 3 times daily, with outpatient monitoring of adverse effects. The starting dosage was 0.5 mg/kg/d for 1 week, then 1 mg/kg/d for the following week, then 2 mg/kg/d for the remaining duration of treatment. Serial examinations and external photography documented the size of the hemangiomas. Complete ophthalmic examinations included assessing for amblyopia with cycloplegic refraction and visual diagnostic testing. Amblyopia was treated with part-time occlusion therapy.

Results.—Nineteen periocular hemangiomas from 17 children (71% girls) were studied. The median age at the start of treatment was 4.5 months (interquartile range, 2.2-5.6 months). The median treatment duration was 6.8 months (interquartile range, 4.1-7.2 months). Treatment with oral propranolol reduced the size of all hemangiomas. Median change in the surface area was 61% (interquartile range, 32%-64%) of the original size. Mild rebound growth that did not necessitate retreatment was found in 2 patients (12%). One patient (6%) experienced a benign episode of bradycardia. Seven patients (41%) had amblyopia.

Conclusions.—Oral propranolol for treatment of infantile hemangiomas was effective in all patients, with 33% reduction in astigmatism and 39% reduction in surface area. Vision equalized in all but 1 child, who receives ongoing amblyopia therapy. Our results suggest that early treatment with propranolol is remarkably effective in treating and preventing loss of visual acuity associated with periocular infantile hemangiomas.

▶ The use of oral propranolol for the treatment of infantile hemangiomas is becoming recognized as the treatment of choice. This is a retrospective study of 19 hemangiomas in 17 patients, which is one of the largest groups studied to date. All 19 patients demonstrated a reduction in size of the hemangioma with the initiation of oral propranolol (Figs 1 and 3 in the original article).

In addition to confirming that oral propranolol works in the treatment of infantile hemangiomas, another important point from this study is that these patients were treated on an outpatient basis with a standardized dose of propranolol. Other authors have suggested the need for inpatient initiation of propranolol treatment. All these patients were treated safely as outpatients. The dosage of propranolol is outlined in the article.

Although additional studies are still needed, the use of propranolol has become the treatment of choice for infantile hemangiomas. I would still recommend consultation with a pediatric cardiologist before initiating propranolol as an outpatient as well as for monitoring during treatment.

R. B. Penne, MD

Clinical Relevance of Thyroid-Stimulating Immunoglobulins in Graves' Ophthalmopathy

Ponto KA, Kanitz M, Olivo PD, et al (Univ Med Ctr, Mainz, Germany; Diagnostic Hybrids Inc, Athens, OH)
Ophthalmology 118:2279-2285, 2011

Purpose.—Thyroid-stimulating immunoglobulins (TSIs) likely mediate Graves' ophthalmopathy (GO). The clinical relevance of these functional autoantibodies was assessed in GO.

Design.—Cross-sectional trial.

Participants.—A total of 108 untreated patients with GO.

Methods.—Thyroid-stimulating immunoglobulins, assessed with a novel bioassay, bind to the thyrotropin receptor (TSHR) and transmit signals for cyclic adenosine monophosphate (cAMP)-dependent activation of luciferase gene expression. The cAMP/cAMP response element-binding protein/cAMP-regulatory element complex induces luciferase that is quantified after cell lysis. The TSI levels were correlated with activity and severity of GO and compared with a TSHR binding inhibitory immunoglobulin (TBII) assay.

Main Outcome Measures.—Thyroid-stimulating immunoglobulins, activity and severity of GO, diplopia, and TBII.

Results.—Thyroid-stimulating immunoglobulins were detected in 106 of 108 patients (98%) with GO. All 53 hyperthyroid patients were TSI positive versus 47 patients (89%) who were TBII positive. All 69 patients with active GO were TSI positive, whereas only 58 of 69 patients (84%)

were TBII positive. Thyroid-stimulating immunoglobulins correlated with the activity (r=0.83, $P < 0.001$) and severity (r=0.81, $P < 0.001$) of GO. All 59 patients with GO with diplopia were TSI positive, and 50 of 59 patients (85%) were TBII positive. Among patients with moderate-to-severe and mild GO, 75 of 75 (100%) and 31 of 33 (94%) were TSI positive compared with TBII positivity in 63 of 75 (84%) and 24 of 33 (73%), respectively. The TSI levels were higher in moderate-to-severe versus mild GO (489% ± 137% vs. 251% ± 100%, $P < 0.001$). Chemosis and GO activity predicted TSI levels alone ($P < 0.001$, multivariable analysis). The TSI levels were higher in patients with chemosis (527% ± 131%) than in patients without chemosis (313% ± 127%, $P < 0.001$).

Conclusions.—Thyroid-stimulating immunoglobulins show more significant association with clinical features of GO than TBII and may be regarded as functional biomarkers for GO (Table 3).

▶ The search for a marker to use to monitor the disease activity of patients with Graves' ophthalmopathy (GO) points to thyroid-stimulating immunoglobulins (TSI) as that marker. This study looks at 108 patients with untreated GO and relates TSI levels and thyrotropin receptor (TSHR)-binding inhibitory immunoglobulin (TBII) levels to disease activity and severity.

This study looks at 2 things in relation to TSI and GO. A more specific assay to measure thyrotropin receptor antibodies that are stimulating is compared with the commercially available test of TBII. At the same time, this study confirms that disease severity and activity correlate with these levels. Not surprising, the assay of TSI, which is specific for the stimulating immunoglobulin, correlates better than TBII, which measures all forms of antibodies that bind to the TSHR, both stimulating and binding/blocking antibodies. The TSI levels were positive in 100% of patients with mild-to-severe GO (Table 3). In addition, the patients with moderate-to-severe GO had statistically significant higher levels of TSI when compared with patients with mild disease.

TABLE 3.—Prevalence of Thyrotropin Receptor Stimulating Immunoglobulins and Thyrotropin Receptor Binding Inhibitory Immunoglobulins with Respect to the Clinical Activity Score and to the Seven Individual Parameters

	n	TSI Positive, (SRR% ≥140%), n (%)	TBII Positive, (≥1 IU/L), n (%)	P Value
Active GO	69	69 (100)	58 (84)	0.196
Inactive GO	39	37 (95)	29 (74)	
Redness of the conjunctiva	89	88 (99)	71 (80)	0.172
Swelling of the eyelids	87	87 (100)	69 (79)	0.024
Chemosis	52	52 (100)	44 (85)	0.440
Pain, spontaneously	24	24 (100)	20 (83)	0.877
Pain, when moving the eye	20	20 (100)	16 (80)	0.922
Redness of the eyelids	20	20 (100)	13 (65)	0.194
Redness/swelling of the caruncle	18	18 (100)	16 (89)	0.726

GO = Graves' ophthalmopathy; TBII = TSHR binding inhibitory immunoglobulin; TSHR = thyrotropin receptor; TSI = thyroid-stimulating immunoglobulins.

The downside of this study is it only looked at the patients' disease and TSI/ TBII levels once. We did not get data to show how these levels changed as the disease activity changed. Showing that the TSI levels increased or decreased as the disease activity increased or decreased would make this more valuable. We also need to know if the change in levels precede or follow the disease activity changes on an individual basis.

This study continues to add to our knowledge of GO. Whether this new assay for TSI will become the gold standard is unclear. We certainly have more information to work with, but we still have a long way to go in predicting the course of GO and better treating it.

R. B. Penne, MD

The Effect of Orbital Decompression Surgery on Lid Retraction in Thyroid Eye Disease
Cho RI, Elner VM, Nelson CC, et al (Univ of Michigan, Ann Arbor)
Ophthal Plast Reconstr Surg 27:436-438, 2011

Purpose.—To determine the effect of orbital decompression surgery on lid retraction as a function of proptosis reduction in the setting of thyroid eye disease.

Methods.—Retrospective interventional case series of all consecutive medial and lateral orbital decompressions performed by the authors for thyroid eye disease from 1999 to 2008. Primary outcome measures included postoperative proptosis and lid retraction.

Results.—One hundred sixty-five eyes of 89 patients were included. The average amount of proptosis reduction at final follow up (average 30 months) was 4.6 mm. The average improvement in upper lid retraction was 0.9 mm, and the average improvement in lower lid retraction was 0.8 mm. There was a statistically significant correlation (0.12, p = 0.005) between the amount of proptosis reduction and lower lid elevation. No such correlation (−0.010, p = 0.90) was seen for upper lid position. In cases where inferior rectus recession was performed subsequent to decompression surgery (n = 20), the effect of proptosis reduction on lower lid position was negated (correlation −0.01, p = 0.980).

Conclusion.—A statistically significant correlation exists between the amount of proptosis reduction from orbital decompression surgery and improvement in lower lid retraction. No such correlation exists between proptosis reduction and upper lid retraction. Inferior rectus recession negates the positive effect of orbital decompression on lower lid position (Fig 1, Table 1).

▶ This retrospective case review study looks at the changes in upper and lower eyelid position after orbital decompression surgery. All these surgeries were either medial wall or medial and lateral wall decompressions. The results showed that the larger the reduction in proptosis, the larger the improvement in the lower lid retraction (Fig 1). The upper lid position did not show a similar correlation,

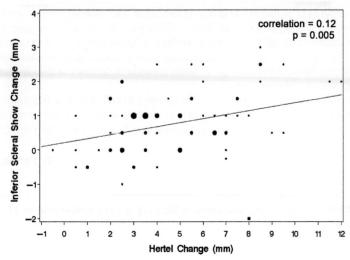

FIGURE 1.—Scatter plot showing positive correlation between proptosis reduction and lower eyelid elevation at final follow-up. Positive values represent postoperative improvement. Dot size is proportional to number of observations at each data point. (Reprinted from Cho RI, Elner VM, Nelson CC, et al. The effect of orbital decompression surgery on lid retraction in thyroid eye disease. *Ophthal Plast Reconstr Surg.* 2011;27:436-438, with permission from The American Society of Ophthalmic Plastic and Reconstructive Surgery.)

TABLE 1.—Demographics and Surgical Data

Characteristic	Eyes (n = 165)
Age at TED diagnosis, years (range)	44 (12–81)
Gender (M:F), patients (n = 89)	25:64
Operative eye (right:left:both)	5:8:76
Time between TED diagnosis and first surgery, months (range)	55.5 (3–309)
Walls decompressed, n (%)	
Medial	18 (10.9)
Lateral	23 (13.9)
Medial and lateral	124 (75.2)
Fat removal	48 (29.1)
Subsequent surgeries, n (%)	
Strabismus	53 (32.1)
Medial rectus recession	48 (29.1)
Inferior rectus recession	20 (12.1)
Upper lid retraction	48 (29.1)
Lower lid retraction	24 (14.5)
Lateral tarsorrhaphy	2 (1.2)
Radiation therapy	6 (3.6)
Follow-up interval, patients (n = 89)	
3 months, n (%)	87 (97.7)
Final, n (%)	64 (71.9)
Interval, months (range)	30 (5–95)

M:F, male:female.

although there was some improvement in upper lid retraction after decompression as well (Table 1).

I do orbital decompressions that are either orbital floor or orbital floor plus medial wall. I often see an improvement in lower eyelid retraction and have always attributed it to the inferior shift of the globe associated with the floor decompression. The result of this study notwithstanding, there is an additional factor of the proptosis reduction reducing the lower eyelid retraction. This also confirms the need to do surgery on patients with thyroid eye disease in the proper order. How much the lower lids change is not so critical because we don't do eyelid surgery until after any orbital decompressive surgery and any required muscle surgery has been completed.

R. B. Penne, MD

Smoking and Strabismus Surgery in Patients with Thyroid Eye Disease
Rajendram R, Bunce C, Adams GGW, et al (Moorfields Eye Hosp, London, UK; et al)
Ophthalmology 118:2493-2497, 2011

Objective.—To investigate the relationship between smoking status at presentation and the use of strabismus surgery in the management of patients with thyroid eye disease.

Design.—Retrospective review of a noncomparative series of patients with thyroid eye disease.

Participants.—All patients with thyroid eye disease under the care of a single consultant at Moorfields Eye Hospital between 1997 and 2002 (inclusive).

Methods.—Retrospective review of clinical case notes.

Main Outcome Measures.—Survival analysis of patients in cohort and the frequency of strabismus surgery in relation to smoking status at ophthalmic presentation. A subanalysis of patients who underwent orbital decompression and those that did not was undertaken.

Results.—Of 501 patients seen during the study period, 425 (85%) of 501 sets of notes were available for review, and initial smoking status was recorded for 89% (378/425) of patients, of whom approximately one half (196/378; 52%) were active smokers. Of the smokers, 51 (26%) of 196 underwent strabismus surgery, compared with only 19 (14%) of 138 nonsmokers at presentation. When adjusted for age, the hazards ratio of having strabismus surgery during management for smokers at presentation versus nonactive smokers was 2.19. In the group who did not undergo orbital decompression, this hazard ratio increased to 4.86.

Conclusions.—Within this thyroid eye disease cohort, the proportion of smokers at presentation was much larger than that of the general population. There was an increased use of strabismus surgery in active smokers at presentation than in nonactive smokers. This finding was independent of the orbital decompression surgery. The results are consistent with those of previous reports of more severe thyroid eye disease in smokers and raise the possibility that smoking cessation early in the disease may reduce the severity of the changes and the number of rehabilitative strabismus operations needed.

▶ This article proves again that patients who smoke and have thyroid eye disease (TED) have a longer, more difficult course with more surgery than those who do not. The specific aim of this retrospective chart review was at the need for strabismus surgery in smokers versus nonsmokers. It was shown that patients with TED who are smokers at the time of presentation have a 2-fold increased chance of requiring strabismus surgery.

There were other interesting findings in this study. Because smoking increases the severity of TED, more of these smoking patients will require orbital decompression surgery. Because it is known that patients who undergo orbital decompressive surgery are more likely to need strabismus surgery, it could be argued that it was the orbital decompression that increased the need for strabismus surgery not the smoking. These investigators looked at patients not having decompressions, and there was still a statistically significant increased risk of requiring strabismus surgery in smokers compared with nonsmokers. Another finding was that 86% of patients with TED in the study were either current smokers (52%) or had stopped smoking within the preceding 5 years. This is another article proving the importance of patients with TED trying to stop smoking. I believe this is the most effective thing a patient with TED who smokes can do to treat their TED. It is very important for every physician to communicate this to patients who smoke and have TED.

R. B. Penne, MD

Medical Management Versus Surgical Intervention of Pediatric Orbital Cellulitis: The Importance of Subperiosteal Abscess Volume as a New Criterion
Todman MS, Enzer YR (Rhode Island Hosp and the Warren Alpert Med School of Brown Univ, Providence)
Ophthal Plast Reconstr Surg 27:255-259, 2011

Purpose.—To investigate age and frontal sinusitis as indications for the surgical management of pediatric orbital cellulitis with subperiosteal abscess (SPA) and to create an SPA volume criterion that would favor nonsurgical management.

Methods.—A retrospective chart review was performed to find all patients age 18 years and younger who presented to Hasbro Children's Hospital with orbital cellulitis secondary to sinusitis with an SPA from 2005 to 2009. SPA volume was measured using a CT ruler at the largest axial, coronal, and sagittal dimensions. Student t testing was used for statistical analysis.

Results.—Twenty-nine patients were included: 8 (27.6%) were managed surgically and 21 (72.4%) were managed medically. The mean age of patients undergoing surgical management was 7.0 years old versus medical management 6.1 years old and was statistically similar ($p < 0.001$). The age range of patients undergoing surgical management was 17 months to 11 years versus 4 months to 13.4 years for medical management. The mean volume of abscesses needing surgery were larger (3,446.3 mm^3) than abscesses not needing surgery (420.5 mm^3) ($p < 0.04$). Volumes of <1,250 mm^3 did not require surgical management ($p < 0.001$). The frontal sinuses were visualized on CT scan in 17 patients; frontal sinusitis was found in 11 of 17 (64.7%) patients; of these 11 patients, 4 (36.4%) underwent surgical drainage and only 2 (18.2%) showed positive culture results. The 2 (18.2%) patients who had positive culture results had an SPA volume that was ≥1,250 mm^3.

Conclusions.—The volume of SPA seemed to be the most important criterion in determining medical versus surgical management. The volumes of abscesses needing surgery were larger than the volumes of abscesses not needing surgery. Volumes of <1,250 mm^3 did not require surgical management. Most cases of SPA with concurrent frontal sinusitis do not require surgical intervention. The cases of frontal sinusitis requiring surgical intervention always had concurrent SPA volumes of ≥1,250 mm^3. Patients both under 9 years old and ≥9 years old required surgical intervention with SPA volumes of <1,250 mm^3 being a consistent determining factor (Fig A-E, Table 1).

▶ Management of a pediatric subperiosteal abscess (SPA) often comes down to whether to drain the SPA or to treat it medically. The classic article by Garcia and Harris[1] in 2000 gave outlines on how to decide. Surgical drainage was suggested

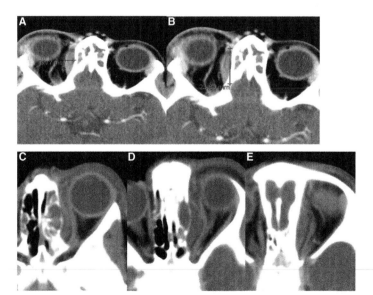

FIGURE.—A–E, Axial views of SPA at the largest axial, coronal, and sagittal dimensions. (Reprinted from Todman MS, Enzer YR. Medical management versus surgical intervention of pediatric orbital cellulitis: the importance of subperiosteal abscess volume as a new criterion. *Ophthal Plast Reconstr Surg.* 2011;27:255-259, with permission from The American Society of Ophthalmic Plastic and Reconstructive Surgery, Inc.)

TABLE 1.—Subperiosteal Culture Results

Patient No./Sex	Age (Years Old)	Microbial Culture Results	Days of Medical Management Before Surgical Drainage	Reasons for Surgical Drainage	Volume of SPA (mm³)	Presence of Frontal Sinusitis
1/M*	4.6	n/a	n/a		17	Y
2/M*	5.0	n/a	n/a		26	Y
3/M*	13.4	n/a	n/a		58	Y
4/M*	8.8	n/a	n/a		84	N
5/F*	6.1	n/a	n/a		90	No view
6/M*	5.4	n/a	n/a		108	No view
7/F*	0.3	n/a	n/a		118	No view
8/M	6.0	No growth	5	Minimal EOM restriction, worsening proptosis, repeat imaging with increase in size of SPA	129	Y
9/M*	1.8	n/a	n/a		160	No view
10/F*	2.2	n/a	n/a		203	No view
11/M*	3.0	n/a	n/a		225	No view
12/F*	8.8	n/a	n/a		297	Y
13/M*	10.0	n/a	n/a		338	N
14/F*	1.0	n/a	n/a		432	No view
15/M*	3.7	n/a	n/a		466	No view
16/M*	1.3	n/a	n/a		476	No view
17/F*	11.0	n/a	n/a		513	No view
18/M*	6.0	n/a	n/a		614	Y
19/M*	7.0	n/a	n/a		696	Y
20/F*	8.4	n/a	n/a		720	N
21/F	3.0	No growth	6	VA unreliable, proptosis, repeat imaging with no improvement in size of SPA	991	No view
22/M*	11.0	n/a	n/a		1000	Y
23/F	11.0	No growth	5	Minimal EOM restriction, pain with eye movement, proptosis	1103	Y
24/M*	10.0	n/a	n/a		1230	N
25/M	10.5	Staphylococcus aureus	4	EOMs nearly fully restricted in upgaze, intracranial abscess noted on repeat CT scan	1251	Y

26/F	5.0	Methicillin-resistant S. aureus	3	Nearly full EOM restriction, persistent fevers	1296	N
27/M	1.4	Streptococcus pneumoniae	2	Full EOM restriction, persistent fevers	1633	No view
28/M	8.0	Streptococcus pyogenes	1	VA 20/80 with nearly full EOM restriction	5032	N
29/M	10.8	Streptococcus pyogenes	2	Nearly full EOM restriction	8020	Y

EOM, extraocular movement; n/a, not applicable; SPA, subperiosteal abscess; VA visual acuity.
*Drainage was not performed.

in children 9 years or older, in instances of frontal sinusitis, nonmedial SPA, chronic sinusitis, aerobic infection, optic nerve or retina compromise, recurrent SPA, or SPA of dental origin. Many ophthalmologists simply remember that children younger than 9 years may not need drainage but often forget the other criteria outlined. This article looks at abscess volume as a criterion for drainage with the suggestion that volumes less than 1250 mm^3 are less likely to require drainage (Fig A-E).

This was a retrospective chart review, and it did find that SPA volumes less than 1250 mm^3 are less likely to require drainage. Three patients with SPA volumes less than 1250 mm^3 did require drainage. All 5 patients with SPA volumes greater than 1250 mm^3 did require drainage (Table 1). I believe this is a helpful criterion, but, as discussed in the article, it cannot be the only criteria. It would appear from this study that if the volume is greater than 1250 mm^3, drainage will be needed. If the volume is less, then drainage is less likely but could still be needed. As with much of medicine, we use guidelines, but the ultimate decision on treatment is often the "art of medicine."

This article emphasizes the importance of abscess volume in treatment of pediatric SPA. I will place more emphasis on volume in future treatment decisions but will still use the other guidelines outlined by Garcia and Harris.

R. B. Penne, MD

Reference

1. Garcia GH, Harris GJ. Criteria for nonsurgical management of subperiosteal abscess of the orbit: analysis of outcomes 1988–1998. *Ophthalmology.* 2000; 107:1454-1458.

Results of Lacrimal Gland Botulinum Toxin Injection for Epiphora in Lacrimal Obstruction and Gustatory Tearing
Wojno TH (The Emory Clinic, Atlanta, GA)
Ophthal Plast Reconstr Surg 27:119-121, 2011

Purpose.—To describe the author's experience with the use of botulinum toxin (Botox, Allergan Inc., Irvine, CA, U.S.A.) injection in the palpebral lobe of the lacrimal gland for symptomatic epiphora due to lacrimal obstruction or gustatory tearing.

Methods.—This is a retrospective review of 46 patients treated by the author with botulinum toxin injection in the palpebral lobe of the lacrimal gland for symptomatic epiphora due to lacrimal obstruction or gustatory tearing from 2001 through 2008. All patients were injected with 2.5 units of botulinum toxin, and the patients' subjective responses were assessed 1 to 2 weeks later. If there was insufficient response, they were reinjected with an additional 2.5 units of botulinum toxin and re-evaluated in 1 to 2 weeks. The response to the treatment and complications were evaluated.

Results.—Overall, 74% of patients treated felt that tearing was mostly or completely improved. The only complication was temporary ptosis in 11% of the patients.

TABLE 3.—Overall Results

Overall Result	Initial 2.5-Unit Treatment	Additional 2.5-Unit Treatment	Overall Improvement
Completely improved	27 (60%)	—	34 (74%)
Improved	11 (24%)	11	8 (17%)
Little improvement	8 (17%)	8	4 (9%)
Total	46* (100%)	19	46 (100%)

*Twenty-four women; 22 men.

Conclusion.—Botulinum toxin injection in the palpebral lobe of the lacrimal gland can be used effectively and safely for symptomatic epiphora due to lacrimal obstruction and gustatory tearing. Although beneficial results are temporary, patient satisfaction in select patients is high (Table 3).

▶ Tearing that cannot be corrected by lacrimal surgery or gustatory tearing can be very frustrating to patients. Patients may be unable to have surgery from a medical standpoint or may have multiple surgery failures. This article offers an alternative, although temporary, to decrease this constant tearing. This article describes the injection of 2.5 U of botulinum toxin directly into the palpebral lobe of the lacrimal gland in 46 patients as a simple office procedure. The results showed that 74% of patients felt the tearing was mostly or completely improved. The onset of maximal improvement was 1 to 2 weeks. As expected, the effects were temporary with a duration of 3 months. The one side effect that must be discussed is that 11% of patients developed a temporary ptosis. The other downside of this treatment is that the use of botulinum toxin was off-label, so this warrants discussion. Likewise, this will not be reimbursed by insurance.

I have used this injection a few times, but the use has been limited by what I perceive as a higher rate of ptosis. I used a larger amount of Botox, which may be the reason, and will try this dosage. The other issue, as noted above, is obtaining this small amount of botulinum toxin when the patient's insurance does not cover it. It is not a problem if a practice does a lot of cosmetic botulinum toxin injections, as 2.5 U costs less than $15. However, needing to open a full bottle of botulinum toxin, even if it is only 50 units, is much more costly.

R. B. Penne, MD

Comparison of nonlaser nonendoscopic endonasal dacryocystorhinostomy with external dacryocystorhinostomy
Walker RA, Al-Ghoul A, Conlon MR (Univ of Saskatchewan, Saskatoon, Canada; Univ of Calgary, Alberta, Canada)
Can J Ophthalmol 46:191-195, 2011

Objective.—To compare the success rate of nonlaser nonendoscopic dacryocystorhinostomy (EN-DCR) with that of external DCR (EX-DCR).

Design.—Retrospective chart review.

Participants.—Eighty-eight patients that underwent 102 consecutive EN-DCR or EX-DCR between November 1, 1995, and September 1, 2003.

Methods.—All DCRs were performed by a single ophthalmologist. The surgical protocol remained constant, and surgical success was defined as a lack of symptoms that indicated DCR or normal canalicular irrigation.

Results.—Eighty-eight patients were reviewed, equating to 102 cases of DCR (56 EX-DCR and 46 EN-DCR). The average age of patients was 63.2 ± 18.2 years old (range, 19–93 years), and the average duration of surgery was 32.1 minutes for EX-DCR and 23.3 minutes for EN-DCR ($p < 0.0001$). Three cases of intraoperative bleed requiring nasal packing were documented in EX-DCR and 2 cases in EN-DCR. The success rates were 89.8% and 90.2% for EX-DCR and EN-DCR, respectively. There was no statistical difference between these 2 numbers. The average follow-up time was 12.8 months (median, 5 months; range, 2–97 months).

Conclusions.—We found that the endonasal approach to DCRs was quicker than the external approach and the success and complication rates of both methods were comparable.

▶ This is one of a number of recent articles that compares the success rate of external dacryocystorhinostomy (DCR) with a transnasal approach. This was a retrospective study that showed the success rate was essentially the same with the 2 approaches. The success rate was defined by lack of epiphora and an open lacrimal system on irrigation. The success rate was 89.8% and 90.2% with external DCR and transnasal DCR, respectively. This was a nonendoscopic trans-nasal approach, but this approach is really comparable to an endoscopic trans-nasal approach.

It appears from this article and others that the success rates in these 2 types of DCR approaches have become the same. As with many procedures, individual patient selection is now the criteria for deciding which procedure to use. I do both external and endoscopic DCRs (with ear, nose and throat). I am doing more endoscopic DCRs than I used to and am happy that I can now tell patients that the success rate is similar. I still use the external approach for patients with canalicular narrowing and suspected tumor. I do transnasal procedures combined with ear, nose, and throat under general anesthesia, while I often do external DCR under local anesthesia with sedation. So some patients are better done with seda-tion. Finally, the total cost is much higher for the endoscopic approach because of the endoscopic equipment, and all patients have stereotactic imaging used for the surgery. If patients have to pay a large portion of the cost, this may affect the surgical choice.

The bottom line is we have equalized the success rates between external and nonlaser transnasal DCR surgery. There remain many variations on how the surgery is done, and these factors will influence which approach is best for an individual patient.

R. B. Penne, MD

A meta-analysis of primary dacryocystorhinostomy with and without silicone intubation

Feng Y-F, Cai J-Q, Zhang J-Y, et al (The Affiliated Eye Hosp of Wenzhou Med College, Zhejiang, China; Yuying Children's Hosp of Wenzhou Med College, Zhejiang, China; Ruian People's Hosp of Wenzhou Med College, Zhejiang, China)
Can J Ophthalmol 46:521-527, 2011

Objective.—To examine possible differences in success rates of primary dacryocystorhinostomy (DCR) with and without silicone intubation, and to find out whether the use of silicone tubes is beneficial.

Design.—A literature search was conducted in the PubMed, EMBASE, and Cochrane Controlled Trials Register to identify potentially relevant controlled trials.

Methods.—Language was restricted to English. The surgical techniques were categorized into external DCR (EX-DCR), endonasal laser-assisted DCR (LA-DCR), and nonlaser endoscopic endonasal DCR techniques (EN-DCR). The main outcome measure was success rates after DCR-with and DCR-without silicone intubation. The statistical analysis was carried out using a RevMan 5.0 software.

Results.—Of 188 retrieved trials from the electronic database, 9 trials (5 randomized controlled trials and 4 cohort studies) involving 514 cases met our inclusion criteria. There was no statistically significant heterogeneity

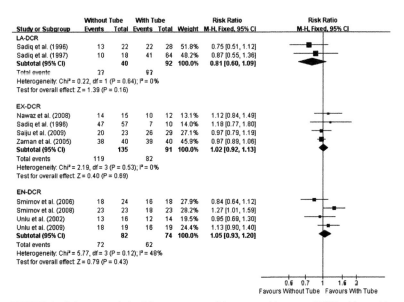

FIGURE 4.—Subgroup analysis of the success rate of dacryocystorhinostomy (DCR) with or without silicone intubation. CI, confidence interval; EN-DCR, endoscopic endonasal dacryocystorhinostomy; EX-DCR, external dacryocystorhinostomy; LA-DCR, endonasal laser-assisted dacryocystorhinostomy; RR, relative risk. (Reprinted from Feng Y-F, Cai J-Q, Zhang J-Y, et al. A meta-analysis of primary dacryocystorhinostomy with and without silicone intubation. *Can J Ophthalmol.* 2011;46:521-527, with permission from Canadian Ophthalmological Society.)

TABLE 1.—Summary of Characteristics of Included Studies

Author	Country	Study Design	Surgical Technique	Mean Age (Year)	Mean Follow-Up (Months)	No. of Patients (Eyes)	Gender (M/F)	Withdrawal (Eyes)	Silicone Removed	Outcomes Measured
Sadiq et al.[19]*	UK	Cohort	LA-DCR	LA: 65.8	4	49 (50)	20/29	0	NA	Sx
Sadiq et al.[19]*	UK	Cohort	EX-DCR	EX: 60.8	4.5	67 (67)	24/43	0	NA	Sx
Sadiq et al.[20]	UK	Cohort	LA-DCR	63.5 (range, 19–91)	12	85 (97)	28/57	15	3 months	Sx
Unlu et al.[21]	Turkey	Cohort	EN-DCR	43.0 (range, 23–66)	15	25 (30)	5/25	NA	8 weeks	Sx, EDT, endosc
Smirnov et al.[22]	US	Cohort	EN-DCR	59 (range, 19–80)	4	36 (42)	11/25	0	NA	Sx, irrig
Zaman et al.[23]	Pakistan	RCT	EX-DCR	30–60	12	80 (80)	30/50	0	6 months	Sx, irrig
Smirnov et al.[24]	US	RCT	EN-DCR	64	6	42 (46)	9/37	0	2 months	Sx, EDT
Unlu et al.[25]	Turkey	RCT	EN-DCR	55.4 (range,32–73)	99.6	42 (44)	9/29	6	8 weeks	endosc, EDT, Jones
Saiju et al.[26]	US	RCT	EX-DCR	41 (range,18–82)	6	100 (100)	22/78	48	6 weeks	Sx, irrig
Nawaz et al.[27]	Pakistan	RCT	EX-DCR	45 (range,20–65)	12	27 (27)	23/4	0	4 months	Sx, inf

Note: EDT, endoscope dye test; EN-DCR, endoscopic endonasal dacryocystorhinostomy; Endosc, patent ostium on nasal endoscopy; EX-DCR, external dacryocystorhinostomy; Irrig, irrigation; inf, infection; Jones, Jones I test; LA-DCR, endonasal laser-assisted dacryocystorhinostomy; NA, not available; SD, standard deviation; Sx, symptomatic relief; UK, United Kingdom; US, United States.

Editor's Note: Please refer to original journal article for full references.

*The study included 2 surgical techniques, LA-DCR and EX-DCR.

between the studies. The pooled risk ratio was 0.99, with a 95% confidence interval (0.91−1.08). There was no significant difference in the success rates between the DCR with and without silicone intubation ($p = 0.81$). Sensitivity analysis and subgroups analyses suggested that the result was comparatively reliable.

Conclusions.—Based on this meta-analysis that included 5 randomized controlled trials and 4 cohort studies, no benefit was found for silicone tube intubation in primary DCR. Further well-organized, prospective, randomized studies involving larger patient numbers are required (Fig 4, Table 1).

▶ This article brings up an interesting question concerning dacryocystorhinostomy (DCR) surgery. It is generally accepted that any DCR surgery, whether external, endoscopic, or laser assisted, will involve tube placement. The question is asked if there is any proof that silicone intubation improves the results. For such an accepted part of DCR surgery, there does not seem to be any real good evidence that surgery with silicone intubation is more successful than without.

The authors review the literature and do a meta-analysis of the cases found in the literature comparing DCR surgery with and without silicone intubation (Fig 4, Table 1). The conclusion is that there is no difference in the results with and without silicone intubation.

What this entire study really means is that we really need a large randomized study of at least 276 patients according to the authors to look for that answer. Until then, I will continue to use silicone tubes as their use is, for now, the standard of care. Hopefully, we can answer this question for this relatively commonly performed procedure in the near future.

R. B. Penne, MD

Late failure of dacryocystorhinostomy
McMurray CJ, McNab AA, Selva D (Royal Victorian Eye and Ear Hosp, Melbourne, Australia)
Ophthal Plast Reconstr Surg 27:99-101, 2011

Purpose.—The authors describe a group of patients with initially successful dacryocystorhinostomy surgery with late recurrence of epiphora. The causes of late failure and its management are documented.

Methods.—A retrospective chart review of primary dacryocystorhinostomy cases was undertaken. Inclusion criteria were an initially successful primary dacryocystorhinostomy and recurrence of symptoms at least 12 months after surgery, together with clinical evidence of impaired lacrimal drainage. Patients' subsequent procedures were detailed and outcomes determined.

Results.—Thirteen cases of late failure of dacryocystorhinostomy were identified (8 of 1,158 surgeries by A.A.M., 4 of 378 by D.S., 1 patient whose initial dacryocystorhinostomy was done by another surgeon). Most patients were female (85%), and average age at initial surgery was 57.9 years. Most cases had nasolacrimal duct obstruction as the initial cause of epiphora (10 of 13 or 76.9%). The mean time to recurrence of symptoms after initial surgery was 46.9 months (range, 15-97 months). Pre- and intraoperative findings at second lacrimal surgery identified the cause of epiphora in late failure to be common canalicular obstruction in 11 of 13 patients (84.6%). Eleven of the 13 patients avoided repeat dacryocystorhinostomy, instead undergoing probing (with or without common canalicular membranotomy/membranectomy) and silicone intubation. Twelve of the 13 patients (92.3%) remained asymptomatic at final follow-up (range, 4-131 months).

Conclusions.—Although late failure after primary dacryocystorhinostomy is rare, this newly described group appears to be a distinct clinical entity, with lacrimal system obstruction often occurring at the common canaliculus. In the large majority of cases, a less invasive surgical solution than repeat dacryocystorhinostomy is effective in resolving symptoms.

▶ This study describes 13 patients who had late failure of their dacryocystorhinostomy (DCR) surgery. This is defined as initially successful surgery with an open lacrimal system that then closes 12 months or longer after the DCR. What is important in this article is that 11 of the 13 patients did not need a repeat DCR but had a membrane over the area of the common internal canaliculus that could simply be snipped, and then tubes were placed. This spared the patients a repeat DCR in all but 2 patients. This knowledge is of great value in approaching these patients. Although this late failure is rare, trying this approach before doing another DCR may well save the patient a more involved surgery.

R. B. Penne, MD

Silent sinus syndrome: dynamic changes in the position of the orbital floor after restoration of normal sinus pressure
Sivasubramaniam R, Sacks R, Thornton M (The Canberra Hosp, Australian Capital Territory, New South Wales, Australia; Concord General Hosp, New South Wales, Australia; St Vincent's Univ Hosp, Dublin, Ireland)
J Laryngol Otol 125:1239-1243, 2012

Background.—Silent sinus syndrome is characterised by spontaneous enophthalmos and hypoglobus, in association with chronic atelectasis of the maxillary sinus, and in the absence of signs or symptoms of intrinsic sinonasal inflammatory disease. Traditionally, correction of the enophthalmos involved reconstruction of the orbital floor, which was performed simultaneously with sinus surgery. Recently, there has been increasing evidence to support the performance of uncinectomy and antrostomy alone, then orbital floor reconstruction as a second-stage procedure if needed.

Methods.—We performed a retrospective review of 23 cases of chronic maxillary atelectasis managed in our unit with endoscopic uncinectomy and antrostomy alone. All patients were operated upon by the same surgeon.

Results.—Twenty-two of the 23 patients had either complete or partial resolution. One patient had ongoing enophthalmos, and was considered for an orbital floor reconstruction as a second-stage procedure.

Conclusion.—Our case series demonstrates that dynamic changes in orbital floor position can occur after sinus re-ventilation. These findings support the approach of delaying orbital floor reconstruction in cases of silent sinus syndrome treated with sinus re-ventilation, as such reconstruction may prove unnecessary over time (Fig 1).

▶ Silent sinus syndrome (SSS) is an uncommon process in which the maxillary sinus drainage becomes obstructed and negative pressure within the sinus over time results in maxillary sinus atelectasis. As the maxillary sinus shrinks, the orbital floor drops, resulting in enophthalmos and hypoglobus. This paper is a retrospective case review of 23 cases of SSS. Of the 23 cases, 22 required only endoscopic uncinectomy and antrostomy and did not require orbital surgery. Seventy-eight

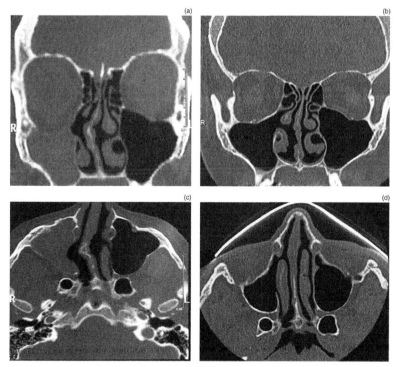

FIGURE 1.—(a) Coronal and (b) following uncinectomy and middle meatal antrostomy, parts (c) axial computed tomography views of a hypoplastic right maxillary antrum in a patient with silent sinus syndrome and (d) show corresponding views indicating remodelling of the orbital floor and orbital medial wall, 10 years post-surgery. (Reprinted from Sivasubramaniam R, Sacks R, Thornton M. Silent sinus syndrome: dynamic changes in the position of the orbital floor after restoration of normal sinus pressure. *J Laryngol Otol.* 2012;125:1239-1243, with permission from JLO (1984) Limited.)

percent of patients had complete resolution of their enophthalmos and hypoglobus after sinus surgery alone, and 17% had partial resolution.

The surgical management of SSS appears to be changing again. When I was training in the 1980s, the teaching was to drain and open the sinuses and then treat the enophthalmos. That then changed to some surgeons recommending operating on the sinus and the enophthalmos at the same surgical sitting. This article shows that with time most patients only require the sinus drainage and that the position of the orbital floor will improve over time if the sinus is opened

This article suggests a change in how SSS is approached surgically. The weakness in this article is that there is no formal measurement of enophthalmos either before or after surgery. Likewise no formal CT scan was done in all patients postoperatively to confirm the hypothesis that the orbital floor goes back into position after sinus drainage (Fig 1 shows 1 patient).

I have always suggested doing these procedures separately and have almost always done orbital reconstruction after the sinus surgery was completed. However, my surgery was usually done within 3 to 4 months after the sinus surgery, and this article suggests that the improvement may not start for 6 months and may take as long as 18 months to fully improve. This article at the very least requires that we discuss this potential improvement in eye position after sinus surgery alone for SSS. This will make me more likely to wait at least 1 year for improvement and hopefully will stimulate additional studies of this uncommon orbital problem.

R. B. Penne, MD

Treatment of severe idiopathic orbital inflammation with intravenous methylprednisolone
Bijlsma WR, Paridaens D, Kalmann R (Univ Med Ctr Utrecht, The Netherlands; Rotterdam Eye Hosp, the Netherlands)
Br J Ophthalmol 95:1068-1071, 2011

Background.—Prednisone pulse therapy is used to treat active noninfectious orbital inflammatory disease to attain faster clinical improvement and to shorten the duration of prednisone treatment. This study addresses the use of intravenous methylprednisolone (IVMP) pulse therapy, in addition to oral prednisone (OP), in the treatment of severe idiopathic orbital inflammation (IOI).

Methods.—This was a multicentre retrospective cohort study. Patients with severe IOI treated with IVMP pulse and OP therapy (IVMP+OP) were compared with patients with IOI who were treated only with OP. Main outcome measures were duration of prednisone treatment, symptom-free outcome and complications.

Results.—Between 2000 and 2007, 12 patients with severe IOI were treated with IVMP+OP and 15 patients were treated with OP only. The median treatment duration was 160 (range 34–680) days in the IVMP+OP

TABLE 1.—Patients with Severe Idiopathic Orbital Inflammation (IOI) Treated with Intravenous Methylprednisolone and Oral Prednisone (IVMP+OP) Versus Patients Treated with OP Only

Characteristics	OP Only (n = 15)	IVMP+OP (n = 12)	p Value*
Male (n (%))	3 (20)	3 (25)	1.0
Age (years) (mean±SD)	49±19	47±13	0.80
Clinic A† (n (%))	9 (60)	8 (67)	1.0
History (n (%))			
IOI	2 (13)	0 (0)	0.49
Autoimmune	2 (13)	1 (8.3)	1.0
Time with symptoms (days) (n (range))	35 (5−180)	14 (2−370)	0.14
Presentation (n (%))			
Pain	11 (73)	9 (75)	1.0
Soft tissue swelling	13 (87)	12 (100)	0.49
Proptosis	10 (67)	8 (67)	1.0
Optic nerve dysfunction	1 (6.7)	1 (8.3)	1.0
Diplopia	12 (80)	10 (83)	1.0
Bilateral	2 (13)	3 (25)	0.63
Localisation (n (%))			0.53
Dacryoadenitis	2 (14)	3 (30)	
Myositis	5 (36)	4 (40)	
Other	7 (50)	3 (30)	
Histology (n (%))			0.57
Typical	5 (83)	4 (67)	
Sclerosing	1 (17)	1 (17)	
Other	0 (0)	1 (17)	
Prednisone treatment (mg)			
Median dose±SD	18±13	15±8.3	0.44
Median cumulative dose (range)	2300 (600−10000)	5100 (2400−18000)	0.011
Median cumulative exclusive IVMP (range)		2100 (640−15000)	0.81
Median days (range)	110 (27−730)	160 (34−680)	0.24
Median days <10 mg (range)	21 (0−540)	42 (0−420)	0.38
Median days 10−30 mg (range)	84 (11−620)	85 (21−330)	0.32
Median days >30 mg (range)	15 (0−75)	8.5 (3−150)	0.94
Median days IVMP (range)		3 (3−7)	
Maintenance (n (%))	2 (13)	0 (0)	0.49
Other treatment (n (%))			
Radiotherapy	0 (0)	3 (25)	0.075
Immunosuppressives	2 (13)	2 (17)	1.0
Surgery	1 (6.7)	1 (8.3)	1.0
Outcome			
Median follow-up days (range)	750 (350−1700)	430 (14−2200)	0.064
Recurrence (n (%))	4 (27)	2 (17)	0.66
Major prednisone complications (n (%))	0 (0)	0 (0)	1.0
Symptom-free (n (%))	13 (87)	8 (73)	0.62

To calculate percentages, cases with missing information on variables were excluded.
*Fisher exact test was used for two proportions, χ^2 test for multiple proportions, t test for means and Mann−Whitney test for medians.
†This study was performed at two centres, clinic A and clinic B.

group and 110 (range 27−730) days in the OP-only group. In patients who had severe IOI, 73% in the IVMP+OP group and 87% in the OP-only group were symptom-free after treatment. No patients developed complications related to prednisone therapy.

Conclusion.—In our study there was no advantage of treating patients with severe IOI with IVMP + OP in terms of shortened treatment duration, lower cumulative dose or decrease in persistent symptoms. We suggest that the indication of IVMP in the treatment of severe IOI is limited to speeding symptom relief and recovery from optic nerve dysfunction (Table 1).

▶ The primary treatment of idiopathic orbital inflammation is systemic steroids. A high percentage of patients will be successfully treated with steroids alone for a variable period. This article studies the use of high-dose intravenous steroids to see how their use may affect the course of the disease.

It should be noted that this is a retrospective study and the number of patients is small at 27. Being a retrospective study, there may have been selection bias in who received intravenous steroids, even though that was not found from the chart review based on severity of symptoms. There was probably some tendency to treat the more severe cases of inflammation with high-dose intravenous steroids. Even with those limitations, this study is worth looking at. The results showed that there was no difference in outcome or total duration of steroid use in the group that received high-dose intravenous steroids first followed by oral steroids versus those that only received oral steroids. The only advantage of the high-dose intravenous steroids was a more rapid resolution of the inflammation with the intravenous steroids.

This article seems to confirm that using higher doses of intravenous steroids should be reserved for patients with severe symptoms. Severe pain, decreased vision, and severe exposure are reasons to consider high-dose intravenous steroids.

R. B. Penne, MD

Lacrimal Gland Ductulitis Caused by Probable *Actinomyces* Infection
Hay-Smith G, Rose GE (Moorfields Eye Hosp, London, UK)
Ophthalmology 119:193-196, 2012

Objective.—To describe the clinical characteristics and management of a group of patients who had chronic mucopurulent conjunctivitis that was probably due to *Actinomyces* infection of the lacrimal gland ductules.

Design.—A retrospective, interventional case series.

Participants.—Seven patients (2 male; 29%) between 34 and 52 years of age (mean, 48.7 years; median, 49 years) who presented to the lacrimal clinic.

Intervention.—Surgical excision of the infective focus (6 cases) or fenestration and expression of infective debris (1 case) from the affected lacrimal gland ductule—typically the most inferolateral of the ductules.

Main Outcome Measures.—The clinical features of this previously unrecognized cause of chronic conjunctivitis and its response to treatment.

Results.—All cases settled rapidly after surgery. There was often a major delay in diagnosis, with the patients having symptoms for between 2 and 42 months before referral (mean, 13.3 months; median, 9 months); 5 patients received prolonged or ineffectual topical medical therapy before referral.

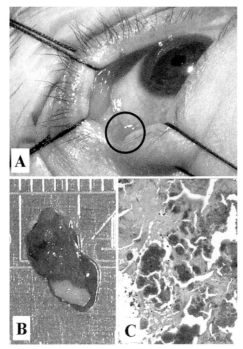

FIGURE 1.—A, Palpebral lobe of the right lacrimal gland at surgery, showing a pyogenic granuloma at the discharging lowest lacrimal gland ductule (ringed). B, Excised lacrimal gland ductule showing purulent debris in its lumen. C, Bacterial debris in the inflamed excised tissues, the debris showing gram-positive bacilli compatible with *Actinomyces* spp. (Gram stain; original magnification, ×40.) (Reprinted from Hay-Smith G, Rose GE. Lacrimal gland ductulitis caused by probable *Actinomyces* infection. *Ophthalmology*. 2012;119:193-196, Copyright 2012, with permission from the American Academy of Ophthalmology.)

Conclusions.—Infective lacrimal gland ductulitis, commonly from *Actinomyces* infection, should be considered in patients with unexplained chronic mucopurulent conjunctivitis; the condition settles rapidly with surgery (Figs 1 and 2).

▶ This article introduces a new cause of chronic purulent conjunctivitis. These are typically patients who have seen multiple doctors and have been on many different drops without improvement. Nasolacrimal duct obstruction, dacryoliths, canaliculitis, and giant fornix syndrome are previously noted causes of this rare condition.

Lacrimal gland ductulitis is an infection of 1 or more of the lacrimal gland ductules with actinomyces. This can be missed if the palpebral lobe of the lacrimal gland is not looked at, and this infection is not suspected. Once identified, this is easily treated by draining/excising the infected ductile and placing the patient on topical antibiotics.

This is another cause to consider when a patient presents with months of mucopurulent discharge that is resistant to treatment. I have never knowingly

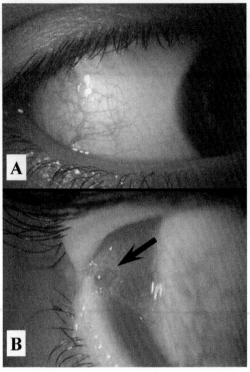

FIGURE 2.—(Case 7; Table 1) Patient referred with 9 months of right ocular irritation, persistent temporal episcleritis (A), and marked chronic mucopurulent ocular discharge. B, The palpebral lobe of the right lacrimal gland is inflamed and the lowest ductule (*arrow*) has a large pyogenic granuloma prolapsing from a markedly dilated orifice. Mucoid, "stringy" purulent debris can be expressed with pressure over the affected lacrimal gland ductule. (Reprinted from Hay-Smith G, Rose GE. Lacrimal gland ductulitis caused by probable *Actinomyces* infection. *Ophthalmology*. 2012;119:193-196, Copyright 2012, with permission from the American Academy of Ophthalmology.)

seen this, but I will now look for it when a patient presents with a chronic purulent conjunctivitis.

R. B. Penne, MD

Orbital Blowout Fractures and Race
de Silva DJ, Rose GE (Moorfields Eye Hosp, London, England, UK)
Ophthalmology 118:1677-1680, 2011

Purpose.—To examine the type of orbital blowout fracture and its variation with race.

Design.—Retrospective review of computed tomography (CT) scans and demography in an unselected cohort of patients with orbital blowout fractures.

Participants.—Patients with a high-resolution CT scan of adequate quality for analysis who presented with an orbital blowout fracture to the Orbital Clinic at Moorfields Eye Hospital. Patients with fractures involving the orbital rim or the cranium, or with penetrating injuries of the globe or orbit, were omitted from the study.

Methods.—Demographic and ethnic information was collected for each patient, and the orbital scans were reviewed by a single observer. On the basis of coronal and axial imaging, a fracture was classified as affecting up to 4 areas: the floor lateral to the infraorbital canal (area 1, "A1"), the floor medial to the canal ("A2"), the maxillo-ethmoidal strut ("inferomedial" strut, "A3"), and the medial wall blowout fracture ("A4"); with fractures involving the inferomedial strut, it was noted whether there was displacement or rotation of the strut. Ethnic origin was classified as Caucasian, Afro-Caribbean, or Asian (Oriental or Indian).

Main Outcome Measures.—The proportion of different walls involved in orbital blowout fractures within 3 ethnic groups.

Results.—A total of 152 patients (125 men, 82%) had imaging adequate for analysis; 103 (68%) were Caucasian, 19 (12%) were Afro-Caribbean,

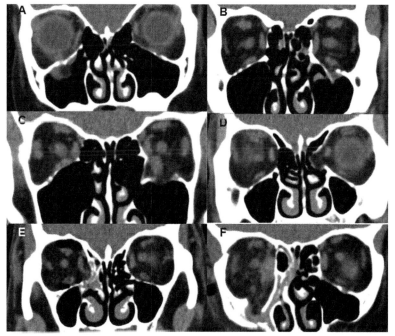

FIGURE 1.—Coronal computed tomography (CT) images showing various types of orbital blowout fracture: **A,** Mild floor fracture medial to the infraorbital nerve (type A2). **B,** Moderate fracture of floor medial to the nerve (A2). **C,** Severe orbital floor fracture with intact maxillo-ethmoidal strut (A1 and A2). **D,** Moderate medial orbital wall fracture (A4). **E,** Moderate medial orbital wall fracture with displaced strut (A3 and A4). **F,** Severe fracture of floor and medial wall, with displaced strut (A1—A4). (Reprinted from de Silva DJ, Rose GE. Orbital blowout fractures and race. *Ophthalmology.* 2011;118: 1677-1680, Copyright 2011, with permission from the American Academy of Ophthalmology.)

TABLE 3.—Type of Orbital Blowout Fracture in Relation to Ethnic Origin (Percentages Down the Columns)

	Ethnic Group			
	Caucasian (103 Patients)	Afro-Caribbean (19 Patients)	Asian (30 Patients)	All (152 Patients)
Isolated orbital floor fractures (A1 or A2)	56/103 (54%)	2/19 (10%)	14/30 (47%)	72/152 (47%)
Isolated medial wall fractures (A4)	10/103 (10%)	7/19 (37%)	2/30 (7%)	19/152 (13%)
Orbital floor and medial wall fractures, sparing strut (A2 + A4)	24/103 (23%)	3/19 (16%)	5/30 (16%)	32/152 (21%)
Orbital floor, medial wall, and strut fractures (A2 + A3 + A4)	13/103 (13%)	7/19 (37%)	9/30 (30%)	29/152 (19%)

and 30 (20%) were Asian. Caucasians most commonly had floor fractures (A1 or A2 in 56 orbits, 54%) compared with 10 of 103 purely medial fractures (A4, 10%); in contrast, medial fractures were the most common type in Afro-Caribbean patients (7/19 cases, 37%), and purely floor fractures occurred in only 2 cases (10%) ($P<0.005$). Asian patients had results similar to those for Caucasian patients, with isolated floor fractures being the most common (14/30 cases, 47%).

Conclusions.—Most blowout fractures involve the orbital floor in Caucasian and Asians, whereas in Afro-Caribbeans the most common site for fracture is the medial wall (Fig 1, Table 3).

▶ This is a simple and interesting study. The authors simply looked at the type of orbital blow out fracture that occurred and compared this with race (Fig 1). The findings are of interest. The study revealed that an isolated orbital floor fracture is by far the most common type of orbital blow out fracture in both white and Asian patients at 54% and 47%, respectively. In contrast, in the Afro-Caribbean patients, only 10% had isolated floor fractures, and 90% had involvement of their medial wall. Thirty-seven percent of Afro-Caribbean patients had isolated medial wall fractures, whereas this number was 10% and 7% for Caucasian and Asian patients, respectively (Table 3).

How these results can be explained is conjecture at this point. It was suggested by the authors that Afro-Caribbean patients have thicker orbital floor bone, and this may be protective from fracture of the orbital floor. I agree with the authors that my experience with orbital floor decompression is that Afro-Caribbean patients have thicker bone. I also cannot recall ever having to repair an isolated medial wall fracture in a white patient.

One weakness of this study is that only patients with symptoms were imaged. Thus, some patients with trauma have had asymptomatic fractures, and these were not seen. Because medial wall fractures don't give infraorbital hypesthesia, those medial wall fractures without entrapment are more likely to be missed. Thus, the numbers could be higher. On a clinical basis, this information does not really change how to approach trauma patients. It is a clinical difference among races that I was not aware of.

R. B. Penne, MD

7 Pediatric Ophthalmology

Smoking and Strabismus Surgery in Patients with Thyroid Eye Disease

Rajendram R, Bunce C, Adams GGW, et al (Moorfields Eye Hosp, London, UK; et al)
Ophthalmology 118:2493-2497, 2011

Objective.—To investigate the relationship between smoking status at presentation and the use of strabismus surgery in the management of patients with thyroid eye disease.

Design.—Retrospective review of a noncomparative series of patients with thyroid eye disease.

Participants.—All patients with thyroid eye disease under the care of a single consultant at Moorfields Eye Hospital between 1997 and 2002 (inclusive).

Methods.—Retrospective review of clinical case notes.

Main Outcome Measures.—Survival analysis of patients in cohort and the frequency of strabismus surgery in relation to smoking status at ophthalmic presentation. A subanalysis of patients who underwent orbital decompression and those that did not was undertaken.

Results.—Of 501 patients seen during the study period, 425 (85%) of 501 sets of notes were available for review, and initial smoking status was recorded for 89% (378/425) of patients, of whom approximately one half (196/378; 52%) were active smokers. Of the smokers, 51 (26%) of 196 underwent strabismus surgery, compared with only 19 (14%) of 138 non-smokers at presentation. When adjusted for age, the hazards ratio of having strabismus surgery during management for smokers at presentation versus nonactive smokers was 2.19. In the group who did not undergo orbital decompression, this hazard ratio increased to 4.86.

Conclusions.—Within this thyroid eye disease cohort, the proportion of smokers at presentation was much larger than that of the general population. There was an increased use of strabismus surgery in active smokers at presentation than in nonactive smokers. This finding was independent of the orbital decompression surgery. The results are consistent with those of previous reports of more severe thyroid eye disease in smokers and raise the possibility that smoking cessation early in the disease may reduce the severity of the changes and the number of rehabilitative strabismus operations needed.

▶ Smoking contributes to many medical conditions. It has been repeatedly reported to be associated with more severe thyroid eye disease. Therefore, it was not surprising that the authors found an increased use of strabismus surgery in active smokers compared to nonactive smokers. Even in patients who had not undergone decompression, smoking was associated with an increased frequency of strabismus surgery. Since strabismus surgery is rarely performed during the active phase of thyroid eye disease, it is important that smoking cease to prevent the long-term outcome of eye muscle fibrosis. Patients with thyroid eye disease need to be made aware of all the potential medical complications both during the active and inactive phases of thyroid eye disease.

L. B. Nelson, MD, MBA

Dynamics of Human Foveal Development after Premature Birth
Maldonado RS, O'Connell RV, Sarin N, et al (Duke Univ School of Medicine, Durham, NC; et al)
Ophthalmology 118:2315-2325, 2011

Purpose.—To determine the dynamic morphologic development of the human fovea in vivo using portable spectral domain-optical coherence tomography (SD-OCT).

Design.—Prospective, observational case series.

Participants.—Thirty-one prematurely born neonates, 9 children, and 9 adults.

Methods.—Sixty-two neonates were enrolled in this study. After examination for retinopathy of prematurity (ROP), SD-OCT imaging was performed at the bedside in nonsedated infants aged 31 to 41 weeks postmenstrual age (PMA) (= gestational age in weeks + chronologic age) and at outpatient follow-up ophthalmic examinations. Thirty-one neonates met eligibility criteria. Nine children and nine adults without ocular pathology served as control groups. Semiautomatic retinal layer segmentation was performed. Central foveal thickness, foveal to parafoveal (FP) ratio (central foveal thickness divided by thickness 1000 μm from the foveal center), and 3-dimensional thickness maps were analyzed.

Main Outcome Measures.—In vivo determination of foveal morphology, layer segmentation, analysis of subcellular changes, and spatiotemporal layer shifting.

Results.—In contrast with the adult fovea, several signs of immaturity were observed in the neonates: a shallow foveal pit, persistence of inner retinal layers (IRLs), and a thin photoreceptor layer (PRL) that was thinnest at the foveal center. Three-dimensional mapping showed displacement of retinal layers out of the foveal center as the fovea matured and the progressive formation of the inner/outer segment band in the opposite direction. The FP-IRL ratios decreased as IRL migrated before term and minimally after that, whereas FP-PRL ratios increased as PRL subcellular elements formed closer to term and into childhood. A surprising finding was the presence of cystoid macular edema in 58% of premature neonates that appeared to affect inner foveal maturation.

Conclusions.—This study provides the first view into the development of living cellular layers of the human retina and of subcellular specialization at the fovea in premature infant eyes using portable SD-OCT. Our work establishes a framework of the timeline of human foveal development, allowing us to identify unexpected retinal abnormalities that may provide new keys to disease activity and a method for mapping foveal structures from infancy to adulthood that may be integral in future studies of vision and visual cortex development.

▶ Although optical coherence tomography (OCT) is currently widely used in ophthalmology practices, it is only rarely used in pediatric ophthalmology. Among the reasons that OCT has not been universally used in pediatric ophthalmology is the need for a child's cooperation and difficulty in placing his or her head in a tabletop chin-rest configuration. The authors' finding of development in the layers of the fovea using OCT correlate with previously documented postmortem histological studies. What was surprising was the OCT finding of cystoid macula edema in many of the premature infants not documented on clinical evaluation. One of the limitations of this study was the authors' inclusion of premature infants who had developed retinopathy of prematurity (ROP) up to stage 2 with infants who did not develop ROP. How much did the ROP contribute to cystoid macula edema is unclear. OCT holds promise as an important test that may elucidate other findings of the fovea in pediatric ophthalmology.

L. B. Nelson, MD, MBA

Changes in exodeviation following hyperopic correction in patients with intermittent exotropia
Chung SA, Kim IS, Kim WK, et al
J Pediatr Ophthalmol Strabismus 48:278-284, 2011

Purpose.—To evaluate changes in the angle of deviation after spectacle correction in patients who had hyperopia and intermittent exotropia (X(T)) and to determine whether the changes and surgical outcomes differ when compared with those of myopic and emmetropic X(T).

Methods.—One hundred fourteen patients with X(T) were recruited and allocated into three groups: X(T) with hyperopia (group I; 38 patients), X(T) with emmetropia (group II; 35 patients), and X(T) with myopia (group III; 41 patients). After at least 6 months wearing spectacles, changes in exodeviation were compared. The results of surgery based on the spectacle-corrected distance angle and the ratios of accommodative convergence over accommodation (AC/A) were also assessed.

Results.—With spectacle correction, the mean exodeviation increased significantly in group I, but did not change in groups II or III. Thirteen patients in group I (34%) showed a more than 10 prism diopters (PD) exotropic shift after wearing spectacles. The mean AC/A ratio in group I was 2.63 (PD/D), whereas in groups II and III the ratios were 4.03 and 4.06, respectively. There was no difference in surgical results among the three groups.

Conclusion.—Although hyperopic correction in patients with X(T) resulted in a limited increase in exodeviation with a subnormal AC/A ratio, one-third of the patients experienced a significant increase in exodeviation. A spectacle correction trial should be considered before surgery in patients with hyperopia and X(T).

▶ Spectacle correction for hyperopia to improve visual acuity may increase both the frequency and size of an associated exodeviation. However, patients with high hyperopia and intermittent exotropia who were prescribed optical correction may actually improve their deviation. It is believed that the improvement in visual acuity with the hyperopic correction, often normalization of accommodation, might lead to this result. In this study, patients who were corrected with a mean cycloplegic retinoscopy of +3.17 diopters had an increased exodeviation, in many by a mere 10 diopters. Therefore, an optical correction of hyperopia to improve the vision in patients with exotropia is useful prior to considering strabismus surgery. If a larger deviation is found, surgery that corrects for the new angle of deviation should result in fewer undercorrections.

L. B. Nelson, MD, MBA

Surgical Management of Residual or Recurrent Esotropia Following Maximal Bilateral Medial Rectus Recession
Morrison DG, Emanuel M, Donahue SP (Vanderbilt Univ School of Medicine, Nashville, TN)
Arch Ophthalmol 129:173-175, 2011

Objective.—To describe the effect of graded unilateral vs bilateral lateral rectus resection in the treatment of residual or recurrent esotropia after maximal medial rectus muscle recession.

Methods.—Retrospective case series of children with residual or recurrent esotropia. All children underwent initial eye muscle surgery for angles of 40 to 60 prism diopters (medial rectus recession of 5.5-6.5 mm; 11.0-11.5 mm from surgical limbus). If significant esotropia persisted or recurred, surgical results from graded lateral rectus resection were recorded.

Results.—Thirty-eight children were identified for the study. Unilateral lateral rectus resection ranging from 4 to 7 mm resulted in mean esotropic corrections of 10.5 to 14.9 prism diopters. Differences in surgical response per millimeter of unilateral lateral rectus resection were not significant. Bilateral lateral rectus resection of 5, 6, and 7 mm resulted in a mean correction of 19.75, 28.75, and 33.5 prism diopters, respectively.

Conclusions.—Graded lateral rectus resection can produce highly variable results on a case-to-case basis, but mean values trend in the expected direction. Residual deviations larger than 15 prism diopters need to be addressed with bilateral surgery.

▶ The authors appropriately pointed out some of the limitations of their study, including that it was retrospective and had a brief follow-up period, and the long-term effects of lateral rectus surgery. However, an important issue that was not addressed is what effect larger unilateral rectus resections would have accomplished. Routinely, I perform unilateral rectus resections of 8 mm for 20 prism diopters of residual esotropia and 9 mm for 25 prism diopters. Both surgical procedures are successful and demonstrate the inadequate unilateral resections performed in this study.

L. B. Nelson, MD, MBA

Long-term Follow-up of Acquired Nonaccommodative Esotropia in a Population-based Cohort

Jacobs SM, Green-Simms A, Diehl NN, et al (Mayo Clinic College of Medicine, Rochester, MN; Mayo Clinic and Mayo Foundation, Rochester, MN)
Ophthalmology 118:1170-1174, 2011

Purpose.—To describe the clinical characteristics and long-term outcomes of children diagnosed over a 30-year period with acquired nonaccommodative esotropia (ANAET).

Design.—Retrospective chart review of a population-based cohort.

Participants.—All pediatric (<19 years of age) residents of Olmsted County, Minnesota, who were diagnosed with ANAET from January 1, 1965, to December 31, 1994.

Methods.—The medical records of all potential patients identified by the resources of the Rochester Epidemiology Project were reviewed.

Main Outcome Measures.—Incidence, clinical characteristics, and long-term motor and sensory outcomes of children with ANAET.

Results.—A total of 174 children were diagnosed during the 30-year period, yielding an incidence of 1 in 287 live births. The median age at diagnosis for the 174 patients was 4.0 years (range, 10 months to 18.2 years), and 61% (107) were male ($P = 0.009$). Although 11% (8/75) of those queried were diplopic, none of the 174 was subsequently diagnosed with an intracranial lesion. During a mean follow-up of 10.9 years (range, 0 days to 37 years), 127 patients (73%) underwent strabismus surgery (mean, 1 surgery; range, 0–3 surgeries). Among the 127 patients who underwent surgery, the median final stereoacuity was 3000 seconds of arc, including 8 patients (6.3%) with ≥50 seconds of arc. Patients who were older (>44 months) at ANAET diagnosis ($P = 0.005$) and without amblyopia at their initial examination ($P < 0.001$) were more likely to achieve excellent final stereopsis.

Conclusions.—In this population-based cohort, ANAET occurred in 1 in 287 children and was more prevalent among male children. Although diplopia was relatively common, none of the children were found to have an intracranial malignancy. Most patients achieved good motor and sensory outcomes, with the best results among those with a later onset of their deviation and no amblyopia.

▶ Acquired nonaccommodative esotropia (ANAET) is a more common ocular motility disorder than the literature indicates. While the authors suggest that brain imaging may not be justified in a subset of patients who lack characteristics suggestive of an underlying intracranial process, occasionally a brain malignancy has been surprisingly noted in these particular children. Therefore, it may be prudent to at least refer patients who lack these characteristics for further neurological evaluation. It is not surprising that those patients who developed ANAET at a later age generally had the best postoperative binocularity. These patients enjoyed some degree of binocularity prior to the onset of ANAET. If these patients' esotropia is reduced to less than 10 prism diopters in a relatively short duration of time, they can reacquire their previous binocular status.

L. B. Nelson, MD, MBA

Deficits in Perception of Images of Real-World Scenes in Patients With a History of Amblyopia
Mirabella G, Hay S, Wong AMF (Univ of Toronto, Ontario, Canada; Private Practice in Huntsville, AL)
Arch Ophthalmol 129:176-183, 2011

Objectives.—To investigate the perception of images of real-world scenes in patients with amblyopia and to compare their performance with that of visually normal participants by viewing conditions (monocular vs binocular) and by treatment outcomes (successfully vs unsuccessfully treated vs normal eyes).

Methods.—Thirty-nine healthy and 26 amblyopic individuals who had undergone previous amblyopia treatment were recruited to perform a match-to-sample task that used images of real-world scenes. Rates of correct, incorrect, and no responses and mean reaction time were recorded.

Results.—Performance during monocular viewing showed that the mean correct response rate was 59% in the amblyopic eyes, 62% in the fellow eyes, and 67% in the normal eyes ($P = .008$). During binocular viewing, the correct response rate remained reduced at 58% in amblyopic patients compared with 68% in participants with normal vision ($P = .03$). Performance by treatment outcomes showed that the mean correct response rate was 59% in the unsuccessfully treated group, 64% in the successfully treated group, and 67% in the normal group ($P = .002$). There was no difference in performance among amblyopia subtypes.

Conclusions.—Real-world scene perception is impaired in amblyopia, with the poorest performance during amblyopic monocular and binocular viewing. Despite successful treatment of the amblyopic eye to normal acuity levels, perception of images in real-world scenes remains deficient in patients with a history of amblyopia.

▶ Monocular amblyopia and binocular viewing appear to adversely affect real-world scene perception. This seems to be present even when the amblyopic eye has relatively good vision. However, these findings do not explain the observation of the high performance of many outstanding athletes who have amblyopia. Whether their performance could have been even better if they did not have amblyopia remains unknown. Further research as to the cause of the subnormal real-world scene perception of amblyopia patients, especially binocular viewing, needs to be undertaken to determine the cause of these findings.

L. B. Nelson, MD, MBA

Outcomes of surgery in long-standing infantile esotropia with cross fixation
Keskinbora KH, Gonen T, Horozoglu F
J Pediatr Ophthalmol Strabismus 48:77-83, 2011

Background.—This is a retrospective study to determine the outcomes of the surgical correction in long-standing infantile esotropia with cross fixation.

Methods.—Medical charts of a group of patients with esotropia who had cross fixation and underwent surgery for strabismus between January 1991 and December 2004 were reviewed. The mean follow-up time was 4.7 years. Binocularity was measured by the Worth 4-dot test and Titmus stereo test. Twenty-six patients underwent surgery for strabismus. Twenty-one patients aged 8 to 26 years with a minimum 3-year postoperative follow-up were included. Five patients were excluded because they were lost to follow-up after surgery.

Results.—Bimedial recession and resection of one lateral rectus muscle were performed in all patients. Recession of the inferior oblique muscle with anteriorization was performed in patients who had inferior oblique overaction. Orthotropia was attained in 14 patients, whereas residual esotropia was diagnosed in 5 patients. Two patients were diagnosed as having exotropia. Two patients required a second surgery for dissociated vertical deviation. Overall, 9 of the 21 patients had indications of binocular function and 12 remained the same in their stereoacuity.

Conclusion.—Surgical correction of long-standing infantile esotropia with cross fixation in young adults may improve binocular function and allow long-term alignment stability.

▶ Congenital esotropia is a large-angle esodeviation that is present by 6 months old. Once any accommodative component and amblyopia are corrected, the accepted treatment is strabismus surgery to realign the visual axes with the goals of attaining not only immediate satisfactory postoperative alignment but also stable long-term alignment with establishment of binocularity. The authors have elucidated the factors that may influence the outcome of treatment, including the age of surgical alignment, the duration of misalignment prior to surgery, and the development of associated features of congenital esotropia.

Although early surgery for congenital esotropia has been the mainstay of treatment, how early has remained controversial. Factors other than age of surgical alignment may influence the degree of binocularity; one factor that may be important besides age is the duration of misalignment. It seems that a shorter duration of misalignment more favorably affects the quality of stereopsis than solely the age at which alignment occurred. Further studies are needed to establish the critical factors to achieve stable, binocular vision in children with congenital esotropia.

L. B. Nelson, MD, MBA

An evidence-based approach to physician etiquette in pediatric ophthalmology
Reddy AK, Coats DK, Yen KG
J Pediatr Ophthalmol Strabismus 48:336-339, 2011

Purpose.—Little objective evidence exists to guide physician etiquette in pediatric ophthalmology. This article describes the preferences of families visiting a pediatric ophthalmology clinic for the first time.

Methods.—Review of 149 questionnaires completed by the families of patients visiting a pediatric ophthalmology clinic in a tertiary care center. The Fisher exact and chi-square tests were used to compare subpopulations.

Results.—Most respondents preferred that their physician wear a white coat. Men preferred a handshake to a verbal greeting $(P=.0264)$ and professional to business casual attire for both male and female physicians $(P=.01,$ both). African-American parents were more likely to prefer being addressed by surname than other races $(P=.008)$. No statistically significant differences were found comparing the preferences of parents with an advanced education (bachelor and graduate degrees) to those without.

Conclusion.—Pediatric ophthalmologists may wish to consider wearing white coats and business casual attire in clinic and addressing parents informally as "mom" or "dad" or by their first name, although etiquette should ultimately be determined on an individual patient basis.

▶ Parents' initial impression of their child's encounter with a pediatric ophthalmologist forms the basis for how parents interact at that visit and subsequently with their child's pediatric ophthalmologist. The way their pediatric ophthalmologist greets them affects the trust and confidence they have in the decision-making ability of their physician. I was surprised that almost 58% of parents in this study preferred that their pediatric ophthalmologist wear a white coat. I always felt that a white coat was intimidating for young children. Perhaps the parents who preferred a white coat were generalizing about their preference for attire for all of their encounters with physicians of other specialties as well. It would be interesting to know if these parents who preferred a white coat also preferred a more formal introduction to the pediatric ophthalmologist. It would also be of interest to know what percentage of pediatric ophthalmologists currently wear a white coat when examining their patients and how they greet and address their parents.

L. B. Nelson, MD, MBA

Long-term follow-up of children with acute acquired concomitant esotropia
Sturm V, Menke MN, Knecht PB, et al (Univ Hosp of Hamburg, Germany; Univ Hosp of Zurich, Switzerland)
J AAPOS 15:317-320, 2011

Purpose.—To study the clinical features and surgical outcome of type 2 (Burian-Franceschetti) acute acquired concomitant esotropia (AACE).

Methods.—Retrospective analysis of children with AACE type 2. All patients underwent strabismus surgery to restore ocular alignment. All children underwent a complete assessment including medical history and pre- and postoperative ophthalmological and orthoptic examinations. Postoperative follow-up was at least 12 months in all cases.

Results.—A total of 25 consecutive patients were included. All but 2 patients (92%) were aligned within 8^Δ or less of orthotropia. Of the 25, 15 (60%) regained normal stereovision. In 6 additional cases (24%) some level of binocular vision (Titmus test, 200″ to 3000″) was demonstrated. All of the patients who finally achieved normal stereopsis had lower levels of binocularity on the first postoperative day. The mean interval between surgery and first occurrence of full stereovision was 18 months (range, 2 to 58 months).

Conclusions.—General features of AACE type 2 are concomitance of strabismus, absence of an accommodative component even in the presence of hyperopic refractive errors, and no neurological pathology. The potential for normal binocular vision plays a key role in defining this entity. The reemergence of full stereopsis may take several years.

▶ Acute acquired concomitant esotropia (AACE) is a rare condition that should always have a neurological evaluation to rule out any intracranial abnormality. Many patients with this condition can ultimately have good binocularity if treatment is instituted immediately. An accommodative component should always be undertaken before surgical intervention. I was surprised that in this study, there was an average 23-month interval between onset of the condition and surgical management. Many children with AACE have binocularity before its onset, so it is not surprising that a majority of the children in this study had some degree of binocularity postoperatively.

L. B. Nelson, MD, MBA

Surgical Outcomes in Convergence Insufficiency-Type Exotropia

Yang HK, Hwang J-M (Seoul Natl Univ Bundang Hosp, Seongnam, Korea)
Ophthalmology 118:1512-1517, 2011

Purpose.—To determine the efficacy of different types of strabismus surgeries in patients with convergence insufficiency (CI)-type exotropia, according to their response to diagnostic monocular occlusion.

Design.—Retrospective cohort study.

Participants.—Sixty-five patients with CI-type exotropia with near-distance differences of ≥10 prism diopters (PD) who underwent strabismus surgery.

Methods.—Patients were divided into 3 groups according to their response to monocular occlusion: (1) true-CI group: near-distance differences ≥10 PD before and after occlusion; (2) masked-CI group: near-distance differences <10 PD before occlusion and ≥10 PD after occlusion; and (3) pseudo-CI group: near-distance differences ≥10 PD before occlusion and <10 PD after occlusion. Either bilateral lateral rectus recession based on near measurements with 1 mm augmentation (BLR) or unilateral medial rectus resection based on the near deviation with lateral rectus recession based on the distant deviation (RR) was performed.

Main Outcome Measures.—Cumulative probabilities of success, near-distance differences of exodeviation, rate of recurrence per person-year, and risk factors of recurrence.

Results.—There were 24 children in the true-CI group, 19 children in the masked-CI group, and 22 children in the pseudo-CI group. The cumulative probabilities of success at 2 years after BLR versus RR were 61% versus 100% in the true-CI group, 58% versus 100% in the masked-CI group, and 77% versus 71% in the pseudo-CI group. The RR procedure was significantly more successful than the BLR procedure in the true-CI and masked-CI groups.

Conclusions.—Successful outcome in CI-type exotropia was closely related to the patients' response to monocular occlusion. In patients with CI-type exotropia maintained after monocular occlusion, unilateral resection-recession based on near-distance measurements is recommended.

▶ Surgery for convergence insufficiency-type exotropia, in which the near deviation is less than 15 prism diopters, is rarely indicated. Most often these patients who undergo surgery can have a postoperative overcorrection at distance with diplopia. These patients who have ocular symptoms at near vision, such as intermittent asthenopia or diplopia, can often be successfully managed with prism glasses.

L. B. Nelson, MD, MBA

High prevalence of amblyopia risk factors in preverbal children with nasolacrimal duct obstruction
Matta NS, Silbert DI (Family Eye Group, Lancaster, PA)
J AAPOS 15:350-352, 2011

Purpose.—To report the percentage of children under the age of 3 with nasolacrimal duct obstruction (NLDO) and amblyopia risk factors who develop clinical evidence of amblyopia over time.

Methods.—Records of children under 3 years of age presenting to a pediatric oculoplastic specialist with NLDO between January 1, 2001, and August 8, 2009, were retrospectively reviewed to identify those who also had amblyopia risk factors. Amblyopia was diagnosed based on visual acuity and treatment history.

Results.—A total of 375 children under the age of 3 had NLDO. Of these, 82 (22%) had amblyopia risk factors, and 70 received a follow-up examination. Average age at first visit was 12 months (1-27 months). In all patients with anisometropia and unilateral NLDO, the side with the NLDO had higher hyperopia. Of the 70 with risk factors, 44 (63%) were later treated for amblyopia: 29 with spectacles alone, 2 with occlusion therapy, 13 with spectacles and occlusion therapy. Six patients required strabismus surgery. In all patients with anisometropia and unilateral NLDO, the side with the NLDO had higher hyperopia.

Conclusions. The percentage of children identified with amblyopia risk factors who later develop clinical amblyopia was much higher than the 1.6% to 3.6% expected in a cohort of normal children.

▶ Occasionally, when a child presents with a nasolacrimal duct obstruction, a parent will question me as to the necessity of using cycloplegic drops as part of my examination. I explain to the parents the reasons for the drops, including doing a thorough ophthalmologic examination, is to rule out any other possible ocular abnormality. I explain that not infrequently I do find, as these authors did, signs of amblyopia. What is unclear is why, when amblyopia is present in a child with a nasolacrimal duct obstruction, it often involves the affected eye. It certainly may be related to early defocus caused by the presence of mucus in the eye, as the authors suggested. Further research needs to be done to attempt to elucidate the reasons for this correlation.

L. B. Nelson, MD, MBA

Adjunctive Effect of Acupuncture to Refractive Correction on Anisometropic Amblyopia: One-Year Results of a Randomized Crossover Trial

Lam DSC, Zhao J, Chen LJ, et al (Chinese Univ of Hong Kong, China; Joint Shantou International Eye Ctr of Shantou Univ and the Chinese Univ of Hong Kong, China; et al)

Ophthalmology 118:1501-1511, 2011

Objectives.—To evaluate the safety and adjunctive effect of acupuncture added to refractive correction for anisometropic amblyopia in younger children.

Design.—Prospective, randomized, controlled, crossover trial.

Participants.—We included 83 children aged 3 to <7 years with untreated anisometropic amblyopia and baseline best-corrected visual acuity (BCVA) of 20/40 to 20/200 in the amblyopic eye.

Methods.—Participants were randomized to receive spectacles alone (group 1; n = 42) or spectacles + acupuncture (group 2; n = 41) for 15 weeks, and were then crossed over to receive the other regimen for another 15 weeks. The BCVA in both eyes was measured at baseline and every 5 (± 1) weeks for the initial 45 weeks and at 60 (± 1) weeks.

Main Outcome Measures.—BCVA in the amblyopic eye at 15, 30, and 60 weeks.

Results.—The mean baseline BCVA in the amblyopic eye was 0.50 and 0.49 logarithm of the minimum angle of resolution (logMAR) in groups 1 and 2, respectively. After 15 weeks of treatment, the BCVA had improved by a mean of 2.2 lines in group 1 and 2.9 lines in group 2. The mean difference in BCVA between groups was 0.77 lines (95% confidence interval (CI), 0.29−1.3; $P = 0.0020$) with baseline adjustment. BCVA of ≤0.1 logMAR was achieved in 14.6% of the patients in group 1 and 57.5% in group 2 ($P<0.00010$). After the regimens were crossed over at 30 weeks, group 1 had a mean of 1.2 (95% CI, 0.98−1.48; $P = 2.0 \times 10^{-12}$) lines additional improvement from the 15-week BCVA, whereas in group 2 the mean improvement was 0.4 (95% CI, 0.19−0.63; $P = 0.0010$) lines. The proportions of responders, resolution, and participants achieving a BCVA of ≤0.1 logMAR at 30 weeks were similar between groups. After completion of acupuncture, only 1 participant had >1 line of VA decrease to 60 weeks. Acupuncture was well-tolerated by all children, and no severe adverse effect was encountered.

Conclusions.—Acupuncture is a potentially useful complementary treatment modality that may provide sustainable adjunctive effect to refractive correction for anisometropic amblyopia in young children. Further large-scale studies seem warranted.

▶ Amblyopia is an asymptomatic condition that requires a visual acuity evaluation for detection. In children with anisometropia amblyopia, refractive correction alone may not result in resolution of the amblyopia. Occlusion therapy remains the mainstay of treatment in amblyopia. However, occlusion therapy does have adverse effects, such as poor compliance, skin irritation, and psychological problems. Acupuncture may offer an alternative treatment for anisometropia amblyopia. Further studies on using acupuncture for anisometropia amblyopia are needed to determine the maximum achievable visual acuity. Also, it remains to be studied whether acupuncture is effective in treating amblyopia that results from strabismus or other causes. The regimen of acupuncture administered 5 times a week may cause compliance issues.

L. B. Nelson, MD, MBA

Clinical review of periorbital capillary hemangioma of infancy
Jalil A, Maino A, Bhojwani R, et al
J Pediatr Ophthalmol Strabismus 48:218-225, 2011

Purpose.—To explore the role of intralesional steroid injections (ILSI) and oral steroids in the management of periocular hemangioma of infancy (HOI).

Methods.—In this retrospective study, treatment options studied were observation, ILSI, and oral steroids. All children received adjunctive amblyopia treatment if required. The main indications for treatment were cosmetic, worsening astigmatism, and visual axis obscuration. Success was defined as complete HOI regression before the age of 5 years (cosmetic group), reduction of astigmatism of at least 1 diopter cylinder (DC) (astigmatism group), or no evidence of amblyopia at the last follow-up (visual axis obscuration group).

Results.—Twenty-four of 41 children (58.5%) had amblyopia at presentation. Eighteen children formed the observation group, 17 children received ILSI, and 6 children received oral steroids. Successful outcome was achieved in all except 2 patients in the cosmetic group and 6 of 7 in the visual axis obscuration group. Mean astigmatic correction of all cases was 1.65 ± 1.34 DC before treatment and 0.91 ± 1.17 DC after treatment, the change being statistically significant ($P < .001$).

Conclusion.—Observation appears to be a highly effective strategy if coupled with amblyopia therapy, especially for mild cases. Intralesional and oral steroids appear to be equally effective for lesions requiring treatment, but their exact role cannot be clearly determined in the presence of a spontaneously resolving lesion.

▶ Capillary hemangiomas often increase, sometimes significantly, during the first 6 months of life and then gradually diminish. Conservative treatment is usually best because there is a strong tendency for this kind of lesion to undergo spontaneous regression. Treatment must be considered when complications develop, such as deprivation amblyopia. All current available treatment modalities are associated with possible adverse local or systemic side effects. The authors are strong advocates of intralesional steroid injections for the treatment of periorbital capillary hemangiomas. However, they discuss in detail the pros and cons of this treatment modality. The authors briefly discuss the recent use of β-blockers as an alternative treatment. Although the use of oral propranolol has successfully treated hemangiomas in infants, there are associated system adverse effects. The application of topical timolol has been a safe and effective treatment for superficial periocular hemangiomas and may have fewer systemic effects. Further prospective studies using topical β-blockers are still needed.

L. B. Nelson, MD, MBA

Ocular Consequences of Bottle Rocket Injuries in Children and Adolescents
Khan M, Reichstein D, Recchia MF (Vanderbilt Univ Med Ctr, Nashville, TN)
Arch Ophthalmol 129:639-642, 2011

Objective.—To describe the spectrum of ocular injuries and associated visual morbidity in the pediatric and adolescent population caused by bottle rockets.

Methods.—Retrospective review of consecutive medical records of patients 18 years or younger seen during a recent 4-year period. Outcome measures were ocular injuries at time of visit, interventions required, visual acuity at most recent follow-up, and most recent anatomic findings.

Results.—Eleven eyes from 10 patients (8 boys and 2 girls aged 5-17 years) were identified. Significant ocular injuries included corneal epithelial defect (7 eyes), hyphema (6 eyes), traumatic iritis (2 eyes), iridodialysis (4 eyes), cataract (4 eyes), retinal dialysis (1 eye), and vitreous hemorrhage (2 eyes). Eight eyes required primary intervention (lensectomy in 4 eyes, corneal debridement in 2 eyes, globe exploration in 1 eye, and retinal laser photocoagulation in 1 eye). Three patients required additional procedures. These secondary interventions included pars plana vitrectomy (1 eye), muscle surgery for sensory strabismus (1 eye), corneal debridement (1 eye), and intraocular lens placement (1 eye). Most recent visual acuity (10 eyes with follow-up) was 20/30 or better in 4 eyes and 20/200 or worse in 6 eyes (for 1 eye, the patient was unavailable for follow-up). Permanent visual impairment was typically due to traumatic maculopathy.

Conclusion.—Bottle rockets can cause significant ocular injury in children, often with permanent loss of vision.

▶ Bottle rocket injuries in children and adolescents can have devastating effects on visual outcomes. Unfortunately, only 5 states ban the sale of all consumer fireworks. Better educational policies need to reach the public regarding the serious repercussions of fireworks-related ocular injuries to participants and bystanders. Perhaps more studies like this one that demonstrate the devastating effects on the visual outcome from bottle rocket injuries will persuade legislators in the other states to ban the sale of bottle rockets.

L. B. Nelson, MD, MBA

Varying Difficulty of Snellen Letters and Common Errors in Amblyopic and Fellow Eyes

Mathew JA, Shah SA, Simon JW (Albany Med College, NY)
Arch Ophthalmol 129:184-187, 2011

Objective.—To investigate the varying difficulty of Snellen letters in children with amblyopia.

Methods.—We tabulated the letter-by-letter responses of amblyopic and nonamblyopic fellow eyes on random, computer-generated Snellen lines. Participants were 60 children, aged 5 to 13 years, with a history of amblyopia. Main outcome measures were relative difficulties of Snellen letters and common misidentifications.

Results.—Errors were 7.5 times more common with certain letters (*B, C, F, S*) than with others (*A, L, Z, T*), this difference increasing to 17.6-fold at threshold. Similar relative letter difficulty was demonstrated at lines above and at visual acuity thresholds, and both difficult and easy letters were the same for amblyopic and nonamblyopic fellow eyes. Specific misidentification errors were often repeated and were often reciprocal (eg, *B* for *E* and *E* for *B*).

Conclusion.—Since therapeutic decisions in amblyopia management are often based on small differences in visual acuities, the relative difficulties of letters used in their measurement should be considered. The Early Treatment Diabetic Retinopathy Study system should be considered for use in this clinical setting.

▶ Pediatric ophthalmologists are aware that certain letters are routinely more difficulty to recognize for both amblyopic and nonamblyopic patients. The letters the authors found to produce more errors—B, C, F, S—are exactly the letters I have found to cause errors. For instance, very often parents will question why their child missed the letter S on the 20/25 line and yet the child was able to identify the other letters without difficulty. This article confirms the clinical observations of pediatric ophthalmologists. Perhaps a new letter system for the Snellen chart needs to be evaluated to coincide with the authors' findings.

L. B. Nelson, MD, MBA

8 Neuro-ophthalmology

Asymmetric bilateral demyelinating optic neuropathy from tacrolimus toxicity

Venneti S, Moss HE, Levin MH, et al (Univ of Pennsylvania School of Medicine, Philadelphia)

J Neurol Sci 301:112-115, 2011

Objective.—To report the first histopathologic description of optic nerve demyelination from tacrolimus (FK 506) toxicity in the absence of toxic levels of tacrolimus in a patient presenting with asymmetric bilateral visual loss after 5 years of tacrolimus therapy.

Patients.—We report a patient status post cardiac and renal transplantation who developed severe, progressive and asynchronous bilateral visual

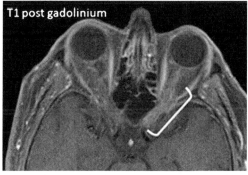

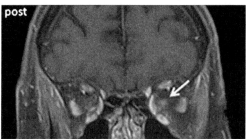

FIGURE 1.—MRI images obtained at time of initial hospitalization. Upper and lower images demonstrate enlargement and enhancement of the proximal left optic nerve (bracket and arrow) on T1 fat saturated post gadolinium sequences. (Reprinted from Venneti S, Moss HE, Levin MH, et al. Asymmetric bilateral demyelinating optic neuropathy from tacrolimus toxicity. *J Neurol Sci.* 2011;301:112-115, Copyright 2011, with permission from Elsevier.)

199

loss after prolonged treatment with tacrolimus. Orbital MRI showed an enlarged left optic nerve that enhanced with gadolinium.

Conclusion.—After extensive negative work up, biopsy of one optic nerve was performed. Microscopic analysis showed extensive demyelination in the absence of vasculitis, neoplastic or infectious etiologies. Our patient illustrates that demyelination of the optic nerve causing asynchronous vision loss can be associated with tacrolimus toxicity in the absence of toxic drug levels (Fig 1).

▶ This is another highly instructive case report that clinicians need to be aware of as more and more patients receive transplanted organs and are treated with tacrolimus for immunosuppression. This case is unique in that the drug levels were never in the toxic range, but there was a 5-year duration of exposure, suggesting a possible cumulative effect of medication in some patients.

The case is well documented and bilateral involvement is required to establish a diagnosis of toxic optic neuropathy, although the involvement may be asymmetric. The MRI images (Fig 1) also demonstrate much more enlargement of the nerve than is usually seen with optic neuritis associated with remitting relapsing multiple sclerosis.

R. C. Sergott, MD

In vivo identification of alteration of inner neurosensory layers in branch retinal artery occlusion

Ritter M, Sacu S, Deák GG, et al (Med Univ of Vienna, Austria)
Br J Ophthalmol 96:201-207, 2012

Background/Aims.—To characterise the extension and progression of alteration of neurosensory layers following acute and chronic branch retinal artery occlusion (BRAO) in vivo using spectral-domain optical coherence tomography.

Methods.—In this observational case series, eight eyes with acute BRAO and nine eyes with chronic BRAO were analysed using a Spectralis Heidelberg Retina Angiograph (HRA)+optical coherence tomography system including eye tracking. Patients with acute BRAO were examined within 36 ± 5 h after primary event and at weekly/monthly intervals thereafter. Segmentation measurements of all individual neurosensory layers were performed on single A-scans at six locations in affected and corresponding non-affected areas. The thickness values of the retinal nerve fibre layer together with the ganglion cell layer (NFL/GCL), inner plexiform layer (IPL), inner nuclear layer together with outer plexiform layer (INL/OPL), outer nuclear layer (ONL), and photoreceptor layers together with the retinal pigment epithelium (PR/RPE) were measured and analysed.

Results.—Segmentation evaluation revealed a distinct increase in thickness of inner neurosensory layers including the NFL/GCL (35%), IPL (80%), INL/OPL (48%) and mildly the ONL by 21% in acute ischaemia

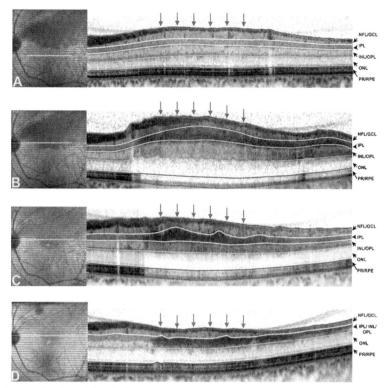

FIGURE 1.—Spectral-domain OCT scans of a case with acute branch retinal artery occlusion (BRAO), 24 h after the first symptoms (A, B) and 2 weeks (C) and 2 months (D) thereafter. For analysis of retinal layers, scans in the area of BRAO (B, C, D) and as a normal counterpart, in the anatomically corresponding area in the non-involved half of macula (A) were selected. Retinal layers were manually segmented as illustrated, and layer thickness was measured at six locations within the selected scans (locations indicated by the six perpendicular arrows). Swelling of the inner retina is most notable in the increased thickness of the inner plexiform layer (IPL) followed by the inner nuclear layer/inner plexiform layer (INL/IPL) and nerve fibre layer/ganglion cell layer (NFL/GCL) (A, B). The IPL could not be distinguished from the INL/IPL at month 2 (D). The outer nuclear layer (ONL) shows a slight increase in thickness in the acute phase (A), and the photoreceptor/retinal pigment epithelium (PR/RPE) complex retained stable thickness values during the entire follow-up (B, C, D). (Reprinted from Ritter M, Sacu S, Deak GG, et al. In vivo identification of alteration of inner neurosensory layers in branch retinal artery occlusion. *Br J Ophthalmol.* 2012;96:201-207, with permission from BMJ Publishing Group Ltd.)

compared with corresponding layers in non-ischaemic areas. Regression of intraretinal oedema was followed by persistent retinal atrophy with loss of differentiation between IPL and INL/OPL at month 2. In contrast, the ONL and subjacent PR/RPE retained their physiological thickness in patients with chronic BRAO.

Conclusion.—In vivo assessment of retinal layer morphology allows a precise identification of the pathophysiology in retinal ischaemia (Figs 1-3).

▶ The next technologic breakthrough with optical coherence tomography imaging for retinal diseases, glaucoma, and neuro-ophthalmic syndromes is

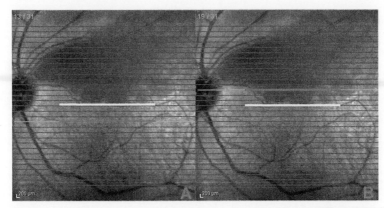

FIGURE 2.—Infrared fundus images with the 31 superimposed spectral-domain OCT scan lines of the patient shown in figure 1 at acute presentation. The central foveal scan is indicated by the yellow line represented by scan No 16. Scan No 19 showed the highest macular oedema, and as this scan is three scans apart from the central fovea, scan No 13 was selected as the normal counterpart in the non-involved macular region. The selected scans in the normal counterpart (A) and the affected region (B) are indicated with a red line. For interpretation of the references to color in this figure legend, the reader is referred to web version of this article. (Reprinted from Ritter M, Sacu S, Deák GG, et al. In vivo identification of alteration of inner neurosensory layers in branch retinal artery occlusion. *Br J Ophthalmol.* 2012;96: 201-207, with permission from BMJ Publishing Group Ltd.)

the accurate, precise, and reproducible measurements of individual retinal layers in specific disease processes. The authors very cleverly use the clinical event of branch retinal artery occlusion in both its chronic and acute state to define the response of the retina to ischemic injury. As expected, the inner retina was significantly thinned (Figs 1-3), but the outer retina was spared. Knowledge of these findings will permit the diagnosis of a pre-existing branch retinal artery occlusion that was not seen at the time of acute presentation. The clinical course of these changes will provide the basis for rational clinical trials for the treatment of retinal ischemia.

R. C. Sergott, MD

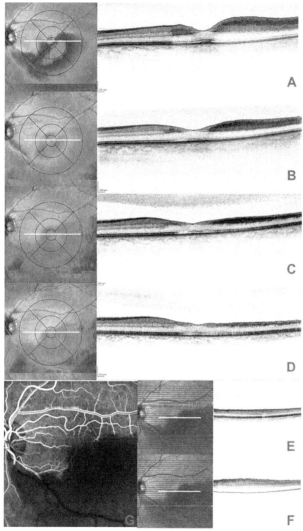

FIGURE 3.—(A—D) Occlusion of the infertior temporal artery in the left eye, showing an oedematous area along the inferior temporal branch and a partially compromised fovea. Serial spectraldomain OCT macular thickness maps and high resolution A scans across the fovea recorded at day 0 (A), month 1 (B), month 2 (C) and month 3 (D). The scans show an increase in retinal thickness in the inferior macula as a result of oedema in the inner retinal layers. The oedema subsequently resolved at month 1 (B) with decreasing macular thickness at month 2 (C). (E, F) Infrared fundus images with the superimposed OCT scan-lines and the selected B-scans for segmentation measurements at baseline. The central foveal scan is indicated by the yellow line, and the selected scans in the normal counterpart (E) and the affected region (F) are indicated with a red line. (G) Fluorescein angiography showing asymmetry in vascular filling in the early phase of the examination. For interpretation of the references to color in this figure legend, the reader is referred to web version of this article. (Reprinted from Ritter M, Sacu S, Deák GG, et al. In vivo identification of alteration of inner neurosensory layers in branch retinal artery occlusion. *Br J Ophthalmol.* 2012;96:201-207, with permission from BMJ Publishing Group Ltd.)

Clinical Characteristics in 53 Patients with Cat Scratch Optic Neuropathy

Chi SL, Stinnett S, Eggenberger E, et al (Duke Eye Ctr and Duke Univ Med Ctr, Durham, NC; Michigan State Univ, East Lansing; et al)
Ophthalmology 119:183-187, 2012

Objective.—To describe the clinical manifestations and to identify risk factors associated with visual outcome in a large cohort of patients with cat scratch optic neuropathy (CSON).

Design.—Multicenter, retrospective chart review.

Participants.—Fifty-three patients (62 eyes) with serologically positive CSON from 5 academic neuro-ophthalmology services evaluated over an 11-year period.

Methods.—Institutional review board/ethics committee approval was obtained. Data from medical record charts were collected to detail the clinical manifestations and to analyze visual outcome metrics. Generalized estimating equations and logistic regression analysis were used in the statistical analysis. Six patients (9 eyes) were excluded from visual outcome statistical analysis because of a lack of follow-up.

Main Outcome Measures.—Demographic information, symptoms at presentation, clinical characteristics, length of follow-up, treatment used, and visual acuity (at presentation and final follow-up).

Results.—Mean patient age was 27.8 years (range, 8−65 years). Mean follow-up time was 170.8 days (range, 1−1482 days). Simultaneous bilateral involvement occurred in 9 (17%) of 53 patients. Visual acuity on presentation ranged from 20/20 to counting fingers (mean, 20/160). Sixty-eight percent of eyes retained a visual acuity of 20/40 or better at final follow-up (defined as favorable visual outcome). Sixty-seven percent of patients endorsed a history of cat or kitten scratch. Neuroretinitis (macular star) developed in 28 eyes (45%). Only 5 patients had significant visual complications (branch retinal artery occlusion, macular hole, and corneal decompensation). Neither patient age nor any other factor except good initial visual acuity and absence of systemic symptoms was associated with a favorable visual outcome. There was no association between visual acuity at final follow-up and systemic antibiotic or steroid use.

Conclusions.—Patients with CSON have a good overall visual prognosis. Good visual acuity at presentation was associated with a favorable visual outcome. The absence of a macular star does not exclude the possibility of CSON.

▶ Cat scratch fever has recently been receiving more and more attention as the ability to diagnose the condition has increased with serological testing. This article offers a comprehensive review of the possible clinical presentations, baseline and follow-up visual acuities, and an analysis of the treatment results. Readers should carefully examine Table 3 in the original article, which illustrates data supporting the thesis that neither antibiotic nor corticosteroid treatment significantly altered the ultimate visual outcome. Another important point is that the absence of a macular star does not exclude the diagnosis.

R. C. Sergott, MD

Traumatic Optic Neuropathy After Maxillofacial Trauma: A Review of 8 Cases

Urolagin SB, Kotrashetti SM, Kale TP, et al (KLE VK Inst of Dental Sciences, Karnataka, India)

J Oral Maxillofac Surg 70:1123-1130, 2012

Purpose.—To study the incidence and prognostic factors of traumatic optic neuropathy in maxillofacial trauma cases.

Material and Method.—Eight patients diagnosed with traumatic optic neuropathy among 354 cases of maxillofacial trauma treated from December 2008 through May 2011 were included in this retrospective study. Factors at the time of trauma, clinical findings, computed tomographic findings, and interventional modalities were studied for any improvement in vision.

Results.—Of 354 maxillofacial trauma cases, 8 cases (2.25%) were diagnosed with traumatic optic neuropathy. Patients' ages ranged from 21 to 60 years. The causes of trauma were road traffic accidents in 7 patients and surgery for zygomaticomaxillary complex (ZMC) fractures in 1 patient. All patients had ZMC fracture; 1 patient had Le Fort II, mandible condyle, and ramus fractures and 2 had associated cranial bone fracture. Six patients were administered steroid therapy; 1 patient showed improvement in visual acuity. Two patients underwent decompression by a lateral orbital approach; 1 patient showed an improvement in visual acuity. In 2 other patients, a spontaneous recovery was observed. Four of the 8 patients underwent open reduction and fixation of the maxillofacial fractures. Of the remaining patients, 1 patient had a nondisplaced ZMC fracture that was treated without surgical intervention and the other 3 patients refused any surgical intervention.

Conclusions.—The present findings showed the occurrence of traumatic optic neuropathy in association with ZMC, Le Fort II, and cranial bone fractures. Additional risk factors such as a history of a loss of consciousness, injury to the superolateral orbital region, fracture of the optic canal, evidence of orbital hemorrhage, and evidence of blood within the posterior ethmoidal cells should be considered during the evaluation.

▶ Traumatic optic neuropathy remains a major unsolved and untreatable problem in neuro-ophthalmology. This study focuses on optic nerve injury occurring in the setting of maxillofacial trauma.

This article confirms the lack of improvement with corticosteroids and the ability for spontaneous improvement. In fact, past studies support the concept that corticosteroids may be harmful for this condition in terms of increased morbidity and mortality. We desperately need more information about the mechanism of injury in these cases in terms of acute axonal and neuronal changes. We currently do not recommend corticosteroids for these patients and consider repair of any optic canal fracture only when there is significant and unequivocal evidence of compression of the optic nerve.

R. C. Sergott, MD

Objective perimetry using a four-channel multifocal VEP system: correlation with conventional perimetry and thickness of the retinal nerve fibre layer
Horn FK, Kaltwasser C, Jünemann AG, et al (Univ of Erlangen-Nürnberg, Germany)
Br J Ophthalmol 96:554-559, 2012

Purpose.—There is evidence that multifocal visual evoked potentials (VEPs) can be used as an objective tool to detect visual field loss. The aim of this study was to correlate multifocal VEP amplitudes with standard perimetry data and retinal nerve fibre layer (RNFL) thickness.

Method.—Multifocal VEP recordings were performed with a four-channel electrode array using 58 stimulus fields (pattern reversal dartboard). For each field, the recording from the channel with maximal signal-to-noise ratio (SNR) was retained, resulting in an SNR optimised virtual recording. Correlation with RNFL thickness, measured with spectral domain optical coherence tomography and with standard perimetry, was performed for nerve fibre bundle related areas.

Results.—The mean amplitudes in nerve fibre related areas were smaller in glaucoma patients than in normal subjects. The differences between both groups were most significant in mid-peripheral areas. Amplitudes in these areas were significantly correlated with corresponding RNFL thickness (Spearman R=0.76) and with standard perimetry (R=0.71).

Conclusion.—The multifocal VEP amplitude was correlated with perimetric visual field data and the RNFL thickness of the corresponding regions. This method of SNR optimisation is useful for extracting data from recordings and may be appropriate for objective assessment of visual function at different locations.

Trial Registration Number.—This study has been registered at http://www.clinicaltrials.gov (NCT00494923).

▶ Any time that clinicians can replace a subjective test with an objective test of structure or function, diagnostic accuracy improves as well as the ability to detect change over time in longitudinal studies.

The authors correlated multifocal visual-evoked potentials (VEP) with spectral domain optical coherence tomography and standard perimetry (Fig 2 in the original article). Even patients who perform visual field testing flawlessly on one occasion can develop significant variability in test-taking performance at subsequent examinations. The multifocal VEP technology offers a potential method to acquire more objective data. Whether this testing method is feasible for large numbers of patients remains to be seen, but it is worth watching in the future.

R. C. Sergott, MD

Amiodarone-associated Optic Neuropathy: A Critical Review
Passman RS, Bennett CL, Purpura JM, et al (Northwestern Univ Feinberg School of Medicine, Chicago, IL; Univ of South Carolina, Columbia; et al)
Am J Med 125:447-453, 2012

Although amiodarone is the most commonly prescribed anti-arrhythmic drug, its use is limited by serious toxicities, including optic neuropathy. Current reports of amiodarone-associated optic neuropathy identified from the Food and Drug Administration's Adverse Event Reporting System and published case reports were reviewed. A total of 296 reports were identified: 214 from the Adverse Event Reporting System, 59 from published case reports, and 23 from adverse events reports for patients enrolled in clinical trials. Mean duration of amiodarone therapy before vision loss was 9 months (range 1-84 months). Insidious onset of amiodarone-associated optic neuropathy (44%) was the most common presentation, and nearly one third were asymptomatic. Optic disk edema was present in 85% of cases. Following drug cessation, 58% had improved visual acuity, 21% were unchanged, and 21% had further decreased visual acuity. Legal blindness (<20/200) was noted in at least one eye in 20% of cases. Close ophthalmologic surveillance of patients during the tenure of amiodarone administration is warranted.

▶ Adverse and serious adverse events from medication therapy always need to be considered in the differential diagnosis of any optic neuropathy. Although bilateral involvement is inevitable, patients may often present with predominately unilateral, asymmetric findings. A comprehensive history of all medication use is essential, and with amiodarone and other medications, detection of the inciting agent may be complicated by reporting of medications by brand names. Amiodarone has a much longer tissue half-life than its half-life in plasma. Therefore, the medication can be stopped promptly in consultation with a cardiologist. In the past, amiodarone was often the only medication available to control a patient's arrhythmia, but now more drugs are available. Patients on amiodarone are also at significantly increased risk for nonarteritic ischemic optic neuropathy, a disorder that only rarely, if ever, is simultaneous and bilateral, except in the case of acute blood loss.

Clinical Significance:

• Amiodarone-induced optic neuropathy is rare but serious.
• Diagnosis is based on 4 parameters: onset of visual loss, degree of visual deficit, time to resolution, and ocular involvement. Amiodarone-induced optic neuropathy is insidious in onset, has a range of visual deficits, resolves over months, and is often bilateral.

• Although rare, risk of severe vision loss and permanent blindness mandate that patients on amiodarone be followed by an ophthalmologist.

R. C. Sergott, MD

Demyelination Affects Temporal Aspects of Perception: An Optic Neuritis Study

Raz N, Dotan S, Chokron S, et al (Hadassah Hebrew Univ Med Ctr, Jerusalem, Israel; Rothschild Ophthalmological Foundation, Paris, France)
Ann Neurol 71:531-538, 2012

Objective.—Visual Evoked Potentials (VEPs) following optic neuritis (ON) remain chronically prolonged, although standard visual tests indicate full recovery. We hypothesized that dynamic visual processes, such as motion perception, may be more vulnerable to slowed conduction in the optic nerve, and consequently be better associated with projection rates.

Methods.—Twenty-one patients with acute unilateral, first-ever ON were studied during 1 year. Static visual functions (visual acuity, color perception, visual field, and contrast sensitivity), dynamic visual functions (motion perception), and VEPs were assessed repeatedly.

Results.—Visual and electrophysiological measurements reached maximal performance 4 months following the acute phase, with no subsequent improvement. Whereas VEP amplitude and static visual functions recovered, VEP latency remained significantly prolonged, and motion perception remained impaired throughout the 12-month period. A strong correlation was found between VEP latencies and motion perception. Visual performance at 1 month was strongly predictive of visual outcome. For static functions, patients who showed partial recovery at 1 month subsequently achieved full recovery. For dynamic functions, the rate of improvement was constant across patients, independent of the initial deficit level.

Interpretation.—Conduction velocity in the visual pathways correlated closely with dynamic visual functions, implicating the need for rapid transmission of visual input to perceive motion. Motion perception level may serve as a tool to assess the magnitude of myelination in the visual pathways. The constancy across patients may serve as a baseline to assess the efficacy of currently developing neuroprotective and regenerative therapeutic strategies, targeting myelination in the central nervous system.

▶ The authors develop an interesting approach to visual parameters in acute and recovering demyelinating optic neuritis. They confirm previous work, first observed in the Optic Neuritis Treatment Trial, that visual performance 1 month after developing optic neuritis was very predictive of the ultimate visual outcome. Improvement stabilized at 4 months, and their data demonstrate that "dynamic" rather than "static" measures of visual function may be better correlated with persistent abnormalities. Visual-evoked potentials, specifically latency and motion perception, remained abnormal throughout 12 months, suggesting that these 2 parameters may be best suited for developing protocols for clinical trials in an attempt to demonstrate neuroprotection and restoration of neural function. Examining spectral domain optical coherence tomography parameters from these patients would have added an important structural dimension to the study; however, despite not having that information, this article has considerable importance in explaining patients' long-term clinical symptoms after an event of optic neuritis and should be valuable in developing meaningful clinical trials.

R. C. Sergott, MD

Acute retinal necrosis associated optic neuropathy
Witmer MT, Pavan PR, Fouraker BD, et al (Univ of South Florida, Tampa, FL)
Acta Ophthalmol 89:599-607, 2011

Acute retinal necrosis (ARN) syndrome is characterized by severe intraocular inflammation, occlusive vasculopathy and peripheral retinal necrosis. Vision threatening complications of this syndrome include retinal detachment, macular oedema and ischaemia and optic neuropathy. Optic nerve involvement may be the presenting sign of ARN and this condition should be included in the differential diagnosis of acute papillitis. Several mechanisms may lead to ARN associated optic neuropathy including vasculitis, optic nerve ischaemia and direct optic nerve invasion by the herpes virus. We review optic nerve involvement during ARN and present its incidence, pathogenesis, differential diagnosis and treatment (Fig 1, Table 1).

▶ Because acute retinal necrosis (ARN) is a rare syndrome and very difficult to treat, early suspicion and diagnosis is essential. Any patient presenting with

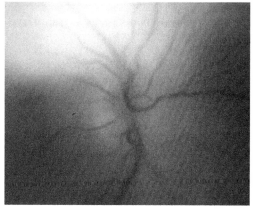

FIGURE 1.—Colour photograph of the right optic nerve head from a patient with ARN, demonstrating optic disc oedema. The veins of the optic nerve are severely dilated. This patient's vitreous biopsy was positive by polymerase chain reaction (PCR) for varicella zoster virus. (Reprinted from Witmer MT, Pavan PR, Fouraker BD, et al. Acute retinal necrosis associated optic neuropathy. *Acta Ophthalmol.* 2011;89:599-607, with permission from Acta Ophthalmologica Scandinavica Foundation.)

TABLE 1.—Percentage of ARN Syndrome Eyes with Optic Neuropathy

Study	No. of Eyes	No. of Patients	No. with Optic Neuropathy	Percentage
Sergott et al. (1989)	17	–	8	47.1
Labetoulle et al. (1995)	14	–	8	57.1
Batisse et al. (1996)	–	23	13	56.5
Muthiah et al. (2007)	31	–	–	>50
Lau et al. (2007)	27	–	3	11.1
Engstrom et al. (1994)*	65	38	11	16.9

Editor's Note: Please refer to original journal article for full references.
*AIDS patients with a diagnosis of Progressive Outer Retinal Necrosis (PORN). All other reported series are ARN syndrome associated.

a swollen optic nerve and papillitis must always be evaluated for the presence of vitreous cells. If vitreous cells are found, then careful attention must be paid to the presence of any whitening of the peripheral retina and narrowing of the retinal arterioles. We also recommend magnetic resonance imaging with and without gadolinium enhancement to search for any optic nerve enlargement/ enhancement as well as any involvement of the meninges. Fig 1 shows a typical case of ARN optic neuropathy (notice the lack of disc hemorrhages). Table 1 provides an overview of the previous publications regarding this syndrome.

R. C. Sergott, MD

Opsoclonus and multiple cranial neuropathy as a manifestation of neuroborreliosis
van Erp WS, Bakker NA, Johannes M, et al (Sint Antonius Ziekenhuis, Nieuwegein, the Netherlands; Univ Med Ctr Groningen, the Netherlands)
Neurology 77:1013-1014, 2011

Background.—Opsoclonus is manifest as involuntary, chaotic dyskinesia of the eyes in random directions that is exacerbated when the patient redirects the gaze and persists even when the eyelids are closed. Strong evidence supports an immune-mediated, paraneoplastic, or parainfectious dysfunction of the central nervous system as the possible pathogenesis of this rare disorder. The many possible presentations of neuroborreliosis include combinations of central and peripheral neurologic symptoms, including opsoclonus-myoclonus syndrome (OMS). A patient with opsoclonus but no myoclonus caused by neuroborreliosis was reported.

Case Report.—Man, 50, had a painful red right eye present for 3 days and diffuse unilateral headache that had lasted about 6 weeks. Physical examination revealed a right-sided conjunctivitis and irregularly jerking, gaze-evoked nystagmus-like conjugated movement of both eyes. A week later the patient awoke with right-sided drooping mouth and eyelid. He had no involuntary jerky limb movements, oscillopsia, or diplopia, and his headache was not associated with other symptoms. He had recently visited areas endemic for Lyme disease, but no tick bite history was reported. Neurologic evaluation found a slight right peripheral facial palsy. When he redirected his gaze, a conjugated, irregular, and unpredictable "dancing" of his eyes was noted in the horizontal, vertical, and diagonal directions. "Shimmering" was observed through the eyelids even after closing the eyes. The pupils were of equal size and had intact light reactions. Routine laboratory investigation results were normal, but a brain magnetic resonance imaging (MRI) scan showed bilateral gadolinium contrast enhancement of cranial nerves III, VII, IX, X, XI, and XII plus right-sided enhancement of nerves IV, V, and VI. Lumbar puncture revealed an opening pressure of 20 cm H_2O, a cerebrospinal fluid (CSF) pleocytosis of 244 leukocytes, a moderately elevated total protein level, and a slightly diminished CSF/serum glucose ratio. Neuroborreliosis was considered, and the patient was given intravenous ceftriaxone 2000 mg twice a day. Three days after hospitalization, the patient's immunoglobulin M and G antibodies for *Borrelia burgdorferi* were elevated in serum and CSF, indicating specific intrathecal antibody production. The CSF culture was negative but antibiotic treatment was continued for 14 days. After 6 weeks the patient was asymptomatic and continued to be up to 18 months after his initial visit.

Conclusions.—This patient had active neuroborreliosis with opsoclonus as a concomitant acute parainfectious manifestation. The radiologic findings may indicate an inflammation of multiple cranial nerves leads to erroneous input to the central motor ocular control mechanisms and thereby contributes to the opsoclonus, or may reflect a separate consequence of the neuroborreliosis.

▶ Neuroborreliosis is often preceded by manifestations of Lyme disease, and this case report adds yet another manifestation of this syndrome—opsoclonus. Opsoclonus presents as a chaotic, involuntary, random eye movement disorder, most often associated with a paraneoplastic syndrome and myoclonus, ataxia, and encephalopathy, which this patient did not have. This specific patient had a parainfectious cause, which responded to antibiotic therapy.

R. C. Sergott, MD

Early Factors Associated with Axonal Loss after Optic Neuritis
Henderson APD, Altmann DR, Trip SA, et al (Univ College London, UK; et al)
Ann Neurol 70:955-963, 2011

Objective.—Acute optic neuritis due to an inflammatory demyelinating lesion of the optic nerve is often seen in association with multiple sclerosis. Although functional recovery usually follows the acute episode of visual loss, persistent visual deficits are common and are probably due to axonal loss. The mechanisms of axonal loss and early features that predict it are not well defined. We investigated clinical, electrophysiological, and imaging measures at presentation and after 3 months as potential markers of axonal loss following optic neuritis.

Methods.—We followed 21 patients after their first attack of acute unilateral optic neuritis for up to 18 months. Axonal loss was inferred from optical coherence tomography measures of retinal nerve fiber layer (RNFL) thickness at least 6 months following the episode. Visual function, visual evoked potential, and optic nerve magnetic resonance imaging measures obtained during the acute episode and 3 months later were investigated for their association with later axonal loss.

Results.—After multivariate analysis, prolonged visual evoked potential latency and impaired color vision, at baseline and after 3 months, were significantly and independently associated with RNFL thinning. Low-contrast acuity measures exhibited significant univariate associations with RNFL thinning.

Interpretation.—The association of RNFL loss with a prolonged visual evoked potential (VEP) latency suggests that acute and persistent demyelination is associated with increased vulnerability of axons. VEP latency and visual function tests that capture optic nerve function, such as color and contrast, may help identify subjects with a higher risk for axonal loss who are thus more suitable for experimental neuroprotection trials.

▶ Although optical coherence tomography (OCT) was once, and in some circles still is, ridiculed for its use in multiple sclerosis and optic neuritis, there is no longer any doubt that this technology has shown us and will continue to show us very important new observations in this debilitating neurodegenerative condition.

This article previews how future clinical and research studies should and will be conducted, that is, combining structure and function. Earlier studies have examined either OCT or visual evoked potential but rarely both entities. This dual approach will enable us to understand more completely the response of the optic nerve to demyelination and to design meaningful trials for neuroprotection.

R. C. Sergott, MD

Diffusion Tensor Imaging in Acute Optic Neuropathies: Predictor of Clinical Outcomes
Naismith RT, Xu J, Tutlam NT, et al (Washington Univ, St Louis, MO)
Arch Neurol 69:65-71, 2012

Objective.—To evaluate directional diffusivities within the optic nerve in a first event of acute optic neuritis to determine whether decreased axial diffusivity (AD) would predict 6-month visual outcome and optic nerve integrity measures.

Design.—Cohort study.

Setting.—Academic multiple sclerosis center.

Patients.—Referred sample of 25 individuals who presented within 31 days after acute visual symptoms consistent with optic neuritis. Visits were scheduled at baseline, 2 weeks, and 1, 3, 6, and 12 months.

Main Outcome Measures.—Visual acuity, contrast sensitivity, visual evoked potentials (VEPs), and thickness of the retinal nerve fiber layer (RNFL).

Results.—An incomplete 6-month visual recovery was associated with a lower baseline AD (1.50 μm^2/ms [95% confidence interval {CI}, 1.36-1.64 μm^2/ms for incomplete recovery vs 1.75 μm^2/ms [95% CI, 1.67-1.83 μm^2/ ms] for complete recovery). Odds of complete recovery decreased by 53% (95% CI, 27%-70%) for every 0.1- unit decrease in baseline AD. A lower baseline AD correlated with worse 6-month visual outcomes in visual acuity ($r = 0.40$, $P = .03$), contrast sensitivity ($r = 0.41$, $P = .02$), VEP amplitude ($r = 0.55$, $P < .01$), VEP latency ($r = -0.38$, $P = .04$), and RNFL thickness ($r = 0.53$, $P = .02$). Radial diffusivity increased between months 1 and 3 to become higher in those with incomplete recovery at 12 months than in those with complete recovery (1.45 μm^2/ms [95% CI, 1.31-1.59 μm^2/ms] vs 1.19 μm^2/ms [95% CI, 1.10-1.28 μm^2/ms]).

Conclusions.—Decreased AD in acute optic neuritis was associated with a worse 6-month visual outcome and correlated with VEP and RNFL measures of axon and myelin injury. Axial diffusivity may serve as a marker of axon injury in acute white matter injury.

▶ Nontraditional MRI scan techniques are not ready for routine clinical work, but these advanced methods are now providing important data about the response of central nervous system pathways to a number of stimuli. The present article is especially important for clinicians and clinical researchers involved with the study of multiple sclerosis and optic neuritis. Using the visual system as a model, the current research enables us to see how the axons of the optic nerve respond to demyelination. Decreased axial diffusivity was associated with incomplete recovery. The lower baseline axial diffusivity also correlated with reduced visual-evoked potential amplitudes and latencies and decreased retinal nerve fiber layer thickness as measured by optical coherence tomography (OCT). Combined with OCT, we believe that diffusion tensor imaging will increase our understanding not only of demyelinating optic neuropathy but also of all other mechanisms of optic nerve injury.

R. C. Sergott, MD

Topiramate Effect in Opsoclonus-Myoclonus-Ataxia Syndrome
Fernandes TD, Bazan R, Betting LE, et al (Universidade Estadual Paulista Júlio de Mesquita Filho, Botucatu São Paulo, Brazil)
Arch Neurol 69:133, 2012

Background.—Opsoclonus-myoclonus-ataxia syndrome (OMS) is rare and mainly affects children, producing abnormal eye movements, limb myoclonia, and cerebellar ataxia. The involuntary, conjugate, arrhythmic, multidirectional, high-amplitude saccades of opsoclonus persist during sleep and are exacerbated by visual fixation. Opsoclonus may occur secondarily to paraneoplastic disease, with about 50% of children who have OMS also exhibiting neuroblastoma. Other associated cancers include breast, ovarian, and lung carcinomas. Among the other causes of OMS are multiple sclerosis, toxic metabolic states, and infectious diseases such as poliomyelitis, salmonella infection, and Coxsackie virus disease. The causative mechanism has not been identified, but a loss of inhibitory γ-aminobutyric acid-n-mediated control leading to disinhibition of the fastigial nucleus in the cerebellum has been proposed as an etiologic focus. The use of topiramate, an antiepileptic drug, may help to manage OMS symptoms.

> *Case Study.*—Woman, 34, had no comorbid conditions but developed severe truncal ataxia and opsoclonus over the course of 4 days. After 20 days she was hospitalized and tested to reveal the cause of her OMS. Tests included cerebrospinal fluid examination; serologic investigations for infectious diseases and collagenosis; brain and spine magnetic resonance imaging; computed tomography of the thoracic, abdominal, and pelvic areas; and screening for gynecologic neoplasia. All results were normal. The patient was given topiramate in a starting dose of 50 mg/day that was titrated to 150 mg/day over 10 days. The patient's symptoms improved remarkably, so the topiramate was gradually reduced to 50 mg/day after a few days. After 1 week, the ataxia and opsoclonus grew worse, prompting a return to the 150-mg/day dosing. Symptoms again improved.

Conclusions.—The mechanisms by which topiramate works are as yet unidentified, but it is hypothesized that this drug inhibits glutamate-mediated neurotransmission and increment of the γ-aminobutyric acid-n-mediated current. This would stabilize hyperexcited neuronal membranes and support GABAergic activity, which would inhibit the cerebellar circuits believed to be the focus in OMS pathophysiology. Topiramate may offer an effective way to manage OMS symptoms.

▶ The opsoclonus-myoclonus-ataxia may develop without an identifiable paraneoplastic or parainfectious cause. In these cryptic cases, treatment must be symptomatic, and the present case adds another potential therapeutic intervention—topiramate. Although having the obvious limitations of single case report, the article does provide strong circumstantial evidence for a therapeutic effect of this medication in this particular case. In addition, topiramate is a relatively low-risk medication in terms of potential side effects and adverse events.

R. C. Sergott, MD

Multiple Cranial Neuropathies Evolving Over a Decade From Occult Perineural Basal Cell Carcinoma

Fletcher WA, Almekhlafi M, Auer RN (Univ of Calgary, Alberta, Canada)
Arch Neurol 69:134-135, 2012

Background.—Between 0.2% and 2% of basal cell carcinomas are complicated by microscopic perineural invasion. The clinical features of perineural spread of basal cell carcinomas are similar to those of squamous cell carcinomas, except with respect to speed of progression. Often the failure to explicitly inquire about a history of skin cancer can lead to a missed diagnosis.

Case Report.—Man, 69, had diplopia and left ptosis of 3 months' duration as well as progressive loss of left trigeminal and facial nerve function over the previous 7 years. The nerve function was initially lost from the upper trigeminal branches and finally culminated in complete hemifacial anesthesia and paralysis. Repeated neurologic assessments and three magnetic resonance imaging (MRI) scans were unable to detect a cause for the problem. Although the patient denied any previous health issues, targeted questioning about skin cancer led to an examination of pathologic records, which revealed the excision of a basal cell carcinoma from the patient's forehead 4 years before he experienced neurologic symptoms. Enhanced MRI revealed the left ophthalmic, maxillary, mandibular, and facial nerves were thickened and enhanced. Mandibular nerve biopsy yielded malignant cells infiltrating the endoneurium and perineurium, with an immunohistochemical profile similar to that of the biopsies of resected basal cell carcinoma taken 10 years previously. The patient underwent radiotherapy of the left oculomotor, trigeminal, and facial nerves. A year later he returned for treatment of the right trigeminal nerve, which was now involved. He died 10 years after first experiencing neurologic symptoms.

Conclusions.—The diagnosis of perineural spread from basal cell carcinoma should be considered in patients who have partial trigeminal nerve dysfunction, particularly if they have experienced progression or also have localized dysfunction of the facial nerve. Often the MRI findings are normal in these patients, but thin-slice scans with gadolinium may reveal subtle intracranial or extracranial nerve involvement. Biopsy of peripheral branches may indicate the diagnosis, avoiding craniotomy. Diagnosis and treatment before MRI abnormalities appear are associated with greatly increased survival rates.

▶ This straightforward, well-documented case presentation emphasizes several important clinical management issues. First and foremost, in any patient with a neuro-ophthalmic problem and a history of cancer, the cancer is the cause of the problem until proven otherwise. This case illustrates that concept perfectly.

Second, clinicians must always be vigilant in seeking details about the removal of any skin lesion in and around the eyes. While squamous cell carcinomas and melanomas are well known to infiltrate cranial nerves, basal cells can infiltrate as well, albeit at a much less common incidence. Finally, normal magnetic resonance imaging (MRI) scans do not eliminate the possibility of infiltration lesion, and biopsy of surgically accessible nerves may be required to make the diagnosis. Figs 1 and 2 in the original article clearly show important MRI and pathological findings in this patient.

R. C. Sergott, MD

Optical coherence tomography segmentation reveals ganglion cell layer pathology after optic neuritis
Syc SB, Saidha S, Newsome SD, et al (Johns Hopkins Univ School of Medicine, Baltimore, MD; et al)
Brain 135:521-533, 2012

Post-mortem ganglion cell dropout has been observed in multiple sclerosis; however, longitudinal *in vivo* assessment of retinal neuronal layers following acute optic neuritis remains largely unexplored. Peripapillary retinal nerve fibre layer thickness, measured by optical coherence tomography, has been proposed as an outcome measure in studies of neuroprotective agents in multiple sclerosis, yet potential swelling during the acute stages of optic neuritis may confound baseline measurements. The objective of this study was to ascertain whether patients with multiple sclerosis or neuromyelitis optica develop retinal neuronal layer pathology following acute optic neuritis, and to systematically characterize such changes *in vivo* over time. Spectral domain optical coherence tomography imaging, including automated retinal layer segmentation, was performed serially in 20 participants during the acute phase of optic neuritis, and again 3 and 6 months later. Imaging was performed cross-sectionally in 98 multiple sclerosis participants, 22 neuromyelitis optica participants and 72 healthy controls. Neuronal thinning was observed in the ganglion cell layer of eyes affected by acute optic neuritis 3 and 6 months after onset ($P < 0.001$). Baseline ganglion cell layer thicknesses did not demonstrate swelling when compared with contralateral unaffected eyes, whereas peripapillary retinal nerve fibre layer oedema was observed in affected eyes ($P = 0.008$) and subsequently thinned over the course of this study. Ganglion cell layer thickness was lower in both participants with multiple sclerosis and participants with neuromyelitis optica, with and without a history of optic neuritis, when compared with healthy controls ($P < 0.001$) and correlated with visual function. Of all patient groups investigated, those with neuromyelitis optica and a history of optic neuritis exhibited the greatest reduction in ganglion cell layer thickness. Results from our *in vivo* longitudinal study demonstrate retinal neuronal layer thinning following acute optic neuritis, corroborating the hypothesis that axonal injury may cause neuronal pathology in multiple sclerosis. Further, these data provide evidence of subclinical disease activity, in both participants with multiple sclerosis and with neuromyelitis optica without a history of optic neuritis, a disease in which subclinical disease activity has not been widely appreciated. No pathology was seen in the inner or outer nuclear layers of eyes with optic neuritis, suggesting that retrograde degeneration after optic neuritis may not extend into the deeper retinal layers. The subsequent thinning of the ganglion cell layer following acute optic neuritis, in the absence of evidence of baseline swelling, suggests the potential utility of quantitative optical coherence tomography retinal layer segmentation to monitor neuroprotective effects of novel agents in therapeutic trials.

▶ The authors demonstrate a loss of ganglion cell thickness following events of acute optic neuritis in remitting relapsing multiple sclerosis (MS) and neuromyelitis optica. In addition, patients with MS without a history of acute optic neuritis also demonstrated ganglion cell loss. The value of segmentation techniques for spectral domain optical coherence technology depends on the ability of the technology to detect different histological layers of the retina. Therefore, caution was not exercised in drawing conclusions about the inner and outer nuclear layers, 2 histological areas that present much more difficult imaging challenges.

R. C. Sergott, MD

Retinal detachment associated with optic disc colobomas and morning glory syndrome
Chang S, Gregory-Roberts E, Chen R (Columbia Univ Med Ctr, NY)
Eye 26:494-500, 2012

We report the diagnosis and treatment of patients with retinal detachment and/or retinoschisis associated with optic nerve coloboma or morning glory syndrome. A retrospective review of patients with optic nerve coloboma or morning glory syndrome with associated retinal detachment or retinoschisis was conducted. For five patients (six eyes), were port the clinical findings, spectral domain optical coherence tomography (OCT) imaging, intraoperative findings, and treatment outcomes. OCT scans demonstrate a bilaminar structure of maculopathy, consisting of inner schisis-like changes and outer layer retinal detachment. In most cases, a retinal break was demonstrated within the optic disc defect with three-dimensional OCT imaging. Glial tissue was sometimes observed within the anomalous defect. Vitrectomy and resection of the tractional tissue in these cases produced good anatomical and visual outcomes. Retinal detachment spontaneously resolved in cases where traction was not present. Traction may contribute to the pathogenesis of retinal detachment associated with colobomatous optic disc anomalies, either directly or by creating a secondary retinal break. OCT imaging assists with understanding the contributing factors to retinal detachment in individual cases of colobomatous optic disc anomalies and can thereby assist with determining the most effective approach to management.

▶ Spectral domain optical coherence tomography (OCT) not only has a definite impact on neuro-ophthalmology in multiple sclerosis with the quantitation of axonal loss, but it also has an impact in the evaluation of unusual structure of the optic disc. This study is a wonderful example of how OCT is taking us beyond the limits of the ophthalmoscope, which ultimately improves our diagnostic and therapeutic strategies. The authors provide beautiful fundus photographic OCT correlations for patients with morning glory syndrome, optic disc colobomas, and retinal detachments (Fig 1 in the original article). The 3-dimensional reconstructions add considerable understanding about the tractional forces at work in these rare but important conditions. In my opinion, any patient with a highly unusual optic disc appearance should have spectral domain OCT imaging to identify any tractional forces that could lead to retinal detachment.

R. C. Sergott, MD

Nonarteritic anterior ischemic optic neuropathy in a child with optic disk drusen
Nanji AA, Klein KS, Pelak VS, et al (Johns Hopkins Univ School of Medicine, Baltimore, MD; Univ of Colorado, Denver)
J AAPOS 16:207-209, 2012

Optic disk drusen are calcific deposits that form in the optic nerve head secondary to abnormalities in axonal metabolism and degeneration. The clinical course is variable, ranging from stable vision to acute or progressive visual loss. We evaluated a healthy 12-year-old boy with a history of asymptomatic bilateral disk drusen who presented with acute painless unilateral visual loss after hiking to an altitude of 11,000 feet. Findings were consistent with nonarteritic anterior ischemic optic neuropathy.

▶ Another very informative case report with important diagnostic and management considerations. Optic disc drusen is most recognized as a "mimicker" of papilledema and a cause of retinal nerve fiber layer visual field defects. In this case, a combination of exposure to increased altitude and dehydration led to an event of ischemic optic neuropathy in a 12-year old (Fig 1 in the original article). I have found over the years that dehydration seems to be associated with nonarteritic ischemic optic neuropathies in some patients, and it is always worth seeking that history not only in optic nerve ischemia but also in any stroke syndrome. This study should prompt clinicians to warn patients with significant optic disc drusen to avoid dehydration or rapid exposure to high altitudes.

R. C. Sergott, MD

9 Imaging

A multi-centre case series investigating the aetiology of hypertrophic pachymeningitis with orbital inflammation
Cannon PS, Cruz AA, Pinto CT, et al (Univ of Adelaide, South Australia, Australia)
Orbit 30:64-69, 2011

Introduction.—To describe our attempt in establishing a definitive diagnosis in patients with hypertrophic pachymeningitis in combination with orbital inflammatory disease and report on the outcome.

Materials and Methods.—This was a retrospective case series of all patients presenting with hypertrophic pachymeningitis in association with orbital inflammation in 4 centres. Ophthalmic and neurological examination data, laboratory data, histology data, treatment plans and clinical outcome data were recorded. Patients underwent orbital/brain computed tomography and magnetic resonance imaging.

Results.—Six patients were identified; the median age was 46.5 years. Headache was the commonest presenting symptom, followed by diplopia and reduced visual acuity. Three patients underwent orbital biopsy, 1 patient underwent dura mater biopsy, 1 patient underwent both and 1 patient underwent nasal biopsy. Four patients were diagnosed with Wegener granulomatosis and 2 patients with tuberculosis. Corticosteroid therapy was initiated in 4 patients, with steroid-sparing drugs added later. Two patients received anti-tuberculosis treatment and 1 patient was commenced on pulsed cyclophosphamide. On follow-up, 1 patient required an exenteration for a painful blind eye and 1 patient's visual acuity remained at no perception to light. One patient had complete resolution of symptoms on treatment, 1 patient had persistent reduced visual acuity and 1 patient was lost to follow-up.

Conclusion.—We postulate that the combination of orbital inflammation and pachymeningitis is strongly suggestive of Wegener granulomatosis, although it may take a number of years to confirm. Tuberculosis should also be considered.

▶ Wegener granulomatosis (WG), also known as *granulomatosis with polyangiitis*, is an uncommon granulomatous vasculitis primarily involving the nasal/oral mucosa, lungs, and kidneys. The c-antineutrophil cytoplasmic antibody blood test is helpful in diagnosis, but biopsy is often required for definitive diagnosis. Central nervous system and orbital involvement have been described in a small percentage of these cases. This multicenter case series investigates the etiology of pachymeningitis and orbital inflammation occurring together, which is rarely reported in the literature. Pachymeningeal inflammation and orbital inflammation share a number of etiologies, including WG, tuberculosis (TB), and fungal infection and sarcoidosis (predilection for involving leptomeninges). Lymphoproliferative disorders and metastasis can mimic this appearance; however, these have been rarely described together. In this study, a definitive diagnosis was established in all cases, contrary to previous case reports, based on which they have postulated that WG and TB should be strongly suspected in cases in which hypertrophic meningitis is associated with orbital inflammation.

K. Talekar, MD
A. Flanders, MD

Carcinoid Tumor Metastases to the Extraocular Muscles: MR Imaging and CT Findings and Review of the Literature
Gupta A, Chazen JL, Phillips CD (Weill Cornell Med College, NY)
AJNR Am J Neuroradiol 32:1208-1211, 2011

Although a relatively rare neoplasm, primary carcinoid tumor has an unusual propensity to metastasize to the orbits. Within the orbit, metastatic EOM lesions have been described in scattered reports in the ophthalmology literature but have received little to no attention in the radiology literature. After a retrospective review, we identified CT and MR imaging studies of 7 patients with carcinoid tumor metastatic to the EOM. Our findings suggest that in patients with known carcinoid tumor, well-defined, round, or fusiform masses of the EOM should strongly suggest metastatic involvement. Our series suggests that bilateral lesions may occur and that any EOM can be involved. Knowledge of this pattern of metastatic disease may spare biopsies in some patients, and with current orbit-sparing therapy for patients with localized orbital disease, early and accurate diagnosis can significantly improve patient outcomes.

▶ Extraocular muscle (EOM) metastases are well described in several neoplasms, including breast, melanoma, prostate, and lung. Carcinoid tumor is a rare neoplasm (approximately 0.5% of all malignancies) that represents 4% to 5% of metastasis to the orbit.[1] There are scattered case reports in literature about this rare entity, with the current series of 7 patients discussing its CT and MRI features. It is important to recognize the propensity of carcinoid tumors to spread to the EOM. MRI and CT remain excellent tools to evaluate orbital lesions, and focal nodular enlargement of the muscle without invasion of the orbital fat or adjacent osseous structures is highly suggestive of EOM metastases in a patient with known malignancy.[2] Confirmation of the diagnosis via tissue sampling or radionuclide scintigraphy with a somatostatin analog or iodine-131 meta-iodobenzylguanidine may be obtained as necessary.

K. Talekar, MD
A. Flanders, MD

References

1. Mehta JS, Abou-Rayyah Y, Rose GE. Orbital carcinoid metastases. *Ophthalmology.* 2006;113:466-472.
2. Capone A Jr, Slamovits TL. Discrete metastasis of solid tumors to extraocular muscles. *Arch Ophthalmol.* 1990;108:237-243.

10 Ocular Oncology

A case-control study: occupational cooking and the risk of uveal melanoma

Schmidt-Pokrzywniak A, Jöckel K-H, Marr A, et al (Univ of Halle-Wittenberg, Germany; Univ of Duisburg-Essen, Germany)
BMC Ophthalmol 10:26, 2010

Background.—A European-wide population based case-control study (European rare cancer study) undertaken in nine European countries examined risk factors for uveal melanoma. They found a positive association between cooks and the risk of uveal melanoma. In our study we examine whether cooks or people who worked in cook related jobs have an increased uveal melanoma risk.

Methods.—We conducted a case-control study during 2002 and 2005. Overall, 1653 eligible subjects (age range: 20-74 years, living in Germany) participated. Interviews were conducted with 459 incident uveal melanoma cases, 827 population controls, 180 ophthalmologist controls and 187 sibling controls. Data on occupational exposure were obtained from a self-administered postal questionnaire and a computer-assisted telephone interview. We used conditional logistic regression to estimate odds ratios adjusting for the matching factors.

Results.—Overall, we did not observe an increased risk of uveal melanoma among people who worked as cooks or who worked in cook related jobs. When we restricted the source population of our study to the population of the Federal State of Northrhine-Westphalia, we observed an increased risk among subjects who were categorized as cooks in the cases-control analysis.

Conclusion.—Our results are in conflict with former results of the European rare cancer study. Considering the rarity of the disease laboratory in vitro studies of human uveal melanoma cell lines should be done to analyze potential exposure risk factors like radiation from microwaves, strong light from incandescent ovens, or infrared radiation.

▶ The cause of uveal melanoma remains unknown. There have been several studies searching for host and environmental factors for uveal melanoma. The most consistent host risk factors include light skin color, light iris color, and tendency to sunburn.[1] The only environmental risk factor, based on a meta-analysis of all published reports, was exposure to arc welding.[2]

A European-wide population-based study in 9 countries examined causes for rare cancers, including uveal melanoma. In the French portion of this study, male cooks showed an odds ratio of 3.8 for uveal melanoma compared with controls. In the German portion of this same study, the risk was increased in both male and female cooks with odds ratio of 3.3. In an English and Welsh cancer registry, a higher incidence of ocular melanoma in female kitchen hands was found. These findings prompted the current investigation.

Some speculate that the cause for the relationship of cooking and ocular melanoma stems from exposure to cooking fumes, microwaves, incandescent oven light, or infrared radiation. In the current study by Schmidt-Pokrzywniak and associates, using 459 uveal melanoma cases and 1194 controls, there was no relationship between cooking and uveal melanoma. Only in one region, the Northrine-Westphalia area, was there a small increased risk for cooks to have ocular melanoma, but this was not found in the entire cohort. This was a powerful study with a large cohort; however, the authors admit that the relative rarity of uveal melanoma and the low frequency of professional cooks might limit the identification of such a relationship.

C. L. Shields, MD

References

1. Weis E, Shah CP, Lajous M, Shields JA, Shields CL. The association between host susceptibility factors and uveal melanoma: a meta-analysis. *Arch Ophthalmol.* 2006;124:54-60.
2. Shah CP, Weis E, Lajous M, Shields JA, Shields CL. Intermittent and chronic ultraviolet light exposure and uveal melanoma: a meta-analysis. *Ophthalmology.* 2005; 112:1599-1607.

Conjunctival Melanoma: Outcomes Based on Tumor Origin in 382 Consecutive Cases
Shields CL, Markowitz JS, Belinsky I, et al (Thomas Jefferson Univ, Philadelphia, PA)
Ophthalmology 118:389-395, 2011

Purpose.—To evaluate prognostic factors based on origin of conjunctival melanoma.
Design.—Interventional case series.
Participants.—Three hundred eighty-two consecutive patients.
Methods.—Retrospective chart review.
Main Outcome Measures.—Melanoma-related metastasis and death.
Results.—The melanoma arose from primary acquired melanosis (PAM; n = 284; 74%), from pre-existing nevus (n = 26; 7%), and de novo (n = 72; 19%). The mean tumor base was 11 mm for melanoma arising from PAM, 6 mm for melanoma arising from nevus, and 10 mm for those arising de novo. At 5 years (10 years), melanoma metastasis occurred in 19% (25%) in melanoma arising from PAM ($P = 0.003$), 10% (26%) in melanoma from nevus ($P = 0.193$), and 35% (49%) in those de novo. Factors predictive of metastasis by multivariable analysis included tumor origin de novo ($P = 0.001$), palpebral location ($P<0.001$), nodular tumor ($P = 0.005$), and

orbital invasion ($P = 0.022$). At 5 years (10 years), melanoma-related death occurred in 5% (9%) in melanoma arising from PAM ($P<0.001$), 0% (9%) in melanoma arising from nevus ($P<0.057$), and 17% (35%) in those arising de novo. Factors predictive of death by multivariable analysis included tumor origin de novo ($P<0.001$), fornix location ($P = 0.04$), and nodular tumor ($P = 0.001$).

Conclusions.—Melanoma arising de novo carries a higher risk of melanoma-related metastasis and death compared with those cases arising from PAM or nevus.

▶ The National Cancer Data Base report identified 84 836 cases of melanoma between 1985 and 1994 in the United States.[1] Of these, 91% were cutaneous, 5% were ocular (presumed uveal), 1% was mucosal, and 2% were unknown primary site. Cutaneous melanoma is divided into 1 of 4 subtypes, including lentigo maligna (21%), superficial spreading (58%), nodular (19%) and acral lentiginous (2%). Survival at 5 years is statistically better with lentigo maligna origin (93%) than with nodular (65%) or acral lentiginous (66%).

Conjunctival melanoma is an uncommon malignancy, but the frequency is rising, similar to cutaneous melanoma. Studies from the United States and Finland have both documented a doubling of age-adjusted incidence of conjunctival melanoma between 1973 and 1999. This malignancy arises from preexisting nevus, primary-acquired melanosis, or de novo (no precursor). In this report, the authors investigate whether the source of melanoma origin affected ultimate outcomes.

They found that melanoma arose from nevus in 7%, primary-acquired melanosis in 74%, and de novo in 19%. Importantly, they found that tumors arising de novo carried a statistical risk for melanoma-related death compared with those from primary-acquired melanosis and nevus, implying more aggressive behavior of de novo tumors. These findings are similar to the above-mentioned prognostic factors for skin melanoma in that better prognosis is found with lentigo maligna melanoma. Lentigo maligna of the skin and primary-acquired melanosis of the conjunctiva are quite similar with 20% chance for melanoma and now evident lower risk for melanoma metastasis and death.

C. L. Shields, MD

Reference

1. Chang AE, Karnell LH, Menck HR. The National Cancer Data Base report on cutaneous and noncutaneous melanoma: a summary of 84,836 cases from the past decade. The American College of Surgeons Commission on Cancer and the American Cancer Society. *Cancer.* 1998;83:1664-1678.

Treatment of eyelid xanthelasma with 70% trichloroacetic acid

Nahas TR, Marques JC, Nicoletti A, et al (Santa Casa de São Paulo, Brazil)
Ophthal Plast Reconstr Surg 25:280-283, 2009

Purpose.—To analyze the results of treatment of eyelid xanthelasma (EX) with 70% trichloroacetic acid (TCA) with regard to efficacy, cosmetic appearance, patient satisfaction, and recurrence rate.

Methods.—Twenty-four patients with EX of up to one third of the affected palpebral area were treated with 70% TCA. All patients were photographed at the start of treatment and 3 months after the last application. The recurrence rate was analyzed at the end of 6 months of treatment.

Results.—The average number of applications of 70% TCA until the xanthelasma resolved was 1.5. Eleven patients (45.8%) had an excellent result, 8 (33.3%) a good result, and 5 (20.8%) had a satisfactory result. The most common complication was hypopigmentation (33.3%). All patients reported an improved final cosmetic result. Six patients (25%) treated with 70% TCA had a recurrence 6 months after treatment.

Conclusions.—The results of prospective treatment of 24 patients with EX with 70% TCA indicated that this is a simple and effective method, achieves a satisfactory cosmetic result, has an acceptable recurrence rate, and high patient satisfaction.

▶ Eyelid xanthelasma is a curious finding. Some claim that it is even visible in the portrait of Mona Lisa as painted by Leonardo da Vinci in 1506. This condition is mostly a cosmetic bother but could indicate underlying hyperlipidemia. It is theorized that a deficiency in lipid oxidation initiates an inflammatory, foreign body reaction that precipitates the lesions. Macrophages appear foamy with intracellular lipid, pushing the nuclei to the periphery.

The treatment of xanthelasma generally involves surgical resection. Others have tried laser ablation, cryotherapy, and use of acids. In one case report, xanthelasma completely disappeared with long-term use of oral statin medication for elevated cholesterol.[1] In this report, the authors use 70% trichloroacetic acid for xanthelasma and found that good or excellent results occurred in 79% of cases. The procedure involved outpatient application of the acid on the wooden end of a cotton swab soaked in the acid. Care to avoid corneal contamination was essential. The skin developed an immediate white burnlike appearance. Follow-up every 2 weeks with reapplication monthly was performed.

The authors correctly claim that there are benefits of trichloroacetic acid therapy including rapid application, outpatient setting, and relatively low cost. There are complications, which they did not experience but include ectropion from scarring and cosmetically unsightly scarring. I would suggest that this procedure be considered in patients considered poor surgical candidates or those who might want to avoid surgery. Based on their illustrations, surgical resection is still the gold standard for this condition, but this therapy comes close.

C. L. Shields, MD

Reference

1. Shields CL, Mashayekhi A, Shields JA, Racciato P. Disappearance of eyelid xanthelasma following oral simavastatin (Zocor). *Br J Ophthalmol.* 2005;89:639-640.

Long-term results of topical mitomycin C 0.02% for primary and recurrent conjunctival-corneal intraepithelial neoplasia
Ballalai PL, Erwenne CM, Martins MC, et al (Federal Univ of São Paulo, Brazil)
Ophthal Plast Reconstr Surg 25:296-299, 2009

Purpose.—To evaluate the efficacy, recurrence rate, and long-term complications of topical mitomycin C (MMC) 0.02% for conjunctival-corneal intraepithelial neoplasia (CCIN).

Methods.—A prospective, nonrandomized, noncontrolled study was conducted of patients with primary or recurrent CCIN treated with topical MMC 0.02%, four times per day, for 28 consecutive days. The main outcome measures were complete resolution of the neoplasia by slit-lamp examination and cytology 1 month after treatment, tumor recurrence, and long-term complications.

Results.—Between June 1999 and September 2005, 23 patients were included. Eighteen had primary CCIN (group 1) and 5 had recurrent CCIN (group 2). The mean follow-up was 46 months in group 1 and 54 months in group 2. All patients were treated with MMC 0.02% for 28 consecutive days. Complete resolution of the lesion was achieved in all patients after 1 month of treatment. Recurrence occurred in 1 patient (4.3%) after 24 months of treatment. Four patients developed corneal erosion (17.4%), 2 of them with primary CCIN and 2 with recurrent CCIN. Corneal erosion occurred 4 to 24 months after treatment and was treated successfully. The probability for corneal erosions by the logrank test was equal for both groups (p = 0.1705).

Conclusions.—The use of topical MMC 0.02% for 28 consecutive days to treat primary or recurrent CCIN was effective and showed a low recurrence rate. Corneal erosion occurred in 17.4% of cases and can occur as late as 24 months after treatment.

▶ Conjunctival/corneal intraepithelial neoplasia (CCIN) can be treated in many ways, including surgical resection or with topical antineoplastic agents or antiviral agents. A popular antineoplastic agent is mitomycin C (MMC). In this report, the authors evaluate a middose MMC for 28 consecutive days for CCIN. This protocol is different from others in that most use the MMC for 1 week, take a 1-week break off medication, resume the medication for another week, then stop, and reassess. The worry about the protocol in this report would be increased complication rate.

The investigators assessed 23 patients with CCIN and found complete resolution of tumor with 1-month treatment in 100% of cases. However, complications of corneal erosion in 4 (17%) were observed, of whom 2 required amniotic membrane grafting to heal the defect. This complication is not unusual with the potent MMC. Long-term, these authors will need to assess limbal stem cell deficiency, as that might not manifest immediately. They propose that perhaps a 2-week lapse between the first 14 days and last 14 days might allow the limbal stems cells to recover and minimize this problem.

Other topical medications that might be equally effective to MMC include topical 5 fluorouracil and topical interferon alfa-2B. Interferon acts against human papillomavirus and slowly heals the malignancy over several months. The complication rates are minimal with interferon. We are fortunate to have so many alternative therapies for CCIN. In the past, multiple surgical resections were often necessary, leading to scarring and vision loss. The topical therapies are, without a question, a major advance in therapy for CCIN.

C. L. Shields, MD

Myopia Over the Lifecourse: Prevalence and Early Life Influences in the 1958 British Birth Cohort
Rahi JS, Cumberland PM, Peckham CS (Univ College London, England)
Ophthalmology 118:797-804, 2011

Purpose.—To investigate the hypothesis that the excessive growth of the eye in myopia is associated with general growth and thus influenced by early life biological and social factors, and that these associations underlie recent secular trends of increasing prevalence and severity of myopia.

Design.—Cohort study.

Participants.—A total of 2487 randomly selected 44-year-old members of the 1958 British birth cohort (27% subsample).

Methods.—Diverse and detailed biological, social, and lifestyle data have been collected by following members since birth through a series of clinical examinations or face-to-face interviews carried out by trained examiners. At 44 years, cohort members underwent autorefraction using the Nikon Retinomax 2 (Nikon Corp., Tokyo, Japan) under non-cycloplegic conditions. A lifecourse epidemiologic approach, based on 4 sequential multivariable "life stage" models (preconceptional; prenatal, perinatal, and postnatal; childhood; and adult), was used to examine the influence of early life biological, social and lifestyle factors, growth patterns, and "eye-specific" factors on myopia.

Main Outcome Measures.—Myopia severity (all, mild/moderate: spherical equivalent -0.75 to -5.99 diopters [D]; severe: ≥-6.00 D extreme vs. emmetropia -0.74 to $+0.99$ D) and myopia onset (early [<16 years] vs. later).

Results.—A total of 1214 individuals (49%; 95% confidence interval, 48.8–50.8) were myopic (late onset in 979 [80.6%]). Myopia was positively associated with low birthweight for gestational age, gender, greater maternal age, higher paternal occupational social class, and maternal smoking in early pregnancy. Myopia was independently associated with proxy markers of near work and educational performance, with some differences by onset and severity. In adults, greater height and higher educational attainment and socioeconomic status were associated with myopia. *Conclusions.*—Trends in the key influences on child health and growth identified as novel putative risk factors in this study are consistent with global trends of increasing myopia: increasing births to older mothers, increasing rates of intrauterine growth retardation and survival of affected children, increasing persistence of smoking in pregnancy, and changing socioeconomic status. Prospects for prevention of myopia would be improved by a paradigm shift in myopia research, with lifecourse and genetic epidemiologic approaches applied in tandem in large unselected populations.

▶ Myopia is the most common eye disease. It is estimated that mild to moderate myopia (−0.75 to −5.99 diopter) affects 25% of the population in Europe and North America, 80% in Asia, and 5% in Africa. Advanced or "pathologic" myopia (−6.00 diopter or greater) affects less than 3% of the population. Over the past decades, there has been an increase in myopia frequency and severity, especially in East Asian populations. Some speculate that the early-life influences on the eye are related to the trends in myopia. These authors investigate some of these life influences in the British Birth Cohort.

In the United Kingdom, these authors found 1 in 3 working-age adults to have myopia. In the cohort of 2487 individuals, 49% were myopic, 42% were emmetropic, and 9% were hypermetropic. Of the 1214 myopic members, 19% showed early-onset myopia before age 16 years, whereas 81% had late-onset myopia. They found that myopia was related to low birth weight, older mother age, higher father social class, and maternal smoking during pregnancy. Postpartum, they also found myopia related to near work and educational performance as well as greater height. For example, late-onset myopia and mild myopia were related to higher standardized reading score at age 7 years and higher general ability test score at 11 years, both markers for intelligence. Regarding sports, however, high myopia was associated with less sporting involvement at ages 11 and 16 years.

The authors conclude that prenatal and early-life influences are important in ocular development and myopic refractive error. They speculate that the global trend for increasing myopia is related to increasing number of older mothers, increasing rates of intrauterine growth retardation, persistence of smoking during pregnancy, declining rates of breastfeeding, and changing socioeconomic status. Furthermore, the average height of a child has consistently increased, also related to increasing myopia. Identification of etiologic causes is important so that potential modification could control the expansion of this globally important disorder.

C. L. Shields, MD

Slow Enlargement of Choroidal Nevi: A Long-Term Follow-Up Study

Mashayekhi A, Siu S, Shields CL, et al (Thomas Jefferson Univ, Philadelphia, PA)

Ophthalmology 118:382-388, 2011

Purpose.—Choroidal nevi are generally considered to be stable lesions, and growth of a choroidal nevus is usually believed to be a sign of malignant transformation. We performed this study to determine whether choroidal nevi enlarge over a long period of follow-up without undergoing malignant transformation.

Design.—Retrospective observational case series.

Participants.—A total of 278 patients with 284 nevi who had at least 7 years of photographic follow-up without clinical signs of transformation into melanoma were included in the study.

Methods.—Data on demographic and clinical information were extracted from patients' charts. Detailed fundus drawings and color fundus photographs were reviewed and compared for evidence of enlargement.

Main Outcome Measures.—Nevus enlargement without clinical evidence of transformation into melanoma.

Results.—Of the 278 patients, 69% were female and more than 99% were White with a median age at presentation of 57 years (range, 4—87 years). The largest nevus basal diameter was a median of 5 mm (range, 0.5—14 mm), and the median thickness was 1.5 mm (range, 0.1—3.6 mm). Only 14 nevi (5%) had subretinal fluid outside the nevus, and 6% showed overlying orange pigment. Overlying retinal pigment epithelial alterations included drusen (61%), atrophy (6%), hyperplasia (10%), and fibrous metaplasia (6%). Of 284 nevi, 31% showed slight enlargement over a mean follow-up of 15 years. The median increase in diameter was 1 mm (mean, 0.9 mm; range, 0.2—3.0 mm), and the median rate of enlargement was 0.06 mm/yr (mean, 0.06 mm/yr; range, 0.01—0.36 mm/yr). None of the lesions that enlarged developed new risk factors that are generally associated with malignant transformation. Frequency of enlargement was 54% in patients aged less than 40 years and 19% in patients aged more than 60 years. On multivariate analysis, younger patient age was the only factor predictive of nevus enlargement ($P<0.001$).

Conclusions.—With long-term follow up, 31% of choroidal nevi showed slight enlargement without clinical evidence of transformation into melanoma. The frequency of enlargement was inversely related to patient age.

▶ The choroidal nevus is a benign tumor that carries a small risk for evolution into melanoma. Quoted figures estimate that 1 in 5000 to 1 in 8800 show evolution to melanoma. This common tumor is witnessed by ophthalmologists on fundu-scopy. Identification of high-risk lesions that show features of > 2 mm thickness, subretinal fluid, orange pigment, margin near the optic disk, or cause symptoms could lead to detection of small melanoma at an early point. Prognosis with uveal melanoma is strongly dependent on size of lesion at detection, so early detection is encouraged.

In most cases, growth of a choroidal nevus implies malignant transformation, particularly if the growth is documented over a short period of several months or 1 year. On the other hand, slight growth of the nevus over 10 years is not as suspicious for malignant transformation and could represent simple evolution of the benign nevus. In this report, the authors followed up 284 choroidal nevi for a minimum of 7 years and most often for 10 or more years. They found that choroidal nevi showed slight enlargement over long periods that could be documented in 54% of patients younger than 40 years and 19% of patients older than 60 years. This suggests that choroidal nevi commonly change or evolve with slight growth over a long period.

The authors caution that similar enlargement over shorter periods could be suggestive of melanoma transformation. It is advised that all choroidal nevi be monitored by annual funduscopy. Consultation with experienced ocular oncologists is advised in challenging cases.

C. L. Shields, MD

Occurrence of sectoral choroidal occlusive vasculopathy and retinal arteriolar embolization after superselective ophthalmic artery chemotherapy for advanced intraocular retinoblastoma
Munier FL, Beck-Popovic M, Balmer A, et al (Jules Gonin Eye Hosp, Lausanne, Switzerland)
Retina 31:566-573, 2011

Background.—Superselective ophthalmic artery chemotherapy (SOAC) has recently been proposed as an alternative to intravenous chemoreduction for advanced intraocular retinoblastoma. Preliminary results appear promising in terms of tumor control and eye conservation, but little is known regarding ocular toxicity and visual prognosis. In this study, we report on the vascular adverse effects observed in our initial cohort of 13 patients.

Methods.—The charts of 13 consecutive patients with retinoblastoma who received a total of 30 injections (up to 3 injections of a single agent per patient at 3-week interval) of melphalan (0.35 mg/kg) in the ophthalmic artery between November 2008 and June 2010 were retrospectively reviewed. RetCam fundus photography and fluorescein angiography were performed at presentation and before each injection. Vision was assessed at the latest visit.

Results.—Enuucleation and external beam radiotherapy could be avoided in all cases but one, with a mean follow-up of 7 months. Sectoral choroidal occlusive vasculopathy leading to chorioretinal atrophy was observed temporally in 2 eyes (15%) 3 weeks to 6 weeks after the beginning of SOAC and retinal arteriolar emboli in 1 eye 2 weeks after injection. There was no stroke or other clinically significant systemic side effects except a perioperative transient spasm of the internal carotid artery in one patient. Vision ranged between 20/1600 and 20/32 depending on the status of the macula.

Conclusion.—Superselective ophthalmic artery chemotherapy was effective in all patients with no stroke or other systemic vascular complications. Unlike intravenous chemoreduction, SOAC is associated with potentially sight-threatening adverse effects, such as severe chorioretinal atrophy secondary to subacute choroidal occlusive vasculopathy or central retinal artery embolism, not to mention the risk of ophthalmic artery obstruction, which was not observed in this series. Further analysis of the risks and benefits of SOAC will define its role within the therapeutic arsenal. Meanwhile, we suggest that SOAC should be given in one eye only and restricted to advanced cases of retinoblastoma, as an alternative to enucleation and/or external beam radiotherapy.

▶ Chemotherapy for retinoblastoma can be given by several pathways, including intravenous, sub-Tenon's fascia, intravitreal, and intra-arterial routes. Intra-arterial chemotherapy (IAC) is exciting, as it allows delivery of a potent but tiny dose of chemotherapy directly into the ophthalmic artery that feeds the eye. The direct delivery technique washes the agent into the eye with relatively good tumor control based on short-term observations.

Our group in Philadelphia has been using IAC for more than 3 years and has found it most useful for groups C and D retinoblastoma. Most children require 3 or more sessions, especially those with advanced disease. We have coined the term *minimal exposure IAC* for those children who need only 1 or 2 doses of melphalan for tumor control. This technique is done on an outpatient basis and requires a morning of surgical intervention for catheterization of the femoral artery into the ophthalmic artery, and the patients tend to do well. Major systemic complications can occur such as stroke, bleeding, ischemia, and organ/vascular puncture.

In this report, Munier and associates evaluate their small cohort of 13 eyes treated with IAC and report the complications of sector choroidal atrophy in 15% of cases and retinal emboli in 8%. They speculate that this was due either to catheter-related intravascular trauma or chemotherapy endothelial toxicity. They cite an important review article that covers this topic in detail.[1] The authors caution that IAC be given to 1 eye only, and that further study is needed.

C. L. Shields, MD

Reference

1. Shields CL, Shields JA. Retinoblastoma management: advances in enucleation, intravenous chemoreduction, and intra-arterial chemotherapy. *Curr Opin Ophthalmol.* 2010;21:203-212.

Prognosis of Uveal Melanoma in 500 Cases Using Genetic Testing of Fine-Needle Aspiration Biopsy Specimens

Shields CL, Ganguly A, Bianciotto CG, et al (Thomas Jefferson Univ, Philadelphia, PA; Univ of Pennsylvania School of Medicine, Philadelphia)
Ophthalmology 118:396-401, 2011

Purpose.—To determine the relationship between monosomy 3 and incidence of metastasis after genetic testing of uveal melanoma using fine-needle aspiration biopsy (FNAB).

Design.—Noncomparative retrospective case series.

Participants.—Five hundred patients.

Methods.—Fine-needle aspiration biopsy was performed intraoperatively immediately before plaque radiotherapy. The specimen underwent genetic analysis using DNA amplification and microsatellite assay. Systemic follow-up was obtained regarding melanoma-related metastasis.

Main Outcome Measures.—Presence of chromosome 3 monosomy (loss of heterozygosity) and occurrence of melanoma metastasis.

Results.—Disomy 3 was found in 241 melanomas (48%), partial monosomy 3 was found in 133 melanomas (27%), and complete monosomy 3 was found in 126 melanomas (25%). The cumulative probability for metastasis by 3 years was 2.6% for disomy 3, 5.3% for partial monosomy 3 (equivocal monosomy 3), and 24.0% for complete monosomy 3. At 3 years, for tumors with disomy 3, the cumulative probability of metastasis was 0% for small (0–3 mm thickness), 1.4% for medium (3.1–8 mm thickness), and 23.1% for large (>8 mm thickness) melanomas. At 3 years, for tumors with partial monosomy 3, the cumulative probability of metastasis was 4.5% for small, 6.9% for medium, and [insufficient numbers] for large melanomas. At 3 years, for tumors with complete monosomy 3, the cumulative probability of metastasis was 0% for small, 24.4% for medium, and 57.5% for large melanomas. The most important factors predictive of partial or complete monosomy 3 included increasing tumor thickness ($P = 0.001$) and increasing distance to optic disc ($P = 0.002$).

Conclusions.—According to FNAB results, patients with uveal melanoma demonstrating complete monosomy 3 have substantially poorer prognosis at 3 years than those with partial monosomy 3 or disomy 3. Patients with partial monosomy 3 do not significantly differ in outcome from those with disomy 3.

▶ Several articles have been written on the importance of genetic testing for uveal melanoma following enucleation. In 1996, a landmark publication identified that chromosome 3 monosomy within the melanoma was a significant predictor of poor patient prognosis. Tumors with that feature showed high risk for ultimate patient mortality. Since then, others have confirmed the importance of chromosome 3 monosomy in retrospective studies.

This study by Shields and associates is different from most previous publications in that it was performed on nonenucleated eyes that were treated with plaque radiotherapy. How did the authors get the tissue for testing in these cases?

They performed fine needle aspiration biopsy that provided only a few cells in each case but was sufficient for performing microarray analysis, yielding a result. They found that cumulative risk for metastasis by 3 years was 2.6% for eyes with no monosomy 3 (disomy 3) but increased to 24% for those with monosomy 3.

The other uniqueness of this study is that the authors stratified results based on tumor size. At 3 years, tumors with monosomy 3 showed metastasis in 0% of small, 24% of medium, and 58% of large melanoma. Size is important with uveal melanoma, so the combination of size and genetics makes for more powerful prediction.

How is this information clinically relevant? Well, patients at high risk for metastasis are placed on systemic chemotherapy protocols to prevent metastatic disease. Those at low risk for metastasis are immensely relieved, achieving a psychological benefit from the testing. Further refinements in the detection of genetic abnormalities and subsequent intervention will hopefully lead to improved prognosis for melanoma patients.

C. L. Shields, MD

Plaque Radiotherapy for Juxtapapillary Choroidal Melanoma: Tumor Control in 650 Consecutive Cases
Sagoo MS, Shields CL, Mashayekhi A, et al (Thomas Jefferson Univ, Philadelphia, PA; et al)
Ophthalmology 118:402-407, 2011

Purpose.—To evaluate treatment of juxtapapillary choroidal melanoma with plaque radiotherapy and to investigate the role of supplemental transpupillary thermotherapy (TTT).

Design.—Retrospective, comparative case series.

Participants.—We included 650 consecutive eyes with juxtapapillary choroidal melanoma within 1 mm of the optic disc.

Methods.—Eyes with juxtapapillary choroidal melanoma receiving plaque radiotherapy over a 31-year period from October 1974 to November 2005 were included in the study. The TTT and no TTT groups were analyzed separately and compared.

Main Outcome Measures.—Local tumor control, metastasis, and tumor-related mortality.

Results.—The median basal tumor diameter was 10 mm (range, 1.5–21) and median thickness was 3.5 mm (range, 0.5–14.8). In 481 eyes (74%), the tumor was directly adjacent to the optic disc and in 169 eyes (26%) the posterior tumor margin was between 0.1 and 1.0 mm from the optic disc. The circumpapillary extent of the tumor was <4 clock-hours in 321 eyes (50%), 4–8 clock-hours in 250 eyes (38%), and >8 clock-hours in 79 eyes (12%). Plaque radiotherapy using iodine-125 in 616 eyes (95%), cobalt-60 in 19 eyes (3%), iridium-192 in 12 eyes (2%), and ruthenium-106 in 3 eyes (<1%) delivered a median radiation dose of 8000 cGy (range, 3600–15 500) to the tumor apex and adjunctive TTT was used in 307 eyes (56%). Kaplan-Meier estimates for tumor recurrence, metastasis, and death were 14%, 11%, and 4% at 5 years and 21%, 24%, and 9% at 10 years, respectively. Eyes treated with additional TTT showed slight (statistically nonsignificant) reduction in recurrence and metastasis. Using multivariable analysis, factors predictive of tumor recurrence included foveolar tumor requiring TTT (hazard ratio, 5.07; *P*<0.001) and greater tumor thickness (hazard ratio, 1.29 per mm increase; *P*<0.001). Factors predictive of metastasis included greater tumor base (hazard ratio, 1.21 per mm increase; *P*<0.001) and increasing intraocular pressure (hazard ratio, 1.11 per mmHg increase; *P* = 0.020).

Conclusions.—Plaque radiotherapy for juxtapapillary melanoma provides local tumor control in approximately 80% of eyes at 10 years. In subjects who received TTT, there was slight but nonsignificant improved local tumor control and lower metastatic rate.

▶ Juxtapapillary melanoma is defined as a choroidal tumor that rests close to the optic disc, often abutting it. There are few treatment options for melanoma in this region, including enucleation or forms of radiotherapy. Occasionally small juxtapapillary melanoma can be treated with transpupillary thermotherapy. In this report, the authors explore the most common conservative method of treatment of these select tumors, using plaque radiotherapy.

When treating melanoma near the disc, there are certain special concerns regarding the radioactive plaque and the placement. The plaque requires a custom design with a notch at the posterior margin to allow for precise placement abutting the optic nerve and surrounding the nerve for a certain number of degrees. If a melanoma overhangs the disc, then the notch must be deeper so that the plaque can nearly encircle the optic nerve to reach adequate radiation parameters to the melanoma. The other concern is regarding precision of placement. These are the most difficult plaques to place, nococcitating perfection in localization of the tumor within the eye, placement of sutures within the sclera to secure the plaque in the postequatorial region, and placement of the "live" plaque in the precise position for treatment.

Many centers prefer to enucleate eyes with juxtapapillary melanoma because the radiation or surgical requirements are too difficult to achieve. However, these authors have shown that tumor control is excellent with approximately 80% of tumors in complete remission by 10 years' follow-up. Metastases occurred in 24% at 10 years, related to larger tumors and higher intraocular pressure.

This information is important as the Collaborative Ocular Melanoma Study, a nationwide collaborative effort to study plaque radiotherapy versus enucleation for choroidal melanoma, did not include juxtapapillary melanoma. Hence, this report fills in the gap of information for this select group. The authors conclude that plaque radiotherapy is a feasible treatment for choroidal melanoma with satisfactory tumor control.

C. L. Shields, MD

Intralesional administration of rituximab for treatment of CD20 positive orbital lymphoma: safety and efficacy evaluation

Laurenti L, De Padua L, Battendieri R, et al (Catholic Univ of the Sacred Hearth, Rome, Italy)
Leuk Res 35:682-684, 2011

B-cell lymphomas constitute the most frequent malignant neoplasm of the ocular adnexal, often presenting with localized disease. Five patients with primary localized CD20 positive B cell non Hodgkin ocular adnexal lymphomas received intralesional rituximab at the dose of 5 mg once a week for one month, followed by 10 mg weekly in case of incomplete response. Four of five patients obtained regression of symptoms and 2 of them showed complete response. No patients experienced side effects besides pain on the site of the injection. Local treatment with Rituximab for OAL is a safe and useful first-line therapeutic option.

▶ Lymphomas are the most common malignant neoplasms of the orbit, particularly in middle-aged and older patients. The most common type is extranodal marginal zone lymphoma of mucosa-associated lymphoid tissue type. Patients with orbital lymphoma are at approximately 10% risk for systemic lymphoma if the disease is unilateral and 70% risk if bilateral.[1] The management of orbital lymphoma includes surgical resection, systemic chemotherapy for patients with multiple sites, or radiotherapy if localized. Standard radiotherapy usually occupies 1 month of treatment with daily applications to the involved site, but CyberKnife radiosurgery, a newer method using 1300 small beams by robotic control, is completed in 4 to 5 days.[2] Regarding chemotherapy, there have been several protocols for lymphoma. More recently, rituximab has been considered as an alternative first-line therapy for localized lymphoma that shows CD20 cellular markers. Rituximab is usually delivered by intravenous route but carries risks of acute infusion reaction and rare toxicity of progressive multifocal encephalopathy. In this report, Laurenti and coworkers locally injected rituximab into orbital lymphoma in 5 cases and found complete remission in 2, stable response in 2, and no response in 1.

Their protocol included induction with 5 mg/wk for 4 weeks and, if complete response was obtained, then a consolidation cycle of 5 mg/wk for 4 weeks was given at 2 months. If the induction cycle produced only partial response, then consolidation with 10 mg/wk for 4 weeks was delivered until complete response for a maximum of 12 injections (3 cycles). All injections were performed in the operating room. Complete remission was achieved with 2 and 3 injections of total dose of 40 mg and 100 mg rituximab, respectively. The only side effect was fever and chills following injection for 3 hours.

This is a novel method for targeted tumor control with minimal side effects. Complete response in 40% is a start but needs to be improved. It is often difficult to compare therapies, but CyberKnife seems to predominate because it offers nearly 100% control, rapidly over 5 days, with minimal side effects and no surgical intervention.

C. L. Shields, MD

References

1. Demirci H, Shields CL, Karatza EC, Shields JA. Orbital lymphoproliferative tumors: analysis of clinical features and systemic involvement in 160 cases. *Ophthalmology.* 2008;115:1626-1631.
2. Bianciotto C, Shields CL, Lally SE, Freire J, Shields JA. Cyberknife radiosurgery for the treatment of intraocular and periocular lymphoma. *Arch Ophthalmol.* 2010;128:1561-1567.

11 Pathology

Histopathologic Observations After Intra-arterial Chemotherapy for Retinoblastoma

Eagle RC Jr, Shields CL, Bianciotto C, et al (Thomas Jefferson Univ, Philadelphia, PA)
Arch Ophthalmol 2011 [Epub ahead of print]

Objective.—To describe histopathologic observations in eyes enucleated after intra-arterial chemotherapy (IAC) for retinoblastoma (Rb).

Methods.—Retrospective histopathologic analysis of 8 eyes.

Results.—The eyes were enucleated for tumor viability (n=4), neovascular glaucoma (n=2), anaphylactic reaction from IAC (n=1), and persistent retinal detachment with poor visualization of the tumor (n=1). Of the 2 eyes judged clinically with complete tumor regression and the 5 with viable tumor, the findings were confirmed on histopathology. The Rb response ranged from minimal (n=1) to moderate (n=1) to extensive (n=4) to complete regression (n=2). Viable vitreous seeds (n=4 eyes), invasion into the optic nerve (n=3), reaching the lamina cribrosa in 2 cases, and invasion into the choroid (n=1) were observed. Histopathologic evidence of ischemic atrophy involving the outer retina and choroid was found in 4 eyes. One eye treated at another center with IAC and enucleated by our team for recurrence was observed to have extensive choroidal and outer retinal atrophy. This case showed orbital vascular occlusion and subendothelial smooth muscle hyperplasia. Intravascular birefringent foreign material was observed in 5 cases within occluded vessels, stimulating a granulomatous inflammatory response. The foreign material comprised cellulose fibers (n=3), synthetic fabric fibers (n=1), or unknown composition (n=2). Thrombosed blood vessels were identified in 5 eyes and involved ciliary arteries in the retrobulbar orbit (n=5), scleral emissarial canals (n=1), small choroidal vessels (n=1), and central retinal artery (n=1).

Conclusion.—Retinoblastoma can be controlled with IAC, but histopathology of enucleated eyes reveals that ocular complications including thromboembolic events can occur (Tables 1-3).

▶ In a recent paper by Abramson et al,[1] the authors reported their successful treatment of 23 patients (28 eyes) with intra-arterial chemotherapy infusions with only 1 eye developing progressive disease, leading to enucleation. The results of pathologic evaluation of the enucleated eye are not stated. A prior,

TABLE 1.—Clinical Features of 8 Eyes With Retinoblastoma Following Treatment With Intra-arterial Chemotherapy

Patient No./Race/Sex/Age, mo	Laterality/Heredity	ICRB Classification	Treatment	Indications for Enucleation	Comments
1/W/F/14	Unilateral/sporadic	E	IAC×2	NVG, VH	Ophthalmic artery obstruction found at IAC No. 2
2/W/F/24	Unilateral/sporadic	E	IAC×2	Persistent RD, no view of fundus	Main Rb regressed; viable vitreous seeds
3/W/M/72	Bilateral/sporadic	Secondary[a]	IAC×4, s/p CRD, cryotherapy	Recurrent Rb in AC and vitreous	Requested IAC AMA
4/A/M/28	Unilateral/sporadic	E	IAC×3	NVG, hyphema, VH, hypotony	Requested IAC AMA; wanted to avoid enucleation
5/W/F/23	Unilateral/sporadic	E	IAC×2	Minimal Rb regression, RD	Minimal Rb regression; intralaminar optic nerve invasion
6/H/F/22	Bilateral/sporadic	Secondary	IAC×2, s/p CRD, EBRT	Minimal Rb regression	IAC as attempt to save only eye; extensive Rb necrosis, residual viable Rb
7/W/M/26	Unilateral/sporadic	E	IAC×6 elsewhere, plaque	Recurrent Rb retina and viable vitreous seeds	IAC at another center AMA, posterior ischemic atrophy noted clinically
8/W/M/28	Unilateral/sporadic	E	IAC×1	Recurrent vitreous seeds	Anaphylaxis

Abbreviations: AC, anterior chamber; AMA, against medical advice; CRD, chemoreduction; EBRT, external beam radiotherapy; F, female; H, Hispanic; IAC, intra-arterial chemotherapy; ICRB, International Classification of Retinoblastoma; M, male; NVG, neovascular glaucoma; Rb, retinoblastoma; RD, retinal detachment; s/p, status post; VH, vitreous hemorrhage; W, white.
[a]Secondary following previous systemic chemoreduction.

TABLE 2.—Histopathologic Findings in 8 Eyes With Retinoblastoma Following Treatment With Intra-arterial Chemotherapy

Feature	No./Total (%)
Tumor regression	
Minimal	1/8 (12.5)
Moderate	1/8 (12.5)
Extensive	4/8 (50.0)
Total	2/8 (25.0)
Treatment regression scar	6/8 (75.0)
Vitreous seeds (viable)	4/8 (50.0)
Tumor differentiation	
Poor	4/6 (83.3)
Poor with well-differentiated foci	2/6 (33.3)
Optic nerve invasion	
Prelaminar	1/8 (12.5)
Intralaminar	2/8 (25.0)
Total	3/8 (37.5)
Choroidal invasion	1/8 (12.5)
Iris neovascularization	5/8 (62.5)
Ischemic chorioretinal atrophy	4/8 (50.0)
Thrombosed vessels	
Any thrombosed vessel	5/8 (62.5)
Orbital artery	5/8 (62.5)
Intrascleral artery	1/8 (12.5)
Choroidal artery	1/8 (12.5)
Central retinal artery	1/8 (12.5)
Birefringent foreign material	
Befriend material identified	5/8 (62.5)
Cellulose fiber	3/8 (37.5)
Synthetic fabric fiber	1/8 (12.5)
Unknown substance	2/8 (25.0)
Orbital pathology	
Orbital pathology identified	5/8 (62.5)
Thrombosed orbital vessels	5/8 (62.5)
Birefringent foreign material	3/8 (37.5)
Intravascular calcification	2/8 (25.0)
Vascular smooth muscle hyperplasia	1/8 (12.5)
Fat necrosis	2/8 (25.0)

smaller pilot study by Abramson et al[2] showed that the 2 eyes enucleated following intra-arterial chemotherapy had no viable tumor.

Since then, several groups have reported on histopathology of the eyes that failed intra-arterial chemotherapy. In one recent study, Vajzovic and colleagues[3] documented viable tumor in all 3 enucleated eyes with progressive disease following superselective intra-arterial melphalan infusion. Moreover, 2 of 3 cases had a viable tumor with high-risk characteristics for the development of metastatic disease on histopathologic evaluation. Eagle et al similarly observed viable tumor in 4 of 8 eyes enucleated following intra-arterial chemotherapy. Additional worrisome pathologic observations included evidence of ischemic atrophy involving the outer retina and choroid in 4 of 8 eyes induced by vascular compromise and the presence of foreign material within the thrombosed vessels.

The results of the studies by Eagle et al and Vajzovic et al cannot be directly correlated with the outcomes of Abramson's study because of differences in patient selection, treatment methods before intra-arterial chemotherapy, and

TABLE 3.—Histopathologic Features (by Case) of 8 Eyes With Retinoblastoma Following Treatment With Intra-arterial Chemotherapy

Feature	Patient No.							
	1	2	3	4	5	6	7	8
Tumor regression	Total	Extensive	Extensive	Total	Minimal	Moderate	Extensive	Extensive
Vitreous seeds	No	Yes	Yes	No	No	No	Yes	Yes
Tumor differentiation	NA	Poor	Poor/WD focus	NA	Poor/WD focus/PRD	Poor	Poor	Poor
Treatment regression scar	Yes	Yes	Yes	Yes	No	Yes	Yes	No
Optic nerve invasion	No	No	No	No	Intralaminar	Prelaminar	Intralaminar	No
Choroidal invasion	No	No	Yes	No	No	Yes (2×0.05 mm)	No	No
Chorioretinal ischemic atrophy	Yes	No	Yes	No	No	Yes	Yes	No
Iris neovascularization	Yes/NVG	No	Yes/NVG	Yes/NVG	Yes/NVG	Yes/NVG	No	No

Abbreviations: NA, not applicable or not available; NVG, neovascular glaucoma; PRD, photoreceptor differentiation; WD, well-differentiated.

differences in intra-arterial chemotherapy dosing and administration protocols. However, the emergent data suggest that randomized trials with standardized treatment protocols and careful patient selection are needed before embracing the intra-arterial chemotherapy for retinoblastoma.

T. Milman, MD

References

1. Abramson DH, Dunkel IJ, Brodie SE, Marr B, Gobin YP. Superselective ophthalmic artery chemotherapy as primary treatment for retinoblastoma (chemosurgery). *Ophthalmology.* 2010;117:1623-1629.
2. Abramson DH, Dunkel IJ, Brodie SE, Kim JW, Gobin YP. A phase I/II study of direct intraarterial (ophthalmic artery) chemotherapy with melphalan for intraocular retinoblastoma initial results. *Ophthalmology.* 2008;115:1398-1404.e1.
3. Vajzovic LM, Murray TG, Aziz-Sultan MA, et al. Clinicopathologic review of enucleated eyes after intra-arterial chemotherapy with melphalan for advanced retinoblastoma. *Arch Ophthalmol.* 2010;128:1619-1623.

Calcification in retinoblastoma: histopathologic findings and statistical analysis of 302 cases
Levy J, Frenkel S, Baras M, et al (Soroka Univ Med Ctr, Beer-Sheva, Israel; Hadassah-Hebrew Univ Med Ctr, Jerusalem, Israel; et al)
Br J Ophthalmol 95:1145-1150, 2011

Aim.—To evaluate the histopathologic factors statistically associated with the presence of calcification in eyes with retinoblastoma.

Methods.—Retrospective, consecutive and observational case series. Three hundred and two enucleated eyes with retinoblastoma examined between the years 1960 and 2008. Five representative histopathologic slides of the pupil—optic nerve section and three cross optic nerve sections were retrospectively reviewed. The presence and degree of calcification as well as other histopathologic features were evaluated. Demographic data including age, gender and country of origin of the case were also reviewed. Univariate and multivariate statistical analyses were performed to search for a possible correlation between calcification and the other histopathologic factors and/or demographic data.

Results.—Calcification was present in 84.9% of cases. Age, tumour size, necrosis, basophilic staining, iris neovascularisation, choroidal, scleral and/or optic nerve invasion were correlated significantly with calcification. Multivariate analysis showed a significant correlation between the presence of calcification and the amount of necrosis and choroidal invasion only.

Conclusions.—In this series, calcification was more frequent in cases with more necrosis and cases with choroidal invasion, a known poor histopathologic risk factor for metastatic disease. The possible clinical implication of the findings from this study deserves additional studies (Fig 1, Tables 1-4).

▶ In this study, the presence of calcification within the retinoblastoma was classified in a semiquantitative fashion into 4 groups: 0, no calcification; 1, few

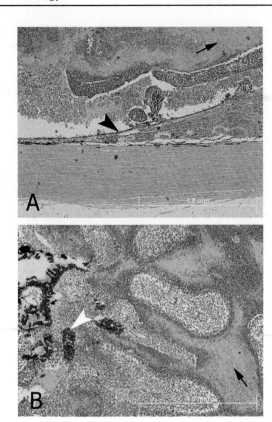

FIGURE 1.—Histological pictures of retinoblastoma with areas of necrosis (arrows, A and B), choroidal invasion with tumor cells invading under the retinal pigment epithelial (RPE) cells (A, black arrowhead) and calcifications (B, white arrowhead). (H&E, ×4). (Reprinted from Levy J, Frenkel S, Baras M, et al. Calcification in retinoblastoma: histopathologic findings and statistical analysis of 302 cases. *Br J Ophthalmol.* 2011;95:1145-1150, Copyright 2011, with permission from BMJ Publishing Group Ltd.)

isolated foci; 2, up to 25% of tumor volume; and 3, 26% and more of the tumor volume is calcified. The authors found a significant correlation between the presence of calcification and the amount of necrosis and degree of choroidal invasion (high-risk characteristic) in multivariate analysis. The significance of this observation from a histopathologic standpoint is questionable for several reasons. Firstly, dystrophic calcification is expected to be directly associated with tumor necrosis and tumor size; thus, the degree of tumor necrosis and tumor size can in themselves serve as prognostic variables. In addition, the authors could not evaluate all pupil-optic nerve sections and calottes for every case; thus, the outcome of the study is questionable, particularly as it relates to the association between the degree of choroidal invasion and calcification. Lastly, the clinical data on the patients were limited; thus, the authors could not assess for potential influence of prior treatment on necrosis or calcification. Thus, a carefully conducted study with uniform histopathologic methodology and meticulous clinical

TABLE 1.—Histopathologic Characteristics of Enucleated Cases With Retinoblastoma

	Number of Cases	%
Tumour size		
<25% of eye area	65	21.5
26–50% of eye area	87	28.8
51–75%	80	26.5
More than 75% of eye area	70	23.2
Focality*		
Monofocal	68	55.3
Multifocal	55	44.7
Tumour pattern†		
Endophytic	16	8.1
Exophytic	25	12.6
Mixed	120	60.6
Diffuse	10	5.1
Total necrosis	27	13.6
Orbital invasion		
Yes	68	22.5
Optic nerve invasion‡		
No invasion	117	42.4
Prelaminar	46	16.7
Laminar	22	8
Retrolaminar	29	10.5
Distal surgical edge	62	22.5
Choroidal invasion§		
Group 1	52	17.2
Group 2	30	9.9
Group 3	27	8.9
Group 4	84	27.8
Scleral invasion		
Group 1	14	4.6
Group 2	7	2.4
Group 3	5	1.7
Group 4	70	23.2
Subretinal seeding¶		
Yes	154	74
Vitreous seeding**		
Yes	156	72.6
Anterior chamber seeding††		
Yes	51	20.5
Iris neovascularisation‡‡		
Group 1	17	6.6
Group 2	50	19.3
Group 3	65	25.1
Group 4	34	13.1
Flexner–Wintersteiner rosettes		
Yes	100	33.1
Homer Wright rosettes		
Yes	99	32.8
Fleurettes		
Yes	6	2
Basophilic staining		
Yes	91	30.1

*Determined in 123 cases.
†Determined in 198 cases.
‡Determined in 276 cases.
§Determined in 193 cases.
¶Determined in 208 cases.
**Determined in 215 cases.
††Determined in 249 cases.
‡‡Determined in 259 cases.

TABLE 2.—Univariate Analysis for Calcifications in Three Categories

Variable	Calcification (in %)			p-Value
	Group 0	Group 1	Groups 2 or 3	
Age				0.001
1–18 months	8.0	33.0	59.0	
19–36 months	12.8	40.4	46.8	
>37 months	32.0	22.0	46.0	
Gender				0.02
Male	11.5	39.2	49.2	
Female	20.6	22.7	56.7	
Side				0.24
Right	19.2	26.9	53.8	
Left	13.9	37.0	49.1	
Size				<0.0001
Group 1	33.8	36.9	29.2	
Group 2	16.1	34.5	49.4	
Group 3	3.8	13.8	82.5	
Group 4	5.6	25.4	69.0	
Focality				0.01
Monofocal	17.6	45.6	36.8	
Multifocal	10.9	25.5	63.6	
Pattern				0.0004
Endophytic	25.0	31.3	43.8	
Exophytic	8.0	36.0	56.0	
Mixed	17.5	32.5	50.0	
Diffuse	50.0	50.0	0	
Total necrosis	0	14.8	85.2	
Orbital invasion				<0.0001
No	16.7	32.1	51.3	
Yes	5.9	11.8	82.4	
Optic nerve invasion				0.0002
Group 0	18.8	38.5	42.7	
Group 1	10.9	26.1	63.0	
Group 2	27.3	18.2	54.5	
Group 3	17.2	31.0	51.7	
Group 4	6.5	11.3	82.3	
No	18.8	38.5	42.7	0.0002
Yes	12.6	20.1	67.3	
Scleral invasion				0.001
Group 0	17.6	33.2	49.3	
Group 1	7.1	28.6	64.3	
Group 2	28.6	14.3	57.1	
Group 3	0	0	100	
Group 4	5.7	14.3	80.0	
No	17.6	33.2	49.3	<0.0001
Yes	7.3	15.6	77.1	
Choroidal invasion				<0.0001
Group 0	27.8	37.0	35.2	
Group 1	1.9	34.6	63.5	
Group 2	13.3	23.3	63.3	
Group 3	7.4	7.4	85.2	
Group 4	7.1	19.0	73.8	
No	27.8	37.0	35.2	<0.0001
Yes	6.7	22.3	71.0	
Subretinal seeding	15.5	34.5	50.0	0.33
Vitreous seeding	19.2	32.1	48.7	0.80
Anterior chamber seeding	11.8	21.6	66.7	0.12
Iris neovascularisation				0.01
Group 0	22.6	33.3	44.1	
Group 1	11.8	41.2	47.1	
Group 2	14.0	34.0	2.0	

(Continued)

TABLE 2.—(*Continued*)

Variable	Group 0	Calcification (in %) Group 1	Groups 2 or 3	p-Value
Group 3	10.8	21.5	67.7	
Group 4	5.9	14.7	79.4	
No	22.6	33.3	44.1	0.01
Yes	10.8	25.9	63.3	
Flexner–Wintersteiner rosettes	11.0	28.0	61.0	0.52
Hommer–Wright rosettes	10.1	30.3	59.6	0.33
Fleurettes	16.7	33.3	50.0	0.92
Mitosis				0.93
Basophilic staining	3.3	16.5	80.2	<0.0001
Necrosis				<0.0001
Retinal seeding	26.5	51.5	22.1	0.43
Optic atrophy	23.5	48.0	28.4	0.30
Cholesterol clefts	0	14.3	85.7	0.01
Cataract	8.7	47.8	43.5	0.20
Angle closure	10.3	44.8	44.8	0.054

TABLE 3.—Univariate Analysis for Calcifications in Two Categories (No/Yes)

Variable	Calcification (in %) No	Yes	p-Value
Age			<0.000
1–18 months	8.0	92.0	
19–36 months	12.8	87.2	
>37 months	32.0	68.0	
Gender			0.07
Male	11.5	88.5	
Female	20.6	79.4	
Side			0.36
Right	19.2	80.8	
Left	13.9	86.1	
Size			<0.0001
Group 1	33.8	66.2	
Group 2	16.1	83.9	
Group 3	3.8	96.3	
Group 4	5.6	94.4	
Focality			0.32
Monofocal	17.6	82.4	
Multifocal	10.9	89.1	
Pattern			0.003
Endophytic	25.0	75.0	
Exophytic	8.0	92.0	
Mixed	17.5	82.5	
Diffuse	50.0	50.0	
Total necrosis	0	100	
Orbital invasion			0.03
No	16.7	83.3	
Yes	5.9	94.1	
Optic nerve invasion			0.09
Group 0	18.8	81.2	
Group 1	10.9	89.1	
Group 2	27.3	72.7	
Group 3	17.2	82.8	
Group 4	6.5	93.5	

(*Continued*)

TABLE 3.—(*Continued*)

Variable	Calcification (in %) No	Yes	p-Value
No	18.8	81.2	0.18
Yes	12.6	87.4	
Scleral invasion			0.07
Group 0	17.6	82.4	
Group 1	7.1	92.9	
Group 2	28.6	71.4	
Group 3	0	100	
Group 4	5.7	94.3	
No	17.6	82.4	0.02
Yes	7.3	92.7	
Choroidal invasion			<0.0001
Group 0	27.8	72.2	
Group 1	1.9	98.1	
Group 2	13.3	86.7	
Group 3	7.4	92.6	
Group 4	7.1	92.9	
No	27.8	72.2	<0.0001
Yes	6.7	93.3	
Subretinal seeding	15.5	84.5	0.18
Vitreous seeding	19.2	80.8	0.56
Anterior chamber seeding	11.8	88.2	0.52
Iris neovascularisation			0.11
Group 0	22.6	77.4	
Group 1	11.8	88.2	
Group 2	14.0	86.0	
Group 3	10.8	89.2	
Group 4	5.9	94.1	
No	22.6	77.4	0.02
Yes	10.8	89.2	
Flexner–Wintersteiner rosettes	11.0	89.0	0.30
Hommer–Wright rosettes	10.1	89.9	0.16
Fleurettes	16.7	83.3	1.0
Mitosis			0.83
Basophilic staining	3.3	96.7	0.0001
Necrosis			<0.0001
Retinal seeding	26.5	73.5	0.62
Optic atrophy	23.5	76.5	0.20
Cholesterol clefts	0	100	0.34
Cataract	8.7	91.3	0.15
Angle closure	10.3	89.7	0.21

data collection are needed to further assess for an existence of an association between the high-risk characteristics and calcification in retinoblastoma.

T. Milman, MD

TABLE 4.—Logistic Regression of Calcification on Penetration Into the Nerve or to the Orbit, Basophilic Staining, Iris Neovascularisation, Penetration Into the Choroid and Necrosis

Variable	N	Initial Model OR	95% CI	p	N	Final Model OR	95% CI	p
Penetration into the nerve or to the orbit								
No	102	1	—	—				
Yes	132	0.68	0.27 to 1.71	0.42				
Basophilic staining								
No	168	1	—					
Yes	66	1.78	0.45 to 6.98	0.41				
Iris neovascularisation								
No	81	1	—	—				
Yes	153	1.09	0.44 to 2.67	0.86				
Penetration into the choroid								
No	97	1	—	—	100	1	—	—
Yes	137	3.24	1.28 to 8.22	0.01	191	3.26	1.53 to 6.96	0.002
Necrosis	234	1.03	1.01 to 1.05	0.01	291	1.02	1.01 to 1.04	0.004

N, number.

Sudden Growth of a Choroidal Melanoma and Multiplex Ligation-Dependent Probe Amplification Findings Suggesting Late Transformation to Monosomy 3 Type

Callejo SA, Dopierala J, Coupland SE, et al (Royal Liverpool Univ Hosp, England, UK; Univ of Liverpool, England, UK)
Arch Ophthalmol 129:958-960, 2011

Background.—It is currently believed that uveal melanomas develop monosomy 3 quite early, with metastatic spread occurring years before becoming apparent. A melanoma with seemingly delayed transformation from disomy 3 to monosomy 3 was reported.

Case Report.—Woman, 65, came for treatment of an inferonasal, pigmented, choroidal tumor in the left eye measuring 10.1 mm wide and 1.6 mm thick. The lesion had scattered drusen but no orange pigment or subretinal fluid. The patient was monitored every 6 months to differentiate between nevus and melanoma. Four years later she had photocoagulation for diabetic retinopathy; the following year she had epiretinal membrane peel. Six years after she was initially seen, the tumor appeared unchanged except for becoming thicker (2.3 mm). She developed an acutely painful left eye, visual acuity at light perception, and intraocular pressure 40 mm Hg 2 years later. The eye was enucleated after finding a collar-stud shape to the tumor, which now measured 14.0 mm basally and 10.5 mm thick. Microscopically the tumor was found to be a choroidal melanoma with extensive necrosis but viable epithelioid cells at the apex and spindle cells at the base. Mitotis rate was 4 per 40 high-power fields. There were no closed connective tissue loops and minimal lymphocytic infiltrate, but melanoma cells were found on the iris surface and extending into the chamber angle. A melanoma satellite penetrated the ciliary body. Microdissection was carried out, then multiplex ligation-dependent probe amplification revealed monosomy 3 and chromosome 6p gains in the melanoma cells from the apex and disomy 3 in those at the base. Six months after surgery the patient had no evidence of metastases.

Conclusions.—This tumor suddenly enlarged after 8 years and became collar-stud shaped, necrotic, and painful. Why it enlarged appears related to its transformation from an indolent disomy 3, spindle-cell type tumor to an aggressive monosomy 3, epithelioid-cell type tumor. Alternatively, it could have been a choroidal nevus that transformed into a monosomy 3 melanoma but one should see nevus cells in the basal area of the tumor and not the melanoma cells that predominated. Nevi also rarely grow slowly. It is equally unlikely that the growth was a response to the panretinal photocoagulation. This case suggests that monosomy 3 can arise at any stage of tumor development and supports the belief that intratumoral genetic heterogeneity exists in most uveal melanomas. A highly malignant clone of melanoma cells may have arisen, based on the sudden growth, the concurrence of epithelioid cells with chromosome 3 loss and chromosome 8q gain in the tumor's apical area, and the absence of these high-grade morphologic and genotypic features in the tumor's basal part, the oldest area of the tumor. Opportunities for preserving the eye and vision may be lost if melanomas are not treated promptly. Further study is needed to clarify whether early treatment of uveal melanoma will prevent conversion to a monosomy 3 later.

▶ It has been suggested that disomy 3 and monosomy 3 uveal melanomas are distinct from their inception.[1] Other investigators noted regional heterogeneity regarding monosomy 3 status in uveal melanomas.[2] Callejo et al report the case of a melanoma that, after 8 years of apparent quiescence, suddenly enlarged, developed a collar-stud shape, became necrotic, and made the eye acutely painful (Fig 1 in original article). Multiplex ligation-dependent probe amplification (MLPA) specifically designed for uveal melanoma, a sensitive and specific technique that examines for genetic gains and losses by means of a multiplex polymerase chain reaction, was used to assess chromosome 3 status. The investigators noted that the apex of the tumor containing epithelioid melanoma cells had monosomy 3, whereas the spindle melanoma cells at the base were demonstrated to be disomy 3 (Fig 2 in original article). Callejo et al hypothesize that after years of apparent dormancy, a choroidal melanoma suddenly enlarged because it had transformed from an indolent, disomy 3, spindle-cell type to an aggressive, monosomy-3, epithelioid type. Another possibility is that a benign choroidal nevus has undergone transformation into a choroidal melanoma, but histopathology of the spindle cell component of the tumor is not consistent with this hypothesis. These findings support prior studies documenting intratumoral genetic heterogeneity in uveal melanomas and suggest that early treatment of uveal melanomas may prevent later conversion into a monosomy-3 genotype and, by implication, metastatic death. Further prospective studies are necessary to confirm these conclusions.

T. Milman, MD

References

1. Damato B, Dopierala JA, Coupland SE. Genotypic profiling of 452 choroidal melanomas with multiplex ligation-dependent probe amplification. *Clin Cancer Res.* 2010;16:6083-6092.
2. Schoenfield L, Pettay J, Tubbs RR, Singh AD. Variation of monosomy 3 status within uveal melanoma. *Arch Pathol Lab Med.* 2009;133:1219-1222.

Clinical and Pathologic Characteristics of Biopsy-Proven Iris Melanoma: A Multicenter International Study

Khan S, Finger PT, Yu G-P, et al (New York Univ School of Medicine; et al)
Arch Ophthalmol 130:57-64, 2012

Objective.—To collaborate with multiple centers to identify representative epidemiological, clinical, and pathologic characteristics of melanoma of the iris. This international, multicenter, Internet-assisted study in ophthalmic oncology demonstrates the collaboration among eye cancer specialists to stage and describe the clinical and pathologic characteristics of biopsy-proven melanoma of the iris.

Methods.—A computer program was created to allow for Internet-assisted multicenter, privacy-protected, online data entry. Eight eye cancer centers in 6 countries performed retrospective chart reviews. Statistical analysis included patient and tumor characteristics, ocular and angle abnormalities, management, histopathology, and outcomes.

Results.—A total of 131 patients with iris melanoma (mean age, 64 years [range, 20-100 years]) were found to have blue-gray (62.2%), green-hazel (29.1%), or brown (8.7%) irides. Iris melanoma color was brown (65.6%), amelanotic (9.9%), and multicolored (6.9%). A mean of 2.5 clock hours of iris was visibly involved with melanoma, typically centered at the 6-o'clock meridian. Presentations included iritis, glaucoma, hyphema, and sector cataract. High-frequency ultrasonography revealed a largest mean tumor diameter of 4.9 mm, a mean maximum tumor thickness of 1.9 mm, angle blunting (52%), iris root disinsertion (9%), and posterior iris pigment epithelium displacement (9%). Using the American Joint Commission on Cancer—International Union Against Cancer classification, we identified 56% of tumors as T1, 34% of tumors as T2, 2% of tumors as T3, and 1% of tumors as T4. Histopathologic grades were G1-spindle (54%), G2-mixed (28%), G3-epithelioid (5%), and undetermined (13%) cell types. Primary treatment involved radiation (26%) and surgery (64%).

TABLE 1.—Iris Melanoma Staging Based on the American Joint Commission on Cancer Staging System[a]

Clinical and Pathologic Staging	Definition
Tumor size	
TX	Primary tumor cannot be assessed
T0	No evidence of primary tumor
T1	Tumor limited to the iris
T1a	Tumor limited to the iris (not more than 3 clock hours in size)
T1b	Tumor limited to the iris (more than 3 clock hours in size)
T1c	Tumor limited to iris with secondary glaucoma
T2	Tumor confluent with or extending into the ciliary body, choroid, or both
T2a	Tumor confluent with or extending into the ciliary body, choroid, or both with secondary glaucoma
T3	Tumor confluent with or extending into the ciliary body, choroid, or both with scleral extension
T3a	Tumor confluent with or extending into the ciliary body, choroid, or both with scleral extension and secondary glaucoma
T4	Tumor with extraocular extension
T4a	Tumor with extrascleral extension ≤5 mm in diameter
T4b	Tumor with extrascleral extension >5 mm in diameter
Regional lymph nodes	
NX	Regional lymph nodes cannot be assessed
N0	No regional lymph node metastasis
N1	Regional lymph node metastasis
Distant metastasis	
MX	Distant metastasis cannot be assessed
M0	No distant metastasis
M1	Distant metastasis
M1a	Largest diameter of the largest metastasis (≤3 cm)
M1b	Largest diameter of the largest metastasis (3.1-8.0 cm)
M1c	Largest diameter of the largest metastasis (>8 cm)
Histopathologic grade	
GX	Grade cannot be assessed
G1	Spindle cell melanoma
G2	Mixed cell melanoma
G3	Epithelioid cell melanoma

Melanoma of the Uvea in Edge et al.[4]
Editor's Note: Please refer to original journal article for full references.
[a]Abstracted from Ophthalmic Sites Part X, Chapter 51: Malignant.

Kaplan-Meier analysis found a 10.7% risk of metastatic melanoma at 5 years.

Conclusions.—Iris melanomas were most likely to be brown and found in the inferior quadrants of patients with light irides. Typically small and unifocal, melanomas are commonly associated with angle blunting and spindle cell histopathology. This multicenter, Internet-based, international study successfully pooled data and extracted information on biopsy-proven melanoma of the iris (Tables 1, 2, and 4-6).

▶ Khan et al present a study that highlights the importance of international collaboration in improving our knowledge of rare eye diseases, such as iris melanoma. A retrospective chart review was conducted at 8 ophthalmic oncology centers (in the United States, Canada, Finland, Sweden, the Netherlands, and England).

TABLE 2.—American Joint Commission on Cancer Staging in This Series of Patients With Iris Melanoma

Staging	Patients, No. (%)
Clinical (n=130)	
TX	9 (6.9)
T0	0 (0.0)
T1	19 (14.6)
T1a	40 (30.8)
T1b	7 (5.4)
T1c	7 (5.4)
T2	32 (24.6)
T2a	12 (9.2)
T3	1 (0.8)
T3a	2 (1.5)
T4	1 (0.8)
Pathologic (n=104)	
TX	23 (22.1)
T0	0 (0.0)
T1	12 (11.5)
T1a	29 (27.9)
T1b	5 (4.8)
T1c	2 (1.9)
T2	15 (14.4)
T2a	5 (4.8)
T3	7 (6.7)
T3a	3 (2.9)
T4	3 (2.9)
Regional lymph nodes (n=130)	
NX	101 (77.7)
N0	29 (22.3)
Distant metastasis (n=130)	
MX	24 (18.5)
M0	97 (74.6)
M1	9 (6.9)
Histopathologic grade (n=131)	
GX	18 (13.7)
G1	71 (54.2)
G2	36 (27.5)
G3	6 (4.6)

An internet-based, password-protected computer program was created to allow for a multicenter online encrypted data entry portal (ScienceTrax, Macon, GA, USA [http://www.sciencetrax.com/Home/]) that provided a secure online framework with technical support (Fig 1 in the original article). This international database allowed for retrospective review of clinical and pathologic characteristics of 131 patients with biopsy-proven iris melanoma.

The authors found that glaucoma was the most common presenting finding. The tumors were typically brown, without color heterogeneity, unifocal, and inferior (between the 3-o'clock and 9-o'clock meridians). The mean diameter was 5.0 mm. Larger tumor size (> 5 mm) was associated with the presence of intrinsic tumor vessels, more than 0.5 clock hours of angle involvement, and epithelioid melanoma cytomorphology (Tables 4 and 5). Most tumors were managed surgically, although larger tumors (> 5mm) were more likely to be managed by radiotherapy (Table 6). Kaplan-Meier analysis found a 10.7% risk of metastatic melanoma at 5 years (Fig 2 in the original article).

TABLE 4.—Tumor Related Characteristics of Patients With Iris Melanoma

Characteristic	Patients, No. (%)
Tumor color (n=131)	
Brown only	86 (65.6)
Tan only	19 (14.5)
Amelanotic only	13 (9.9)
Multicolored	9 (6.9)
Black only	2 (1.5)
Not specified	2 (1.5)
Heterogeneity (n=125)	37 (29.6)
Heterochromia iridis (n=126)	14 (11.1)
Intrinsic tumor vessels (n=124)	70 (56.5)
Episcleral, sentinel, vessel (n=125)	21 (16.8)
Iris feeder vessels (n=124)	9 (7.3)
Glaucoma (n=127)	34 (26.8)
Pigment dispersion (n=120)	53 (44.2)
Ectropion uveae (n=129)	55 (42.6)
Correctopia (n=131)	34 (26.0)
Sector cataract (n=131)	23 (17.6)
Synechiae, anterior or posterior (n=131)	10 (7.7)
Anterior chamber inflammation (n=131)	5 (3.8)
Hyphema (n=129)	4 (3.1)

TABLE 5.—Association of Clinical Factors With Tumor Size in Patients With Iris Melanoma

Clinical Factor	Tumor Diameter, No. of Patients		Unadjusted OR	Adjusted OR[a] (95% CI)	χ^2 Value	P Value
	≥5.0 mm	<5.0 mm				
Age, y						
<50	7	12	1 [Reference]	1 [Reference]		
50-69	18	25	1.2	1.6 (0.4-6.0)	0.55	.46
≥70	11	18	1.0	1.7 (0.4-7.0)	0.48	.49
Sex						
Female	21	36	1 [Reference]	1 [Reference]		
Male	16	20	1.4	2.2 (0.7-6.4)	2.03	.15
Eye color						
Other than blue	12	18	1 [Reference]	1 [Reference]		
Blue only	25	40	0.9	2.2 (0.7-7.6)	1.65	.20
Starting clock hours						
≥9:30	3	6	1 [Reference]	1 [Reference]		
3:00 to <9:30	29	48	1.4	1.8 (0.3-10.9)	0.41	.52
<3:00	6	3	4.5	3.8 (0.4-39.6)	1.22	.27
Tumor color						
Other than brown	13	27	1 [Reference]	1 [Reference]		
Brown only	25	31	1.7	2.4 (0.8-7.5)	2.42	.12
Tumor vessels						
No	12	32	1 [Reference]	1 [Reference]		
Yes	25	25	2.7	4.4 (1.4-13.8)	6.66	.01
Angle involvement,[b] clock hours						
0	6	24	1 [Reference]	1 [Reference]		
0.5-2.0	14	16	2.5	4.8 (1.4-17.2)	5.98	.02
>2.0	13	11	3.3	5.7 (1.3-24.0)	5.60	.02
Histopathologic grade						
GX and G1	21	42	1 [Reference]	1 [Reference]		
G2 and G3	17	16	2.1	2.9 (1.0-8.6)	3.68	.06

Abbreviations: CI, confidence interval; OR, odds ratio.
[a]Mutually adjusted by age, sex, eye color, starting clock hours, tumor color, presence of intrinsic tumor vessels, angle involvement, and histopathologic grade.
[b]$P = .012$ for trend.

TABLE 6.—Analysis of Treatment Strategy, Tumor Size, and Pathologic Tumor Stage for Patients With Iris Melanoma

Treatment	Tumor Size,[a] No. of Patients		P Value[b]
	<5.0 mm (n=57)	≥5.0 mm (n=38)	
No surgery and no radiation	0 (0.0)	0 (0.0)	<.001
Surgery only	42 (73.7)	12 (31.6)	
Radiation only	13 (22.8)	20 (52.6)	
Surgery and radiation	2 (3.5)	6 (15.8)	

Treatment	Tumor Stage, No. of Patients		P Value[b]
	TX or T0 (n=22)	T1, T2, T3, or T4 (n=80)	
No surgery and no radiation	4 (18.2)	0 (0.0)	<.001
Surgery only	9 (40.9)	61 (76.3)	
Radiation only	9 (40.9)	9 (11.3)	
Surgery and radiation	0 (0.0)	10 (12.5)	

[a]The largest tumor diameter measured by use of ultrasonography.
[b]Determined by use of the Fisher exact test (2-tailed).

This study illustrates readily apparent strengths of multicenter collaborative studies and some of the inherent weaknesses. As authors state in their concluding remarks, the strengths of registry-based collaborative studies include recruitment of larger numbers of patients and/or clinical samples in relatively short periods. Collaborative data collection may minimize duplication of ineffective treatments, more quickly validate effective treatments and cancer staging systems (in this case American Joint Commission on Cancer TNM staging for iris melanoma, Tables 1 and 2), and more efficiently allocate resources. In addition, collaborative studies foster communication and cooperation among eye cancer specialists and thereby raise the standards of clinical care. However, the multicenter Internet registry-based study may have potential limitations. For example, the authors of this study do not provide the data on whether the clinical and pathologic staging and grading systems on iris melanoma were standardized and validated to ensure interobserver consistency in clinical and pathologic staging and grading. This is particularly important in iris melanoma, which does not have well-defined pathologic grading criteria. What standards, if any, did the authors use to define spindle-cell—type iris melanomas, mixed-cell—type iris melanomas, and epithelioid iris melanomas?

T. Milman, MD

Ultra-High Resolution Optical Coherence Tomography for Differentiation of Ocular Surface Squamous Neoplasia and Pterygia

Kieval JZ, Karp CL, Abou Shousha M, et al (Univ of Miami, FL)
Ophthalmology 119:481-486, 2012

Objective.—To assess the use of an ultra–high-resolution (UHR) optical coherence tomography (OCT) as an adjuvant diagnostic tool in distinguishing ocular surface squamous neoplasia (OSSN) and pterygia.

Design.—Prospective case series.

Participants.—Thirty-four eyes of 34 patients with conjunctival lesions clinically suspicious for OSSN or pterygia.

Methods.—All patients were photographed and then imaged with a custom-built UHR OCT device. Subsequently, each patient underwent excisional or incisional biopsy with histopathologic diagnosis.

Main Outcome Measures.—Comparison of preoperative UHR OCT images and the corresponding histopathologic specimen; comparison of epithelial thickness between the 2 groups as measured by UHR OCT.

Results.—Preoperative UHR OCT images of OSSN demonstrated similarities to the histopathologic specimens. Both optical and pathologic specimens showed a thickened layer of epithelium, often with an abrupt transition from normal to neoplastic tissue. Likewise, preoperative UHR OCT images of patients with pterygia were well correlated with the histopathologic specimens. As opposed to OSSN, both UHR OCT and pathologic images of pterygia demonstrated a normal thin epithelium, with underlying thickening of the subepithelial mucosal layers. Differences in the measured epithelial thickness on UHR OCT between OSSN and pterygia were statistically significant, with an average epithelial thickness of 346 μm (standard deviation [SD], 167) in OSSN patients and 101 μm (SD, 22) in pterygium patients ($P<0.001$). By receiver operating characteristic curve, the sensitivity and specificity of UHR OCT for differentiating between OSSN and pterygia was found to be 94% and 100%, respectively, using a cutoff value of 142 μm.

Conclusions.—Ultra–high-resolution OCT may show promise as a noninvasive diagnostic tool to evaluate ocular surface lesions. In addition to a statistically significant difference in epithelial thickness, a significant degree of morphologic correlation with the histopathologic results demonstrates its potential in evaluating ocular surface squamous neoplasia and pterygia (Figs 1 and 2, Table 1).

▶ Optical coherence tomography (OCT) has the potential to provide a noninvasive, optical biopsy of the tissue, where morphologic characteristics can be examined in vivo. A study on uterine cervical tissues demonstrated the ability of OCT to distinguish between the normal and dysplastic epithelia. Similar technology is now applied to the evaluation of the ocular surface disease. The custom-built ultra-high-resolution (UHR) units allow axial resolution of 2 to 3 μm and have been shown to enable visualization of the corneal and retinal architecture. In a recent small case series Shousha et al[1] demonstrated that UHR OCT images correlated well with the histopathologic specimens in the cases of ocular surface squamous neoplasia (OSSN) (conjunctival intraepithelial neoplasia/squamous cell carcinoma in situ) following topical chemotherapy and pterygia. Despite the promising results of that study, the authors commented on the need to establish standardized OCT scanning protocols and diagnostic criteria to distinguish between the various ocular surface pathologies.

In the current study from the same group, the authors aim to define further UHR OCT characteristics of OSSN and to provide UHR OCT standards that would

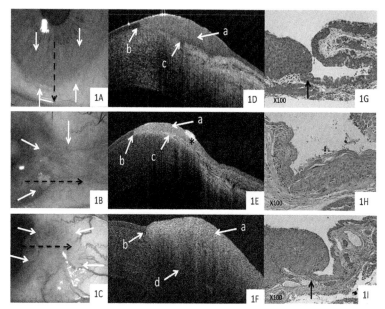

FIGURE 1.—Sample imaging of ocular surface squamous neoplasia. A—C, Anterior segment slit-lamp photographs demonstrating gelatinous, leukoplakic, and papillary ocular surface squamous neoplasia, respectively (white arrows). The black dotted arrows represent the direction and location of the ultra—high-resolution optical coherence tomography (OCT) scans. D—F, Ultra—high-resolution OCT images of the lesions demonstrating a thickened hyperreflective epithelium (arrow a). Note the abrupt transition between abnormal and normal epithelium (arrow b). A plane of cleavage between the lesion and the underlying tissue is also noted (arrow c). However, in Figure 1F, the plane of cleavage in this histologically proven corneal and conjunctival intraepithelial neoplasia is not as evident because of some shadow casted by the thickened lesion (arrow d). A leukoplakic lesion is noted by the asterisks in Figure 1E exhibiting an even brighter hyperreflective focus. G—I, Photomicrographs of histopathologic specimens from these lesions revealing a mucosal epithelium with disorganized cellular maturation extending to the full thickness of the tissue. Note the abrupt transition zone between abnormal and normal epithelium (black arrows). No subepithelial invasion is seen, consistent with the diagnosis of carcinoma in situ (stain, hematoxylin—eosin; original magnification, ×100). (Reprinted from Kieval JZ, Karp CL, Abou Shousha M, et al. Ultra-high resolution optical coherence tomography for differentiation of ocular surface squamous neoplasia and pterygia. *Ophthalmology.* 2012;119:481-486, Copyright 2012, with permission from American Academy of Ophthalmology.)

enable differentiation of OSSN from pterygia (Table 1). The authors found that in OSSN, UHR OCT images demonstrated severely thickened, hyperreflective epithelium with an abrupt transition between the normal and affected epithelium (Figs 1 and 2). The authors noted that assessment of epithelial thickness was particularly valuable. Using the cutoff value of 142 μm, they found that UHR OCT has the sensitivity of 94% and specificity of 100% in its ability to differentiate between OSSN and pterygia.

This study highlights the amazing advances in ocular imaging-based diagnostics. As with any new technology, however, there are limitations with the use of UHR OCT. The authors mention that UHR OCT has the potential for noninvasive diagnosis, which may guide treatment. However, in this study UHR OCT failed to detect a small focus of microinvasive squamous cell carcinoma and to distinguish between squamous cell carcinoma and mucoepidermoid carcinoma. As

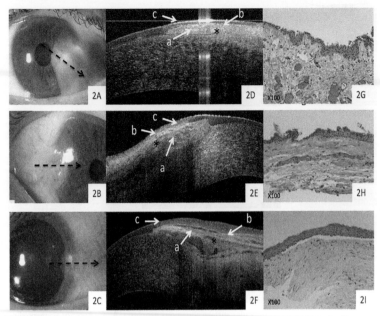

FIGURE 2.—Sample imaging of pterygia. **A−C,** Anterior segment slit-lamp photographs demonstrating a conjunctival and corneal lesion, consistent with a pterygium. The black dotted arrows represent the direction and location of the ultra− high-resolution optical coherence tomography (OCT) scans. **D−F,** Ultra−high-resolution OCT images disclosing thick subepithelial hyperreflective lesions (arrow a) that are separated from the overlying epithelium by a plane of cleavage (arrow b). Areas of hyporeflectivity also are noted in the subepithelial tissue that could represent feeding blood vessels in the pterygium tissue (asterisks). Epithelium overlying those lesions is thin or of a normal thickness and shows only mild hyperreflectivity (arrow c). **G−I,** Photomicrographs of histopathologic specimens from these lesions revealing a normal mucosal epithelium with appropriate maturational sequencing throughout the tissue. The thickened substantia propria with elastotic changes seen in the specimens is consistent with the diagnosis of pterygium (stain, hematoxylin−eosin; original magnification, ×100). (Reprinted from Kieval JZ, Karp CL, Abou Shousha M, et al. Ultra-high resolution optical coherence tomography for differentiation of ocular surface squamous neoplasia and pterygia. *Ophthalmology.* 2012;119:481-486, Copyright 2012, with permission from American Academy of Ophthalmology.)

TABLE 1.—Demographic Information and Lesion Characteristics in Patients with Ocular Surface Squamous Neoplasia and Pterygium

	Ocular Surface Squamous Neoplasia	Pterygium	P Value
No. of eyes (patients)	17 (17)	17 (17)	
Age, yrs (mean±standard deviation)	71 ± 14	47 ± 11	<0.005
Male gender, % (n/N)	65 (11/17)	41 (7/17)	0.30
Involved right eye, % (n/N)	41 (10/17)	59 (7/17)	0.49
Recurrent disease (n/N)	35 (6/17)	12 (2/17)	0.22
Involved quadrant, % (n/N)			
Nasal	24 (4/17)	88 (15/17)	
Temporal	29 (5/17)	12 (3/17)	
Superior	24 (2/17)		
Inferior	12 (2/17)		
More than 2 involved	18 (3/17)		

n/N = number of patients with feature/total number of patients studied.

the authors note, leukoplakic and hyperreflective lesions can cast shadows on the underlying tissue and may obscure a clear diagnosis of underlying pathologic features, including microinvasion. In addition, if epithelial thickness is used as a primary differentiating criterion between the OSSN and pterygium, some cases of mild dysplasia or even carcinomas in situ, lacking appreciable acanthosis, can be misinterpreted as benign lesions. Correlation of UHR OCT with histopathology of a wide range of ocular surface lesions that can mimic OSSN is needed to better define the UHR OCT diagnostic features of OSSN. Lastly, the UHR OCT device used in this study is not yet commercially available, which limits its applicability and validation.

T. Milman, MD

Reference

1. Shousha MA, Karp CL, Perez VL, et al. Diagnosis and management of conjunctival and corneal intraepithelial neoplasia using ultra high-resolution optical coherence tomography. *Ophthalmology.* 2011;118:1531-1537.

Diagnosis and Management of Conjunctival and Corneal Intraepithelial Neoplasia Using Ultra High-Resolution Optical Coherence Tomography
Shousha MA, Karp CL, Perez VL, et al (Univ of Miami, FL)
Ophthalmology 118:1531-1537, 2011

Purpose.—To report a novel diagnostic technique and a case series of conjunctival and corneal intraepithelial neoplasia (CCIN) diagnosed and followed up using prototype ultra high-resolution (UHR) optical coherence tomography (OCT).
Design.—Prospective, noncomparative, interventional case series.
Participants.—Seven eyes of 7 consecutive patients with CCIN treated using topical interferon alfa-2b or 5-fluorouracil and 7 eyes of 6 consecutive patients with history of surgically excised pterygia.
Intervention.—Ultra high-resolution OCT imaging of the ocular surface at primary diagnosis of CCIN and during the follow-up period until resolution of the lesion. Ultra high-resolution OCT images of sites of excised pterygia also were captured and compared with images from resolved CCIN patients.
Main Outcome Measures.—Clinical course and photographs, UHR OCT images, and histopathologic findings.
Results.—Ultra high-resolution OCT was capable of providing a noninvasive optical biopsy of all examined CCIN lesions. Ultra high-resolution OCT images of the lesions disclosed a thickened hyperreflective epithelium and abrupt transition from normal to hyperreflective epithelium in all 7 cases. Ultra high-resolution OCT images showed excellent correlation with histopathologic specimens obtained at primary diagnosis of the cases that had incisional biopsies before treatment. All patients were treated medically and were followed up for clinical resolution. In 4 patients, at clinical

resolution, UHR OCT images also showed normal epithelial configuration at the site of the treated lesions. In 3 patients, despite apparent clinical resolution, the UHR OCT was able to detect residual disease that was clinically invisible. Continuation of treatment resulted in complete resolution of the residual lesions on the UHR OCT images in all cases. Ultra high-resolution OCT images of patients with surgically excised pterygia demonstrated similar findings to resolved CCIN cases.

Conclusions.—Ultra high-resolution OCT is a novel noninvasive technique to diagnose and manage medically treated CCIN. Using UHR OCT to guide medical treatment could prevent the premature termination of topical treatment in the presence of subclinical disease. A larger sample size is needed for further validation of its sensitivity and specificity (Figs 1-3).

▶ Clinical examination, impression cytologic analysis, and histopathologic examination of excised tissue are the currently available techniques for the diagnosis and follow-up of conjunctival intraepithelial neoplasia (CIN). These methods have limitations. Clinical examination is subjective and may miss subclinical microscopic disease. Impression cytologic analysis accesses only superficial layers of cells, which are not representative of the deeper layers. Excisional biopsy, despite being the diagnostic gold standard, carries the risk of inducing conjunctival scarring and limbal stem cell deficiency and may be not representative of the entire lesion. Recent reports have described the use of in vivo confocal microscopy in the diagnosis of CIN. Although in vivo confocal microscopy can provide an impressive cellular-level resolution of the ocular

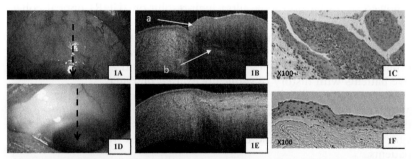

FIGURE 1.—Images from patient 1. **A,** Slit-lamp photograph showing a superior conjunctival and corneal intraepithelial neoplasia (CCIN). The black arrows represent the location of the ultra high-resolution (UHR) optical coherence tomography (OCT) scan. **B,** Ultra high-resolution OCT image of this lesion disclosing a severely thickened limbal hyperreflective epithelial lesion (a). A plane of cleavage between the lesion and the underlying tissue is noted (b). **C,** Photomicrograph of histopathologic results the incisional biopsy specimen from the lesion disclosing faulty epithelial maturational sequencing extending up to full thickness, with no invasion, consistent with CCIN (stain, hematoxylin—eosin; original magnification, ×100). The correlation between the UHR OCT image (**B**), slit-lamp photography (**A**), and histologic results (**C**) demonstrates the capability of the UHR OCT to diagnose CCIN noninvasively. **D,** Slit-lamp photograph showing resolution of CCIN lesions after treatment with interferon. Posttreatment (**E**) UHR OCT image and (**F**) biopsy specimen disclosing a normal limbus and confirming the resolution of the tumor (stain, hematoxylin—eosin; original magnification, ×100). (Reprinted from Shousha MA, Karp CL, Perez VL, et al. Diagnosis and management of conjunctival and corneal intraepithelial neoplasia using ultra high-resolution optical coherence tomography. *Ophthalmology.* 2011;118:1531-1537, Copyright 2011, with permission from the American Academy of Ophthalmology.)

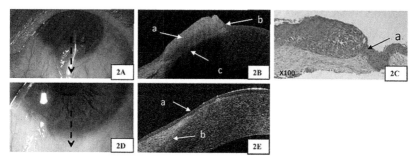

FIGURE 2.—Images from patient 2. A, Slit-lamp photograph showing a gelatinous limbal conjunctival and corneal intraepithelial neoplasia (CCIN) lesion. B, Ultra high-resolution optical coherence tomography (OCT) image disclosing a severely thickened hyperreflective epithelial inferior limbal lesion (a). Abrupt transition between the normal and affected hyper-reflective epithelium is evident (b). A plane between the lesion and the underlying tissue is noted (c). C, Photomicrograph of histopathologic results of the incisional biopsy specimen from the lesion disclosing faulty epithelial maturational sequencing extending up to full thickness, with no invasion of underlying tissue, consistent with CCIN (stain, hematoxylin—eosin; original magnification, ×100). D, Posttreatment slit-lamp photograph of the inferior limbus showing resolution of the CCIN lesion. E, Ultra high-resolution OCT image disclosing normal epithelium (a) with a subepithelial opaque layer (b) that is attributed to subepithelial fibrous tissue and posttreatment corneal pannus. (Reprinted from Shousha MA, Karp CL, Perez VL, et al. Diagnosis and management of conjunctival and corneal intraepithelial neoplasia using ultra high-resolution optical coherence tomography. *Ophthalmology.* 2011;118:1531-1537, Copyright 2011, with permission from the American Academy of Ophthalmology.)

surface, it requires direct contact with the eye.[1] Recent advances in optical coherence tomography (OCT) have enabled exact and rapid cross-sectional imaging of the cornea and conjunctiva without direct contact between the eye and the instrument. The researchers in this study used a custom-built, ultra-high resolution spectral domain OCT (UHR OCT, SD-OCT) prototype, which enables analysis of the topographic characteristics of conjunctival and corneal epithelia and their underlying stroma with an enhanced resolution when compared with conventional time domain OCT. Shousha et al showed that UHR OCT images correlated well with the histopathologic specimens in the cases of incisional biopsies. The thickened hyperreflective epithelium, the abrupt transition from normal to abnormal epithelium, and the plane between the lesion and the underlying tissue could be seen in UHR OCT images and in the histopathologic specimens. In addition, partial and complete response to treatment (incisional biopsy and topical chemotherapy with interferon-α or 5-fluorouracil) was documented with UHR OCT and correlated with histopathology (Figs 1-3). The control group included the eyes with pterygia, which lacked histopathologic and UHR OCT characteristics of CIN (Fig 5 in the original aticle).

As the authors mention, this promising new technology has several important limitations. The UHR OCT device used in this study is not yet commercially available. Standardized protocols to scan the entire ocular surface using UHR OCT and providing a patient map are needed. Correlation of UHR OCT with histopathology of a wide range of ocular surface lesions (not only pterygia) is needed to better define the UHR OCT diagnostic features of CIN. Furthermore, although the authors state this imaging modality is useful in demonstrating resolution of CIN, obviating the need for confirmatory biopsy, they have not evaluated the

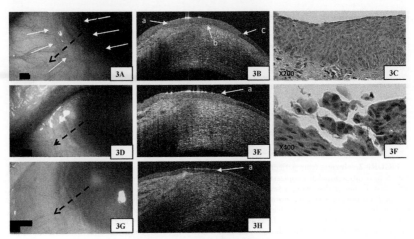

FIGURE 3.—Images from patient 4. A, Slit-lamp photograph showing a conjunctival and corneal intraepithelial neoplasia (CCIN; white arrows). The black arrows represent the location of the Ultra high-resolution optical coherence tomography (OCT) scan. B, Ultra high-resolution OCT image disclosing a thickened hyperreflective epithelial layer (a), Bowman's layer (b), as well as the abrupt transition from normal to hyperreflective epithelium (c). C, Photomicrograph of histopathologic results of examination of the incisional biopsy specimen from the lesion disclosing CCIN (stain, hematoxylin—eosin; original magnification, ×200). D, After 3 months of treatment, the lesion appeared significantly resolved. E, Ultra high-resolution OCT image showing residual CCIN with hyperreflective epithelial layer (a). F, Photomicrograph of histopathologic results of a midtreament biopsy revealing a small foci of atypical cells (stain, hematoxylin— eosin; original magnification, ×400). G, After 3 additional months of interferon treatment the clinical picture remained similar. H, Ultra high-resolution OCT image disclosing normal epithelium (a) and confirming the resolution of the lesion. (Reprinted from Shousha MA, Karp CL, Perez VL, et al. Diagnosis and management of conjunctival and corneal intraepithelial neoplasia using ultra high-resolution optical coherence tomography. *Ophthalmology.* 2011;118:1531-1537, Copyright 2011, with permission from the American Academy of Ophthalmology.)

potential effect of mitomycin-C on UHR OCT characteristics of ocular surface epithelium. In addition, the resolution of the current UHR OCT is approximately 2 μm, and thus cannot detect intracellular features. Although in most cases a discreet layer of epithelial neoplasia was seen with a plane separating from the underlying tissue, this device cannot rule out microinvasion. This concern is particularly pertinent for very thick hyperreflective lesions, which can cast a shadow on the underlying tissue and can obscure the view of the posterior limit of the lesion. Thus, further studies with larger and more varied sample sizes will be needed for validation of these results and evaluation of their sensitivity and specificity in the diagnosis and management of CIN lesions.

T. Milman, MD

Reference

1. Alomar TS, Nubile M, Lowe J, Dua HS. Corneal intraepithelial neoplasia: in vivo confocal microscopic study with histopathologic correlation. *Am J Ophthalmol.* 2011;151:238-247.

An Update on Reporting Histopathologic Prognostic Factors in Melanoma

Ivan D. Prieto VG (Univ of Texas M. D. Anderson Cancer Ctr, Houston)

Arch Pathol Lab Med 135:825-829, 2011

Context.—Accurate diagnosis of melanocytic lesions is essential for the adequate clinical management of patients. Thus, thorough reporting of histopathologic parameters, especially in the initial biopsies, is a critical component of both diagnosis and staging.

Objective.—To review current data on histopathologic prognostic factors for melanoma, with special emphasis on their use and applicability to clinical practice. Special attention is focused on the criteria highlighted by the new 2009 version of The American Joint Committee on Cancer (AJCC) system of melanoma staging and classification.

Data Sources.—Published peer-reviewed literature and personal experience of the authors.

Conclusions.—When reporting melanoma, we recommend that a template be provided, including all the histologic parameters that have been proved significant in determining the tumor staging and prognosis of a patient. The template may also include other details that may be helpful in further analysis of potential complete excisional biopsies or metastatic lesions, such as predominant type of tumor cells, presence or absence of desmoplastic component, or associated benign melanocytic lesions. Although there are several drawbacks in reporting some of these histopathologic parameters (interobserver variability, occasional lack of a perfectly reproducible method for quantifying these criteria), we suggest that at least the essential histopathologic parameters highlighted by the newest version of the AJCC system for melanoma staging and classification should be included in the report (Figs 1-3).

▶ This is an excellent article in which the authors comment on the new developments in melanoma histopathologic prognostic factors and on the recommended guidelines for their reporting. They base their discussion on the 2009 American Joint Commission on Cancer guidelines, which has been incorporated into the new College of American Pathology Checklist on cutaneous melanoma reporting. The authors provide excellent histopathology photomicrographs to illustrate the discussed concepts (Figs 1-3). They also support these data with the recent evidence-based studies and add their own experience and interpretation to the recommended guidelines. This article crystallizes the important histopathologic parameters in melanoma reporting and is a must for a practicing pathologist.

For additional information, I recommend several articles in the same journal issue that focus on the histopathologic, immunohistochemical, and molecular genetic diagnostic parameters of melanocytic lesions.[1-3]

T. Milman, MD

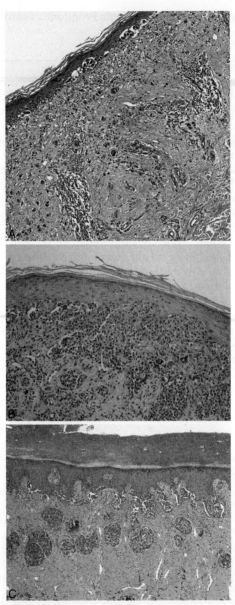

FIGURE 1.—Traditionally described histogenetic subtypes of melanoma. A, Lentigo maligna (thin epidermis, sun damage, predominantly single melanocytes with confluent growth pattern). B, Superficial spreading (predominantly nested with prominent pagetoid upward migration). C, Acral lentiginous type (lentiginous spread and pagetoid upward migration) (hematoxylin-eosin, original magnifications ×20). (Reproduced with permission of College of American Pathologists from Ivan D, Prieto VG. An update on reporting histopathologic prognostic factors in melanoma. *Arch Pathol Lab Med.* 2011;135:825-829, with permission from Copyright Clearance Center, Inc.)

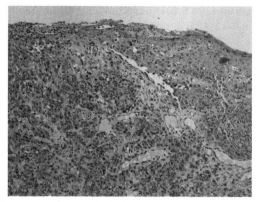

FIGURE 2.—The presence of tumor-related ulceration in melanoma is an independent prognostic factor for survival (hematoxylin-eosin, original magnification ×20). (Reproduced with permission of College of American Pathologists from Ivan D, Prieto VG. An update on reporting histopathologic prognostic factors in melanoma. *Arch Pathol Lab Med.* 2011;135:825-829, with permission from Copyright Clearance Center, Inc.)

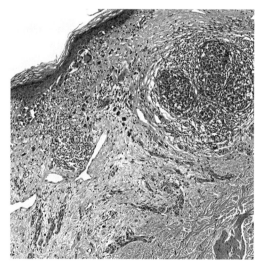

FIGURE 3.—Lentigo maligna melanoma with regression: dermal fibrosis, vascular proliferation, inflammatory infiltrate, and dermal melanor phages, with absence of an invasive component (hematoxylin-eosin, original magnification ×20). (Reproduced with permission of College of American Pathologists from Ivan D, Prieto VG. An update on reporting histopathologic prognostic factors in melanoma. *Arch Pathol Lab Med.* 2011;135:825-829, with permission from Copyright Clearance Center, Inc.)

References

1. Prieto VG, Shea CR. Immunohistochemistry of melanocytic proliferations. *Arch Pathol Lab Med.* 2011;135:853-859.
2. Reed JA, Shea CR. Lentigo maligna: melanoma in situ on chronically sun-damaged skin. *Arch Pathol Lab Med.* 2011;135:838-841.
3. Fox JC, Reed JA, Shea CR. The recurrent nevus phenomenon: a history of challenge, controversy, and discovery. *Arch Pathol Lab Med.* 2011;135:842-846.

Update on Fluorescence In Situ Hybridization in Melanoma: State of the Art
Gerami P, Zembowicz A (Northwestern Univ and the Feinberg School of Medicine, Chicago, IL; Lahey Clinic, Burlington, MA)
Arch Pathol Lab Med 135:830-837, 2011

Context.—Recent advances in understanding the molecular basis of melanoma have resulted in development of fluorescence in situ hybridization (FISH) protocols designed to detect genetic abnormalities discriminating melanoma from nevi. The most extensively studied is a 4- probe multicolor FISH probe panel targeting chromosomes 6 and 11. Validation studies showed promising sensitivity and specificity for distinguishing benign nevi and malignant melanoma by FISH. Recent studies show that a melanoma FISH assay has great potential for becoming an important diagnostic adjunct in classification of melanocytic lesions and in diagnosis of melanoma.
Objective.—To present a comprehensive review of the science and practical aspects of FISH in melanoma for pathologists considering the use of melanoma FISH in their practice.
Data Sources.—Review of the literature and personal experience of the authors.
Conclusions.—Judicious use of a 4-probe multicolor melanoma FISH procedure can enhance accuracy for diagnosis of melanoma and improve classification of melanocytic proliferations (Figs 1 and 2, Table 1).

▶ This is an excellent article for any pathologist, clinician, or surgeon involved in the care of patients with cutaneous melanoma. The authors concisely and clearly

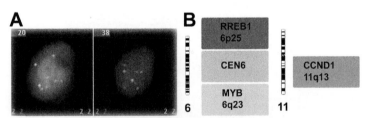

FIGURE 1.—Abbott Molecular's 4-probe melanoma fluorescence in situ hybridization (FISH) test. A, The figure shows a composite of 2 images for 2 representative normal nuclei from a benign nevus. Each of the images shows pairs of red, aqua, yellow, and green dots. Each signal represents a fluorochrome-labeled probe bound to a copy of a complementary DNA of a particular gene (see B for details). The images are from Metafer Slide Scanning System (MetaSystems, Altlussheim, Germany). The numbers in the left upper corner indicate image numbers and the aqua, red, yellow, and green numbers at the bottom of each image indicate number of signals for each probe, calculated by the automatic algorithm. B, The assay uses 4 fluorescent dye—tagged probes, which are hybridized to 5-μm thick, formalin-fixed, paraffin-embedded sections. Three probes bind to loci on chromosome 6, and 1 binds to a locus on chromosome 11. *RREB1* (ras responsive element binding protein 1) probe (labeled with a red fluorochrome) corresponds to 6p25; CEN6 (centromere 6) probe (labeled with an aqua fluorochrome) corresponds to a centromeric region of chromosome 6; *MYB* (v-myb myeloblastosis viral oncogene homologue) probe (labeled with a yellow fluorochrome) corresponds to 6q23; and *CCND1* (cyclin D1) probe (labeled with a green fluorochrome) corresponds to 11q13 (original magnification ×640 under oil immersion [A]). For interpretation of the references to color in this figure legend, the reader is referred to web version of this article. (Reproduced with permission of College of American Pathologists from Gerami P, Zembowicz A. Update on fluorescence in situ hybridization in melanoma: state of the art. *Arch Pathol Lab Med.* 2011;135:830-837, with permission from Copyright Clearance Center, Inc.)

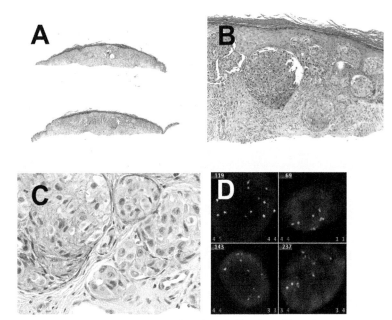

FIGURE 2.—Spitzoid melanoma with tetraploidy from the files of one of the authors (A.Z.). A, A super-ficial shave biopsy specimen of a rapidly growing pigmented lesion from a left ankle lesion in a 17-year-old adolescent girl. B and C, The tumor showed pagetoid spread, consumption of epidermis, and severe cyto-logic epithelioid cell atypia, allowing diagnosis of malignant melanoma. D, Composite fluorescence in situ hybridization (FISH) images of 4 tetraploid nuclei from this case, each showing 3 to 4 signals for *CCND1* (cyclin D1, 11q13, green), *RREB1* (ras responsive element binding protein 1, 6p25, red), *MYB* (v-myb mye-loblastosis viral oncogene homologue, yellow, 6q23) and centromere 6 (aqua). The images are from Metafer Slide Scanning System (MetaSystems, Altlussheim, Germany). The numbers in the left upper corner indicate image numbers and the aqua, red, yellow, and green numbers at the bottom of each image indicate number of signals for each probe, calculated by the automatic algorithm (hematoxylin-eosin, original magnifications ×20 [A], ×100 [B], and ×400 [C]; FISH, original magnification ×640 under oil immersion [D]). For inter-pretation of the references in this figure legend, the reader is referred to web version of this article. (Reproduced with permission of College of American Pathologists from Gerami P, Zembowicz A. Update on fluorescence in situ hybridization in melanoma: state of the art. *Arch Pathol Lab Med.* 2011;135:830-837, with permission from Copyright Clearance Center, Inc.)

TABLE 1.—Abbott Molecular's 4-Probe Melanoma Fluorescence In Situ Hybridization Test

Criterion	Signal	UCSF/Northwestern University Cutoff, %	NeoGenomics Cutoff, %
6p25 gain	>2 *RREB1* (red)	>29	>16
6p25 gain	*RREB1* (red) > CEN6 (aqua)	>55	>53
6p23 loss	*MYB* (yellow) < CEN6 (aqua)	>40	>42
11q13 gain	>2 *CCND1* (green)	>38	>19

Criteria and signal cutoffs were established by University of California in San Francisco UCSF/Northwestern University (Chicago, Illinois) studies and NeoGenomics Laboratories (Irvine, California). By NeoGenomics criteria, the fluorescence in situ hybridization test is considered abnormal if (1) 16% of cells show more than 2 red signals (*RREB1* probe), indicating gain of 6p25 locus; (2) 53% of cells show more red (*RREB1* probe) than aqua (centromere 6 probe) signals, indicating gain of 6p25 locus (*RREB1*); (3) 42% of cells show fewer yellow (*MYB* probe) than aqua (centromere 6) signals, indicating loss of 6q23 locus; and (4) more than 19% of cells show more than 2 green signals (*CCND1* probe), indicating gain of 11p13 locus. For each of these 4 criteria, UCSF/Northwestern cutoffs were 29%, 55%, 40%, and 38%, respectively. *CCND1*, cyclin D1; CEN6, centromere 6; *MYB*, v-myb myeloblastosis virus oncogene homologue; *RREB1*, ras responsive element binding protein 1.

explain the early data on cytogenetic and molecular genetic differences between the various melanoma subtypes and nevi. They follow this discussion with a description of recent advances in the field of molecular genetics of cutaneous and mucosal melanoma. The most notable advance is the development of commercially available Abbot Molecular's 4-Probe Melanoma Fluorescence in Situ Hybridization (FISH) Test (Fig 1, Table 1), which has a sensitivity and specificity of about 70% to 75% in distinguishing melanomas from nevi and can be performed on paraffin-embedded tissue. The authors state that they routinely use Abbott Molecular's melanoma FISH test as a diagnostic adjunct in virtually all borderline cases with sufficient tissue (Fig 2). However, the authors add that they do not automatically reclassify a nevus into melanoma or vice versa based on the results of the FISH test; the ultimate diagnosis is based on careful histopathologic reevaluation in conjunction with ancillary molecular diagnostic testing. Although the field of molecular diagnostics of melanocytic lesions is still evolving, this study offers promising results, which, hopefully, can be translated into broad pathology practice. For additional information on the topic, please read the article in the same journal issue by Soheil Dadras.[1]

T. Milman, MD

Reference

1. Dadras SS. Molecular diagnostics in melanoma: current status and perspectives. *Arch Pathol Lab Med.* 2011:860-869.

DICER1 deficit induces *Alu* RNA toxicity in age-related macular degeneration
Kaneko H, Dridi S, Tarallo V, et al (Univ of Kentucky, Lexington; et al)
Nature 471:325-330, 2011

Geographic atrophy (GA), an untreatable advanced form of age-related macular degeneration, results from retinal pigmented epithelium (RPE) cell degeneration. Here we show that the microRNA (miRNA)-processing enzyme DICER1 is reduced in the RPE of humans with GA, and that conditional ablation of *Dicer1*, but not seven other miRNA-processing enzymes, induces RPE degeneration in mice. *DICER1* knockdown induces accumulation of *Alu* RNA in human RPE cells and *Alu*-like B1 and B2 RNAs in mouse RPE. *Alu* RNA is increased in the RPE of humans with GA, and this pathogenic RNA induces human RPE cytotoxicity and RPE degeneration in mice. Antisense oligonucleotides targeting *Alu*/B1/B2 RNAs prevent *DICER1* depletion-induced RPE degeneration despite global miRNA downregulation. DICER1 degrades *Alu* RNA, and this digested *Alu* RNA cannot induce RPE degeneration in mice. These findings reveal a miRNA-independent cell survival function for DICER1 involving retrotransposon transcript degradation, show that *Alu* RNA can directly

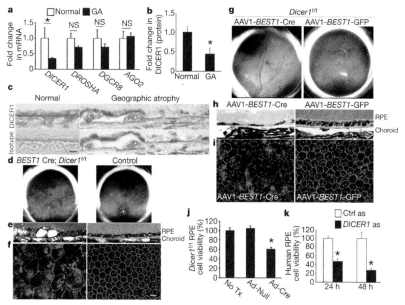

FIGURE 1.—*DICER1* deficit in GA induces RPE degeneration. a, *DICER1* is less abundant in RPE of human eyes with GA ($n = 10$) compared to control RPE ($n = 11$). $P = 0.004$ by Mann–Whitney U-test. *DROSHA, DGCR8* and *EIF2C2* (encoding AGO2) abundance not significantly different ($P > 0.11$ by Mann–Whitney U-test). $n = 10–11$. b, DICER1 quantification, assessed by western blotting (Supplementary Fig. 1), lower in human GA RPE ($n = 4$) compared to control RPE ($n = 4$). $P = 0.003$ by Student t-test. c, Reduced DICER1 (blue) in human GA RPE compared to control eyes. d, e, Fundus photographs (d) and toluidine-blue-stained sections (e) show RPE degeneration in *BEST1* Cre; *Dicer1*$^{f/f}$ mice but not controls. Arrowheads point to basal surface of RPE. f, Flat mounts stained for zonula occludens-1 (ZO-1; red) show RPE disruption in *BEST1* Cre; *Dicer*$^{f/f}$ mice compared to controls. g, h, Fundus photographs (g) and toluidine blue-stained sections (h) show RPE (g, h) and photoreceptor (h) degeneration in *Dicer1*$^{f/f}$ mice following subretinal injection of AAV1-*BEST1*-Cre but not AAV1-*BEST1*-GFP. i, Flat mounts show *Dicer1*$^{f/f}$ mouse RPE degeneration following subretinal injection of AAV1-*BEST1*-Cre but not AAV1-*BEST1*-GFP. Nuclei stained blue with Hoechst 33342. Representative images shown. $n = 16–32$ (d–f); 10–12 (g–i). Scale bars (c, e, h), 10 μm; (f, i) 20 μm. j, Adenoviral vector coding for Cre recombinase (Ad-Cre) treatment reduces *Dicer1*$^{f/f}$ mouse RPE cell viability compared to Ad-Null or untreated (no Tx) cells. k, *DICER1* antisense (as) reduces human RPE cell viability compared to control antisense (Ctrl as)-treated cells. $n = 6–8$. All error bars indicate mean ± s.e.m. For interpretation of the references to color in this figure legend, the reader is referred to web version of this article. (Reprinted from Kaneko H, Dridi S, Tarallo V, et al. DICER1 deficit induces *Alu* RNA toxicity in age-related macular degeneration. *Nature*. 2011;471:325-330, Copyright 2011, with permission from Macmillan Publishers Limited.)

cause human pathology, and identify new targets for a major cause of blindness (Figs 1-5).

▶ A collaboration of 40 researchers published results of their groundbreaking work in *Nature*, providing us with a new insight into the pathogenesis of geographic atrophy. Kaneco et al discovered that patients with geographic atrophy have reduced levels of an enzyme, DICER1, in their retinal pigment epithelium (RPE). Kaneko and colleagues also noted that RPE is severely degenerated in mice lacking DICER1 selectively, similar to the observations in geographic atrophy, further implicating reduced DICER1 levels in the pathogenesis of this disorder (Fig 1).

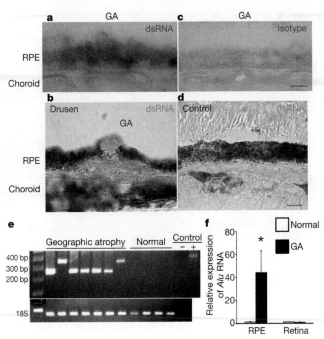

FIGURE 2.—*Alu* RNA accumulation in GA triggered by *DICER* reduction. **a, b,** dsRNA immunolocalized (blue) in RPE (**a, b**) and sub-RPE deposits (drusen; **b**) in human GA. **c, d,** No staining with isotype antibody in GA RPE (**c**) and with anti-dsRNA antibody in control eye (**d**). Scale bars (**a–d**), 10 μm. n = 10 (a–d) **e,** PCR amplification of immunoprecipitated dsRNA yielded amplicons with homology to *Alu* in GA RPE but not normal RPE. Water control (−) showed no amplification and recombinant dsRNA (+) showed predicted amplicon. **f,** Increased *Alu* RNA in GA RPE compared to control (*n* = 7). *P* < 0.05 by Student *t*-test. No significant difference in *Alu* RNA in neural retina. Values normalized to abundance in normal eyes. For interpretation of the references to color in this figure legend, the reader is referred to web version of this article. (Reprinted from Kaneko H, Dridi S, Tarallo V, et al. DICER1 deficit induces *Alu* RNA toxicity in age-related macular degeneration. *Nature.* 2011;471:325-330, Copyright 2011, with permission from Macmillan Publishers Limited.)

DICER1 enzymes, as the name implies, cut long double-stranded RNA molecules into shorter pieces and are, therefore, crucial for gene-silencing pathways that involve small RNAs. An example of small RNAs are interfering RNAs or microRNAs (miRNAs)—the most abundant class of small RNAs in mammals. Although loss of DICER1 intuitively points to a role for miRNAs in geographic atrophy, Kaneko and colleagues refuted this hypothesis, observing that mice lacking 2 other enzymes required for miRNA processing (DROSHA and DGCR8) did not demonstrate degeneration of the RPE, despite severely impaired miRNA function. To explain these observations, the researchers speculated that a different class of double-stranded RNA might be involved in the pathogenesis of geographic atrophy. Their investigations led to a discovery of a marked increase in the levels of Alu RNA sequences (the most common noncoding, repetitive DNA sequences in human genome) in the RPE of patients with geographic atrophy, but not in those of healthy individuals (Fig 2). These findings were also observed in an animal model and in cell culture experiments: Mice

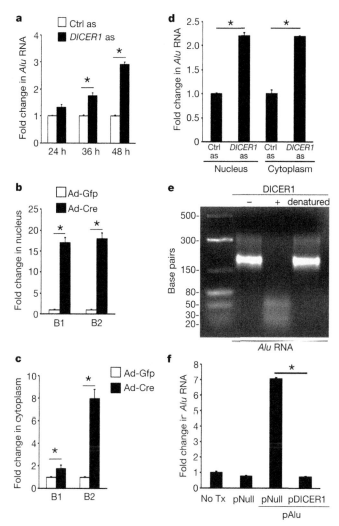

FIGURE 3.—*DICER1* degrades *Alu* RNA. **a,** DICER1 antisense (as) increased *Alu* RNA in human RPE cells. **b, c,** Ad-Cre, but not Ad-GFP, increased B1 and B2 RNAs in *Dicer1*^f/f mouse RPE cells in nucleus (**b**) and cytoplasm (**c**). **d,** DICER1 as upregulated *Alu* RNA in human RPE cell nucleus and cytoplasm. **e,** Agarose gel electrophoresis shows recombinant DICER1 (+), but not heat-denatured DICER1, degrades *Alu* RNA isolated and cloned from human GA RPE. Image representative of six experiments. **f,** *Alu* RNA in human RPE cells upregulated by plasmid coding for *Alu* (pAlu) versus pNull or no treatment (no Tx) at 24 h reduced by pDICER1. *$P < 0.05$. $n = 4–8$ (**a–d, f**). Values normalized to control as-treated (for *Alu*) or Ad-GFP-infected cells (for B elements). (Reprinted from Kaneko H, Dridi S, Tarallo V, et al. DICER1 deficit induces *Alu* RNA toxicity in age-related macular degeneration. *Nature.* 2011;471:325–330, Copyright 2011, with permission from Macmillan Publishers Limited.)

with DICER1 deficiency in the RPE and human DICER1 knockdown RPE cells were found to express increased levels of Alu RNAs (Fig 3). Furthermore, Kaneko et al found that enhancing the expression of Alu RNAs and their direct injection

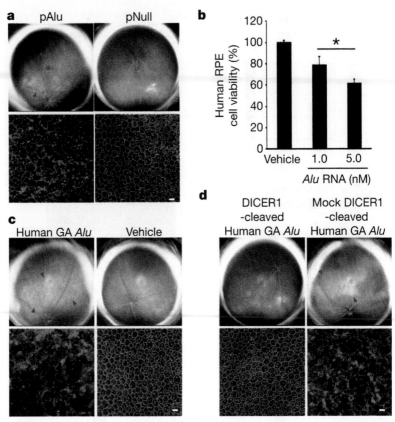

FIGURE 4.—*DICER1* protects RPE cells from *Alu* RNA cytotoxicity. **a,** Subretinal pAlu, but not pNull, induced wild-type mouse RPE degeneration (fundus photographs, top row; ZO-1 stained (red) flat mounts, bottom row). **b,** *Alu* RNA induced human RPE cytotoxicity. Values normalized to pNull or vehicle. *$P < 0.05$ by Student *t*-test. $n = 4–6$. **c,** Subretinal *Alu* RNA isolated and cloned from human GA RPE induced wild-type mouse RPE degeneration. **d,** Subretinal injection of this *Alu* RNA, when cleaved by DICER1, did not induce wild-type mouse RPE degeneration (fundus photographs, top row; flat mounts, bottom row) in contrast to mock-cleaved *Alu* RNA. Degeneration outlined by blue arrowheads (**a, c, d**). Scale bars, 20 μm. $n = 10–15$. For interpretation of the references to color in this figure legend, the reader is referred to web version of this article. (Reprinted from Kaneko H, Dridi S, Tarallo V, et al. DICER1 deficit induces *Alu* RNA toxicity in age-related macular degeneration. *Nature*. 2011;471:325-330, Copyright 2011, with permission from Macmillan Publishers Limited.)

into the eyes of normal mice and in human-cultured RPE, reduced RPE viability and led to its degeneration (Fig 4). In contrast, when the expression of DICER1 was increased or when Alu antisense oligonucleotides were injected, the toxic effects of increased levels of Alu RNAs were no longer seen (Fig 5).

Kaneko et al propose that reduced Dicer1 levels in patients with geographic atrophy result in accumulation of long, toxic, Alu RNAs, leading to RPE cell death and degeneration. Alternatively, small Alu RNAs may play an important role in RPE maintenance, and their absence may contribute to pathogenesis of geographic atrophy. The discovery of the role of DICER1 and Alu RNAs in the

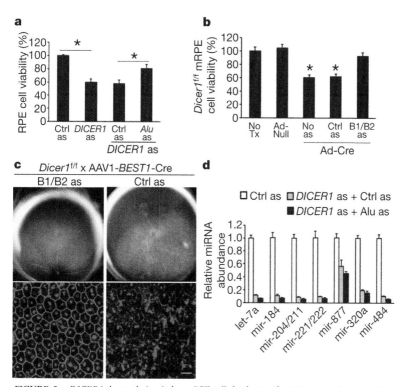

FIGURE 5.—*DICER1* dysregulation induces RPE cell death via *Alu* RNA accumulation. a, Human RPE cytotoxicity induced by DICER1 as rescued by *Alu* RNA antisense. Values normalized or compared to control (Ctrl) antisense. b, Ad-Cre but not Ad-Null induced *Dicer1*^{f/f} mouse RPE cytotoxicity. B1/B2 RNA as, but not control (Ctrl) as, rescued viability. Values normalized to untreated cells (no Tx). * *P* < 0.05 by Student *t*-test. *n* = 4–6 (a, b). c, Subretinal AAV-*BEST1*-Cre induced RPE degeneration (blue arrowheads in fundus photograph, top row; ZO-1 stained (red) flat mounts, bottom row) in *Dicer1*^{f/f} mice 20 days after injection was inhibited by subretinal cholesterol-conjugated B1/B2 as, but not cholesterol-conjugated Ctrl as, 10 days after AAV-*BEST1*-Cre injection. Values normalized to Ctrl as-treatment. *n* = 8. Scale bar, 20 μm. d, DICER1 as induced global miRNA expression deficits in human RPE cells compared to Ctrl as. No significant difference in miRNA abundance between *Alu* as and Ctrl as-treated DICER1 depleted cells. *n* = 3. For interpretation of the references to color in this figure legend, the reader is referred to web version of this article. (Reprinted from Kaneko H, Dridi S, Tarallo V, et al. DICER1 deficit induces *Alu* RNA toxicity in age-related macular degeneration. *Nature.* 2011;471:325-330, Copyright 2011, with permission from Macmillan Publishers Limited.)

pathogenesis of geographic atrophy can be potentially translated into therapeutic strategies aimed at reduction of Alu levels (such as injecting antisense oligonucleotides into the eye) or via increasing DICER1 expression in the eye.

T. Milman, MD

Fluorescein Angiographic and Histopathologic Findings of Bilateral Peripheral Retinal Nonperfusion in Nonaccidental Injury: A Case Series
Bielory BP, Dubovy SR, Olmos LC, et al (Univ of Miami—Miller School of Medicine, FL; Univ of Southern California—Keck School of Medicine, Los Angeles, CA)
Arch Ophthalmol 130:383-387, 2012

Background.—In shaken baby syndrome, one expects to find multilayered retinal hemorrhages, subdural hematomas, and neurologic abnormalities in the setting of an inconsistent history and often other inflicted injuries. Unilateral peripheral retinal nonperfusion can be a late development in nonaccidental injuries (NAIs). A case series of relevant clinicopathologic findings showed bilateral peripheral retinal nonperfusion in three living subjects with NAI. Findings were compared with ocular and systemic findings in 11 full-term autopsy specimens with NAI and five control subjects.

Case Reports.—Case 1: Girl, 2, had a history of NAI involving both eyes. She suffered recurrent pain in her right eye and atypical seizures unresponsive to medication. Computerized tomography (CT) scans showed left frontal lobe damage. When examined under anesthesia, the patient's intraoperative fluorescein angiographic (FA) images showed significant bilateral peripheral retinal ischemia with no neovascular process. An electroretinogram revealed marked depression in the rod and cones response and a selectively impaired b-wave on combined rod-cone electroretinogram response.

Case 2: Boy, 7 months, had a history of NAI and peripheral retinal ischemia in both eyes 1 month before being admitted for an examination under anesthesia. Fundoscopic evaluation showed preretinal hemorrhages and a subretinal demarcation line in both eyes. Significant bilateral peripheral retinal ischemia was found on intraoperative FA.

Case 3: Boy, 1, had a history of NAI and dense vitreous hemorrhage in the right eye. Examination under anesthesia of both eyes and a 23-gauge pars plana vitrectomy of the right eye showed extensive ischemia at the posterior pole and periphery in both eyes.

Autopsy Specimen Findings.—Previous ocular trauma was found in nine cases of children who had sustained NAI and lived for at least 2 months. Iron stain results were negative in control subjects and positive in NAI cases. Four NAI cases had an increased distance of termination of vascular lumen formation from the ora serrata in the nasal and temporal retina compared to the control subjects. CD31 staining of the peripheral retinal vessels was less for cases than controls, and there was decreased lumen formation and increased punctate staining of the mid and far periphery. Cases of NAI also demonstrated increased glial fibrillary acid protein staining of the neural retina compared to controls.

Conclusions.—Bilateral nonperfusion of the peripheral retinal vasculature is a new finding in association with NAI. The biomechanics of NAI related to this finding remains unclear, but vitreoretinal traction plus rotational and acceleration-deceleration forces may produce vascular damage and secondary nonperfusion where there is tight vitreotractional adhesion in the peripheral retina. Apparent glial cell activation is also noted in many cases and may contribute to peripheral retinal nonperfusion. Children with this type of injury should be evaluated using serial fundus examinations and possibly undergo diagnostic imaging.

▶ Multilayered retinal, preretinal and subretinal hemorrhages, perimacular folds, multilayered retinoschisis and internal limiting membrane detachments, and subdural hemorrhages are well-recognized clinical and histopathologic findings in patients with nonaccidental injury (NAI), also known as shaken baby syndrome. Bilateral nonperfusion of the peripheral retinal vasculature is a recently recognized sequela of ocular trauma in NAI. Prior clinical and angiographic case series have shown that peripheral retinal nonperfusion can involve both arterial and venous branches of retinal vasculature and can be associated with preretinal and vitreous hemorrhages and vitreoretinal neovascularization.

In this study, the authors describe the clinical and angiographic findings of 3 live patients with NAI who subsequently developed peripheral retinal nonperfusion documented by fluorescein angiography (Fig 1 in the original article). The authors then discuss the histopathologic findings of autopsy eyes of 11 patients with NAI (9 surviving at least 2 months after documented injury event) and compare these findings to 5 age-matched controls (Figs 2 and 3 in the original article). The authors found that in 8 eyes with NAI (4 patients) there was increased distance between the identifiable vessel lumina and ora serrata and a punctate immunoreactivity for vascular endothelial marker CD31 in the peripheral retina (anterior to the recognizable vascular lumina), suggestive of vessel involution. In addition, NAI eyes demonstrated intraretinal hemosiderin deposition, consistent with prior hemorrhage and glial cell activation, consistent with reactive changes. Interestingly, there was absent immunoreactivity for vascular endothelial growth factor (VEGF) in both NAI and control eyes. The authors speculate that vitreoretinal traction coupled with acceleration-deceleration forces may have led to vascular damage and nonperfusion in the areas of tight vitreoretinal adhesion (vitreous base), and that glial cell activation may have contributed to peripheral retinal nonperfusion. Absence of immunoreactivity for VEGF in the eyes with peripheral retinal nonperfusion is unclear, particularly considering the previously reported association with vitreoretinal neovascularization, but may potentially reflect an early time point in the course of disease, prior to the increase in VEGF expression.

Despite several limitations of this study, including absence of true clinical-pathologic correlation, it reinforces the importance of inclusion of NAI on the differential diagnosis of the peripheral retinal nonperfusion and provides us with histopathologic findings that may reflect clinical observations.

T. Milman, MD

Congenital Fibrovascular Pupillary Membranes: Clinical and Histopathologic Findings
Lambert SR, Buckley EG, Lenhart PD, et al (Emory Univ, Atlanta, GA; Duke Univ, Durham, NC)
Ophthalmology 119:634-641, 2012

Purpose.—To report the clinical and histopathologic findings associated with congenital fibrovascular pupillary membranes.

Design.—Case series.

Participants.—Seven infants were included, 6 with a unilateral congenital pupillary membrane and 1 with classic persistent fetal vasculature (PFV).

Methods.—Patients underwent a membranectomy, pupilloplasty, or lensectomy. Histopathologic examination was performed on the excised membranes.

Main Outcome Measures.—Visual acuity and pupil size.

Results.—Four of the 6 patients with a unilateral congenital pupillary membrane had 1 or more recurrences after a membranectomy and pupilloplasty. The most recent pupil size ranged from 2 to 5 mm in the affected eye. When last tested, the vision in the affected eye was excellent in 4 of the 6 patients. The 2 patients without recurrences of the pupillary membranes

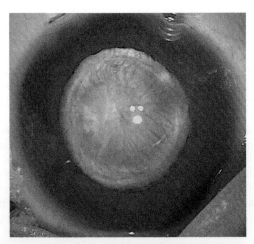

FIGURE 1.—Intraoperative photograph of the right eye of a 7-week-old child with classic persistent fetal vasculature. The lens has been aspirated, revealing a highly vascularized retrolenticular membrane attached to the ciliary processes. (Reprinted from Lambert SR, Buckley EG, Lenhart PD, et al. Congenital fibrovascular pupillary membranes: clinical and histopathologic findings. *Ophthalmology.* 2012;119: 634-644, Copyright 2012, with permission from the American Academy of Ophthalmology.)

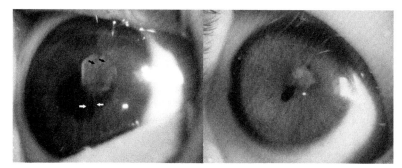

FIGURE 2.—A, Right eye of patient 1 at age 2 weeks after pharmacologic dilation. Fibrovascular membrane blocks the pupil nasally. The membrane is attached to the pupil inferiorly by iris strands (*white arrows*). Radial iris vessels (*black arrows*) extend onto the surface of the membrane. B, Right eye of patient 1 at age 8 months after pharmacologic dilation. The pupil is adherent to the fibrovascular membrane except for 1 small sector inferotemporally. (Reprinted from Lambert SR, Buckley EG, Lenhart PD, et al. Congenital fibrovascular pupillary membranes: clinical and histopathologic findings. *Ophthalmology.* 2012;119: 634-644, Copyright 2012, with permission from the American Academy of Ophthalmology.)

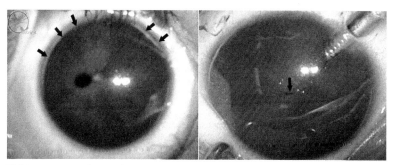

FIGURE 3.—A, Right eye of patient 2 at age 3 months after pharmacologic dilation. All but the temporal margin of the pupil is adherent to white fibrovascular tissue. Posterior embryotoxon is present superiorly (*arrows*). B, Right eye of patient 2 at age 10 months after 2 recurrences of miosis. After pharmacologic dilation, the pupil was still only a narrow slit (*arrow*) and no red reflex was visible. (Reprinted from Lambert SR, Buckley EG, Lenhart PD, et al. Congenital fibrovascular pupillary membranes: clinical and histopathologic findings. *Ophthalmology.* 2012;119:634-644, Copyright 2012, with permission from the American Academy of Ophthalmology.)

underwent multiple iris sphincterotomies at the time of the initial surgery. Histopathologic examination of 2 primary pupillary membranes showed fibrovascular tissue that did not stain for neuron-specific enolase. Smooth muscle actin was only present in vascular walls. In contrast, histopathology of a recurrent pupillary membrane revealed collagenized fibrovascular tissue that was immunoreactive for smooth muscle actin. Finally, histopathology of the retrolenticular membrane excised from an infant with classic PFV was similar to the latter aside from hypercellularity.

Conclusions.—Congenital fibrovascular pupillary membranes in infants are likely a variant of PFV that may recur if incompletely excised. The risk of these membranes recurring may be reduced by excising as much as the

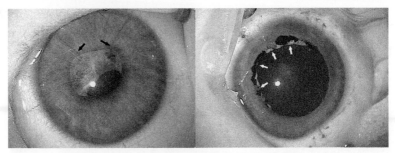

FIGURE 4.—A, Left eye of patient 6 after pharmacologic dilation. Fibrovascular membrane covers most of the pupil. Radial vessels (*arrows*) extend onto the membrane superiorly, and vascular channels can be seen coursing through the membrane. B, Left eye of patient 6 after a membranectomy and pupilloplasty. Multiple sphincterotomies have been made circumferentially around the pupil. A white membrane (*arrows*) that is adherent to the iris pigment epithelium extends beneath the iris for 180 degrees. (Reprinted from Lambert SR, Buckley EG, Lenhart PD, et al. Congenital fibrovascular pupillary membranes: clinical and histopathologic findings. *Ophthalmology*. 2012;119:634-644, Copyright 2012, with permission from the American Academy of Ophthalmology.)

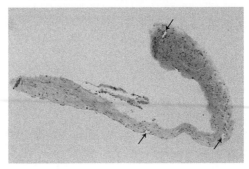

FIGURE 5.—The pupillary membrane excised from case 6 shows fibrovascular tissue composed of vascular channels (*arrows*), spindle-shaped cells, round cells, and extracellular collagen (hematoxylin—eosin 40×). (Reprinted from Lambert SR, Buckley EG, Lenhart PD, et al. Congenital fibrovascular pupillary membranes: clinical and histopathologic findings. *Ophthalmology*. 2012;119:634-644, Copyright 2012, with permission from the American Academy of Ophthalmology.)

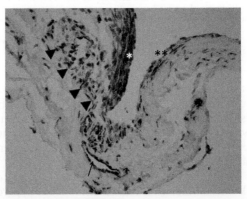

FIGURE 6.—Iris with melanocytes (*) on its surface. Its posterior interface (*arrowheads*) is adherent to fibrovascular tissue. Vascular channels in the fibrovascular tissue are highlighted with smooth muscle actin (*arrow*). Melanocytes from the iris have migrated onto the surface of the fibrovascular tissue in one area (**) (peroxidase anti-peroxidase, 100×). (Reprinted from Lambert SR, Buckley EG, Lenhart PD, et al. Congenital fibrovascular pupillary membranes: clinical and histopathologic findings. *Ophthalmology*. 2012;119:634-644, Copyright 2012, with permission from the American Academy of Ophthalmology.)

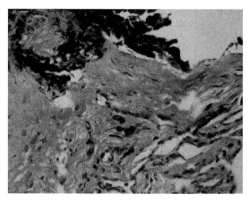

FIGURE 7.—Histopathologic section from retro-irido nodule excised from the right eye of patient 2 at age 10 months. The fibrovascular tissue is collagenized and contains spindle-shaped cells that were immunoreactive for smooth muscle actin consistent with myofibroblasts. The overlying iris pigment epithelium is hypertrophic (hematoxylin—eosin 100×). (Reprinted from Lambert SR, Buckley EG, Lenhart PD, et al. Congenital fibrovascular pupillary membranes: clinical and histopathologic findings. *Ophthalmology.* 2012;119:634-644, Copyright 2012, with permission from the American Academy of Ophthalmology.)

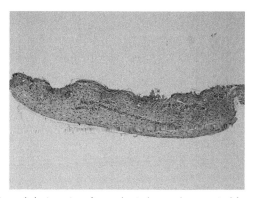

FIGURE 8.—Histopathologic section of a retrolenticular membrane excised from a 7-week-old child with classic persistent fetal vasculature. It contains multiple vascular channels and is hypercellular (hematoxylin—eosin 25×). (Reprinted from Lambert SR, Buckley EG, Lenhart PD, et al. Congenital fibrovascular pupillary membranes: clinical and histopathologic findings. *Ophthalmology.* 2012;119:634-644, Copyright 2012, with permission from the American Academy of Ophthalmology.)

membrane as possible and enlarging the pupil with iris sphincterotomies. A lensectomy should be avoided if possible (Figs 1-8, Tables 1 and 2).

▶ This is a nicely executed clinical-pathologic case series of 6 infants with congenital pupillary membranes and 1 infant with retrolental persistent fetal vasculature (PFV). The authors describe in depth the clinical findings, surgical interventions, postoperative course, and histopathology of the primary and recurrent pupillary membranes. They also speculate on the origin of the pupillary membranes, correlating embryological concepts with the clinical and pathologic findings of the membranes in their series.

TABLE 1.—Clinical Findings

Patient/Affected Eye	Age at Presentation	Ocular Findings	Initial Surgery	No. of Reoperations	Follow-up (mos)	Initial Pupil Size (mm)	Last Pupil Size (mm)	Last Visual Acuity
1/RE	4 days	Miosis, anterior capsular cataract, persistent iris vessels	Synechialysis	1	120	1	2	RE: 20/50 LE: 20/20
2/RE	3 mos	Miosis, corectopia, posterior embryotoxon	Membranectomy, pupilloplasty	2	34	0.5	5	RE: 20/250 LE: 20/20
3/RE	2 mos	Miosis, corectopia, posterior embryotoxon, microphthalmos (9.0 mm)	Membranectomy, pupilloplasty	1	10	1	2.5	RE: CSM LE: CSM
4/LE	5 wks	Miosis, corectopia, anterior capsular cataract, pupillary membrane, posterior embryotoxon	Synechialysis, lensectomy, pupilloplasty	2	7	1	5	RE: CSM LE: CSNM
5/LE	3 mos	Miosis, pupillary membrane, persistent iris vessels	Membranectomy, pupilloplasty	0	11	1	3	RE: CSM LE: CSM
6/LE	2 mos	Miosis, pupillary membrane, persistent iris vessels	Membranectomy, pupilloplasty	0	9	1	3	RE: CSM LE: CSM

CSM = central, steady, and maintained; CSNM = central, steady, and not maintained; LE = left eye; RE = right eye.

TABLE 2.—Histopathologic Findings and Immunohistochemical Staining

Patient No.	Surgical Sample	Pupillary Membrane	Overlying Iris	Smooth Muscle Actin	CD31	Neuron-Specific Endolase	PDGF Beta Receptor	LCA	GFAP
2	Recurrent pupillary membrane	Collagenized fibrovascular tissue	Normal iris pigment epithelium	+ in anterior portion of tissue	Only + in walls of vascular channels	—	+	—	—
4	Vitreous aspirate ×2	Fragments of hypocellular material	NA	NA	NA	NA	NA	NA	NA
5	Primary pupillary membrane	Thin fibrovascular membrane	Absence of iris pigment epithelium iris stroma normal	Only + in walls of vascular channels	Only + in walls of vascular channels	—	+	—	—
6	Primary pupillary membrane	Thin fibrovascular membrane	Normal iris pigment epithelium and iris stroma	Only + in walls of vascular channels	Only + in walls of vascular channels	—	+	—	—
Classic PFV	Retrolenticular membrane	NA	NA	Only + in walls of vascular channels	Only + in walls of vascular channels	—	+	—	—

LCA = leukocyte common antigen; GFAP = glial fibrillary acidic protein; NA = not available; PDGF = platelet-derived growth factor; PFV = persistent fetal vasculature.

The congenital fibrovascular pupillary membranes in this case series were all unilateral and were associated with miosis (6 of 6 patients), corectopia (3 of 6 patients), posterior embryotoxon (3 of 6 patients), anterior capsular cataract (2 of 6 patients), and microcornea (1 of 6 patients) (Table 1, Figs 1 and 4). Histopathology of primary pupillary membranes showed fibrovascular tissue that did not immunostain for neural crest marker neuron-specific enolase. The blood vessels immunoreacted with platelet-derived growth factor (PDGF; pericyte marker) and smooth muscle actin, suggestive of mature vessels formed in utero, as opposed to neovascularization (Table 2, Figs 5 and 6). The histopathologic and immunohistochemical findings were identical to those observed in retrolental PFV (Fig 8), which led the authors to conclude that the congenital fibrovascular pupillary membranes are a variant of PFV.

The authors observed a tendency for membranes to recur (2 of 6 patients) (Figs 2 and 3) and suggested that complete membrane excision with sphincterotomies should be performed to prevent recurrence. However, the 2 patients with recurrent membranes underwent this advocated surgery. Conversely, 1 patient with nonrecurrent membrane underwent synechialysis only, raising questions regarding the optimal management of these membranes. Histopathologically, recurrent membranes were noted to have more collagenous and smooth muscle actin immunoreactive stromal components, consistent with myofibroblastic, reactive changes in the stroma (Fig 7). It is not clear if the recurrent membranes demonstrated immunoreactivity for PDGF.

From the standpoint of prognosis, congenital fibrovascular pupillary membranes appear to be associated with a variable degree of visual impairment or amblyopia, ranging from moderate visual loss to severe visual loss. Visual impairment was more severe in patients with recurrent membranes.

T. Milman, MD

Characterization of Retrokeratoprosthetic Membranes in the Boston Type 1 Keratoprosthesis

Stacy RC, Jakobiec FA, Michaud NA, et al (Massachusetts Eye and Ear Infirmary, Boston)
Arch Ophthalmol 129:310-316, 2011

Objective.—To evaluate retroprosthetic membranes that can occur in 25% to 65% of patients with the Boston type 1 keratoprosthesis (KPro).

Methods.—Two patients with Peter anomaly and 2 with neurotrophic scarred corneas underwent revisions of their type 1 KPros because of visually compromising retroprosthetic membranes. The excised membranes were studied by light microscopy with hematoxylin-eosin, periodic acid—Schiff, and toluidine blue stains. Immunohistochemical and transmission electron microscopic examination were also used.

Results.—Light microscopic examination revealed that the retro-KPro fibrous membranes originated from the host's corneal stroma. These mildly to moderately vascularized membranes grew through gaps in the Descemet membrane to reach behind the KPro back plate and adhere to the anterior iris surface, which had undergone partial lysis. In 2 cases, the fibrous membranes merged at the pupil with matrical portions of metaplastic lens epithelium, forming a bilayered structure that crossed the optical axis. Retro-KPro membranes stained positively for α–smooth muscle actin but negatively for pancytokeratin. Electron microscopy confirmed the presence of actin filaments within myofibroblasts and small surviving clusters of metaplastic lens epithelial cells.

Conclusions.—Stromal downgrowth, rather than epithelial downgrowth, was the major element of the retro- Kpro membranes in this series. Metaplastic lens epithelium also contributed to opacification of the visual axis. Florid membranous inflammation was not a prominent finding and thus probably not a requisite stimulus for membrane development. Further advances in prosthetic design and newer antifibroproliferative agents may reduce membrane formation.

▶ This meticulously worked up and beautifully illustrated clinicopathologic series of 4 patients with failed Boston type 1 keratoprosthesis describes the range of pathologic (histochemical, immunohistochemical, and ultrastructural) findings in explanted retrokeratoprosthetic membranes (Fig 2 in original article). The authors noted a prominent stromal myofibroblast component in all 4 membranes. They observed discontinuity in Descemet's membrane at the edges of the graft-host junction and hypothesized that this is the major mechanism contributing to retro-keratoprosthetic fibrous membrane formation. In addition, Stacy et al observed concomitant transdifferentiated lens epithelial component in 2 membranes from pseudophakic eyes. This finding correlates with clinically observed frequency of keratoprosthetic membranes in pseudophakic eyes, underscoring the potential role for lens epithelial cells in the membrane formation. In a prior clinicopathologic study, Dudenhoefer et al[1] noted a surface epithelial component in Boston retrokeratoprosthetic membranes of patients with autoimmune and inflammatory corneal diseases, suggesting that immune-mediated corneal fistula with fibrovascular and inflammatory membrane formation are predisposed to epithelial downgrowth. The results of these 2 studies can have several practical applications, such as meticulous attention to the maintenance of the integrity of the graft-host junction region during penetrating keratoplasty and keratoprosthesis surgery, potential benefits of removal of the lens capsular material prior to keratoprosthesis placement, and the potential role for aggressive anti-inflammatory and antifibrotic agents in selected patients.

T. Milman, MD

Reference

1. Dudenhoefer EJ, Nouri M, Gipson IK, et al. Histopathology of explanted collar button keratoprostheses: a clinicopathologic correlation. *Cornea.* 2003;22:424-428.

Improving the interaction between the ophthalmology and histopathology departments

Maudgil A, Salvi SM, Tan JHY, et al (Royal Hallamshire Hosp, Sheffield, UK)
Eye 25:998-1004, 2011

Purpose.—The purpose of this study was to improve communication between the ophthalmology and histopathology departments at Royal Hallamshire Hospital, Sheffield, by effectively changing the structure and completion of the histopathology request form through the process of a

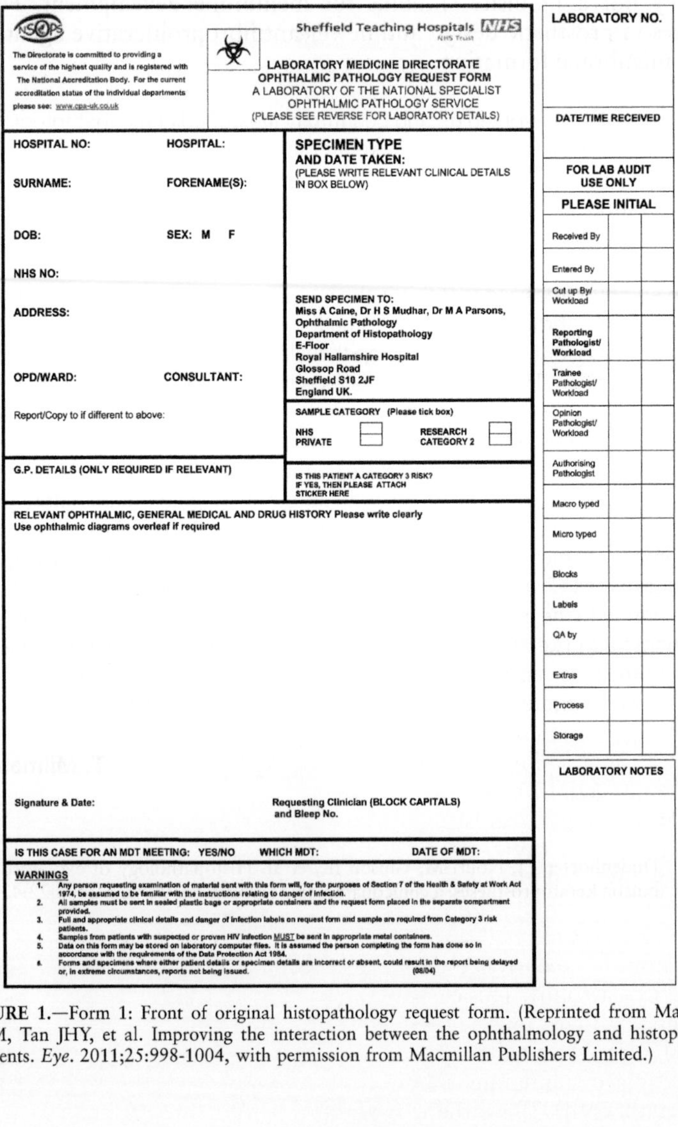

NSOPS

The Directorate is committed to providing a service of the highest quality and is registered with The National Accreditation Body. For the current accreditation status of the individual departments please see: www.cpa-uk.co.uk

Sheffield Teaching Hospitals NHS
NHS Trust

LABORATORY MEDICINE DIRECTORATE
OPHTHALMIC PATHOLOGY REQUEST FORM
A LABORATORY OF THE NATIONAL SPECIALIST OPHTHALMIC PATHOLOGY SERVICE
(PLEASE SEE REVERSE FOR LABORATORY DETAILS)

HOSPITAL NO: HOSPITAL:
SURNAME: FORENAME(S):
DOB: SEX: M F
NHS NO:
ADDRESS:
OPD/WARD: CONSULTANT:
Report/Copy to if different to above:

SPECIMEN TYPE AND DATE TAKEN:
(PLEASE WRITE RELEVANT CLINICAL DETAILS IN BOX BELOW)

SEND SPECIMEN TO:
Miss A Caine, Dr H S Mudhar, Dr M A Parsons,
Ophthalmic Pathology
Department of Histopathology
E-Floor
Royal Hallamshire Hospital
Glossop Road
Sheffield S10 2JF
England UK.

SAMPLE CATEGORY (Please tick box)
NHS PRIVATE ☐ RESEARCH CATEGORY 2 ☐

G.P. DETAILS (ONLY REQUIRED IF RELEVANT)

IS THIS PATIENT A CATEGORY 3 RISK?
IF YES, THEN PLEASE ATTACH STICKER HERE

RELEVANT OPHTHALMIC, GENERAL MEDICAL AND DRUG HISTORY Please write clearly
Use ophthalmic diagrams overleaf if required

Signature & Date: Requesting Clinician (BLOCK CAPITALS) and Bleep No.

IS THIS CASE FOR AN MDT MEETING: YES/NO WHICH MDT: DATE OF MDT:

WARNINGS
1. Any person requesting examination of material sent with this form will, for the purposes of Section 7 of the Health & Safety at Work Act 1974, be assumed to be familiar with the instructions relating to danger of infection.
2. All samples must be sent in sealed plastic bags or appropriate containers and the request form placed in the separate compartment provided.
3. Full and appropriate clinical details and danger of infection labels on request form and sample are required from Category 3 risk patients.
4. Samples from patients with suspected or proven HIV infection MUST be sent in appropriate metal containers.
5. Data on this form may be stored on laboratory computer files. It is assumed the person completing the form has done so in accordance with the requirements of the Data Protection Act 1984.
6. Forms and specimens where either patient details or specimen details are incorrect or absent, could result in the report being delayed or, in extreme circumstances, reports not being issued. (08/04)

LABORATORY NO.		
DATE/TIME RECEIVED		
FOR LAB AUDIT USE ONLY		
PLEASE INITIAL		
Received By		
Entered By		
Cut up By/ Workload		
Reporting Pathologist/ Workload		
Trainee Pathologist/ Workload		
Opinion Pathologist/ Workload		
Authorising Pathologist		
Macro typed		
Micro typed		
Blocks		
Labels		
QA by		
Extras		
Process		
Storage		
LABORATORY NOTES		

FIGURE 1.—Form 1: Front of original histopathology request form. (Reprinted from Maudgil A, Salvi SM, Tan JHY, et al. Improving the interaction between the ophthalmology and histopathology departments. *Eye*. 2011;25:998-1004, with permission from Macmillan Publishers Limited.)

successful audit. This aimed to ensure that comprehensive information was made available to the histopathologist.

Methods.—An audit was performed by review of 710 histopathology request forms, completed by the ophthalmology department, over a 1-year period, between July 2005 and June 2006 inclusive. Results were used to re-model the ophthalmic histopathology request form. New forms were circulated and all forms completed over a 3-month period, between January 2008 and March 2008, were reviewed, thus closing the audit loop.

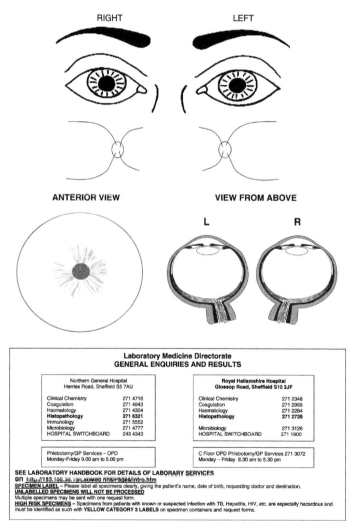

FIGURE 2.—Form 1: Back of original histopathology request form. (Reprinted from Maudgil A, Salvi SM, Tan JHY, et al. Improving the interaction between the ophthalmology and histopathology departments. *Eye.* 2011;25:998-1004, with permission from Macmillan Publishers Limited.)

Results.—On the basis of audit results of 710 histopathology request forms, a new histopathology request form was created, which was easier to complete. Review of the 224 new histopathology request forms showed improved percentages of completion of important sections of the form.

Conclusions.—Through the audit process we have created a new ophthalmic histopathology request form that is more user-friendly for the ophthalmologist and more consistently provides the necessary information for the ophthalmic histopathologist. This has improved efficiency and effectiveness of communication between the specialities, which should contribute

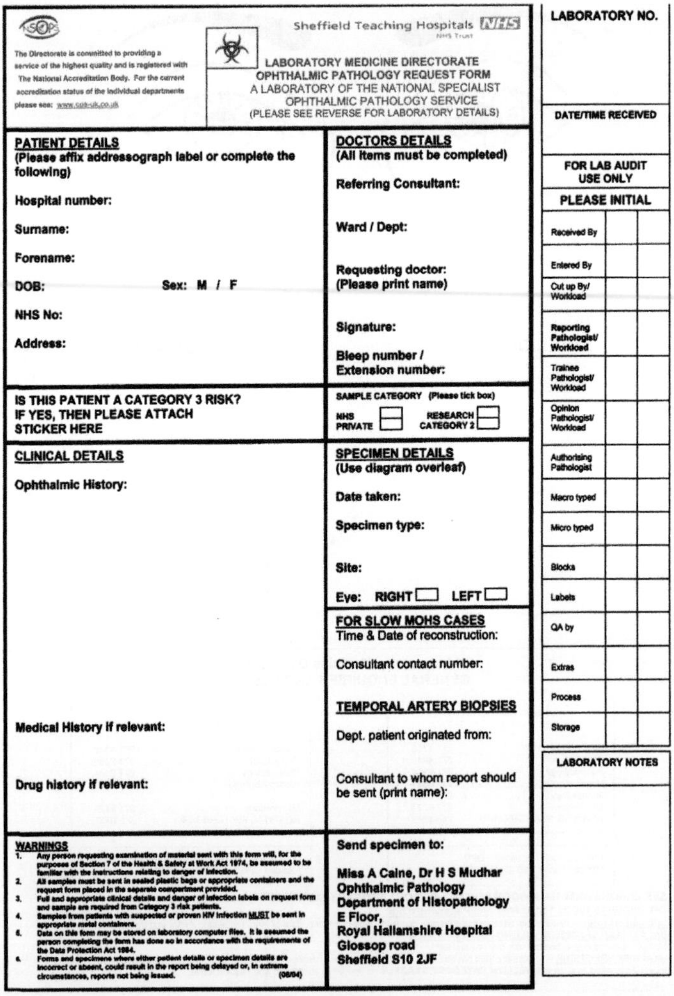

The Directorate is committed to providing a service of the highest quality and is registered with The National Accreditation Body. For the current accreditation status of the individual departments please see: www.cpa-uk.co.uk

Sheffield Teaching Hospitals NHS
NHS Trust

LABORATORY MEDICINE DIRECTORATE
OPHTHALMIC PATHOLOGY REQUEST FORM
A LABORATORY OF THE NATIONAL SPECIALIST OPHTHALMIC PATHOLOGY SERVICE
(PLEASE SEE REVERSE FOR LABORATORY DETAILS)

PATIENT DETAILS
(Please affix addressograph label or complete the following)
Hospital number:
Surname:
Forename:
DOB: **Sex: M / F**
NHS No:
Address:

DOCTORS DETAILS
(All items must be completed)
Referring Consultant:
Ward / Dept:
Requesting doctor:
(Please print name)
Signature:
Bleep number / Extension number:

IS THIS PATIENT A CATEGORY 3 RISK?
IF YES, THEN PLEASE ATTACH STICKER HERE

SAMPLE CATEGORY (Please tick box)
NHS PRIVATE ☐ **RESEARCH CATEGORY 2** ☐

CLINICAL DETAILS
Ophthalmic History:
Medical History if relevant:
Drug history if relevant:

SPECIMEN DETAILS
(Use diagram overleaf)
Date taken:
Specimen type:
Site:
Eye: RIGHT ☐ **LEFT** ☐

FOR SLOW MOHS CASES
Time & Date of reconstruction:
Consultant contact number:

TEMPORAL ARTERY BIOPSIES
Dept. patient originated from:
Consultant to whom report should be sent (print name):

WARNINGS
1. Any person requesting examination of material sent with this form will, for the purposes of Section 7 of the Health & Safety at Work Act 1974, be assumed to be familiar with the instructions relating to danger of infection.
2. All samples must be sent in sealed plastic bags or appropriate containers and the request form placed in the separate compartment provided.
3. Full and appropriate clinical details and danger of infection labels on request form and sample are required from Category 3 risk patients.
4. Samples from patients with suspected or proven HIV infection MUST be sent in appropriate metal containers.
5. Data on this form may be stored on laboratory computer files. It is assumed the person completing the form has done so in accordance with the requirements of the Data Protection Act 1984.
6. Forms and specimens where either patient details or specimen details are incorrect or absent, could result in the report being delayed or, in extreme circumstances, reports not being issued. (08/04)

Send specimen to:
Miss A Caine, Dr H S Mudhar
Ophthalmic Pathology
Department of Histopathology
E Floor,
Royal Hallamshire Hospital
Glossop road
Sheffield S10 2JF

LABORATORY NO.

DATE/TIME RECEIVED

FOR LAB AUDIT USE ONLY

PLEASE INITIAL		
Received By		
Entered By		
Cut up By/ Workload		
Reporting Pathologist/ Workload		
Trainee Pathologist/ Workload		
Opinion Pathologist/ Workload		
Authorising Pathologist		
Macro typed		
Micro typed		
Blocks		
Labels		
QA by		
Extras		
Process		
Storage		

LABORATORY NOTES

FIGURE 3.—Form 2: Front of new histopathology request form. (Reprinted from Maudgil A, Salvi SM, Tan JHY, et al. Improving the interaction between the ophthalmology and histopathology departments. *Eye*. 2011;25:998-1004, with permission from Macmillan Publishers Limited.)

TABLE 1.—Results Comparing Percentage Completion of Form 1 *vs* Form 2

Section of Form	Form 1 Completion (*n* = 710)	Form 2 Completion (*n* = 224)
Patient sticker	93.2%	95.9%
If no sticker, forms without minimum data set?	4 of 48	0 of 9
Ward/OPD	50.6%	96.4%
Referring consultant	80.1%	99.6%
Operating doctor	85.6%	95.9%
Signature	97.2%	97.8%
Contact number	50.3%	82.5%
Sufficient ophthalmic history	84.1%	98.2%
Medical history	9.8%	14.2%
Drug history	3.9%	4.0%
Date taken	64.4%	93.0%
Side	88.2%	98.0%
Diagrams marked	48.2%	71.4%

to minimise the chances of medical error and improved turnaround times for the planning and delivery of patient care (Figs 1-3, Table 1).

▶ Any eye pathologist is familiar with these "diagnoses" on the pathology requisition form: *cornea, vitreous, eyelid.* If we are lucky, the diagnoses are expanded to *cornea, right eye.* It is, indeed, a joyful occasion when instead of an eye the preoperative diagnosis is refined to the blind and painful eye. Unfortunately, occasionally, the eyes submitted with this diagnosis harbor a known-to-a-clinician intraocular tumor, underscoring the lack of communication between the surgeon and pathologist. Although the above observations reflect one extreme of the spectrum, the lack of communication between the treating physician and the pathologist is a real and widespread problem.

The pathologists and ophthalmologists from the Royal Hallamshire Hospital, Sheffield, United Kingdom, tried to address this issue by reviewing and scoring the original histopathology request forms (Figs 1 and 2) for completeness, discussing how the form can be optimized, and creating the new form (Fig 3), which is based on the recommendations of both ophthalmologists and pathologists. After introducing the new form for a 3-month period, the authors noted a significant increase in compliance with filling all the required check points (Table 1). As the authors mention, the improvement in data collection may reflect not just the form modification, but also increased awareness of the need for clear communication between the 2 departments to optimize patient care.

This need for clear communication between the pathologists and ophthalmologists cannot be overemphasized. My mentor frequently educates the ophthalmology residents: "When you consult another physician on your patient, you write him (or her) a nice letter. A pathologist is a consultant! You are referring parts of your patient! If you provide the necessary clinical information, you will get a better service." I cannot say it better than that.

T. Milman, MD

Article Index

Chapter 1: Cataract Surgery

Chapter 2: Refractive Surgery

Chapter 3: Glaucoma

Chapter 4: Cornea

Chapter 5: Retina

Chapter 6: Oculoplastic Surgery

Chapter 7: Pediatric Ophthalmology

Chapter 8: Neuro-ophthalmology

Chapter 9: Imaging

Chapter 10: Ocular Oncology

Chapter 11: Pathology

Author Index

Printed and bound by CPI Group (UK) Ltd, Croydon, CR0 4YY

08/05/2025

01864678-0007